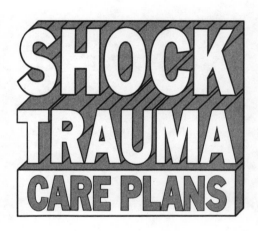

SHOCK TRAUMA CARE PLANS

JULIE MULL STRANGE, RN, CCRN

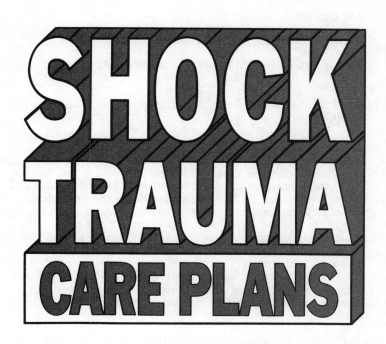

SHOCK TRAUMA CARE PLANS

JULIE MULL STRANGE, RN, CCRN

Springhouse Corporation
Springhouse, Pennsylvania

Publisher: Keith Lassner

Senior Acquisitions Editor: Susan L. Taddei

Art Director: John Hubbard

Editorial Services Manager: David Moreau

Senior Production Manager: Deborah Meiris

Illustrations by Bob Newman. Original concept and photographs by Paula M. Kelly.

The clinical procedures described and recommended in this publication are based on research and consultation with nursing, medical, and legal authorities. To the best of our knowledge, these procedures reflect currently accepted practice; nevertheless, they can't be considered absolute and universal recommendations. For individual application, all recommendations must be considered in light of the patient's clinical condition and, before administration of new or infrequently used drugs, in light of latest package-insert information. The authors and the publisher disclaim responsibility for any adverse effects resulting directly or indirectly from the suggested procedures, from any undetected errors, or from the reader's misunderstanding of the text.

Library of Congress Cataloging-in-Publication Data
Shock trauma care plans.

Includes bibliographies and index.
1. Wounds and injuries—Nursing.   2. Intensive care nursing.   3. Nursing care plans.   I. Strange, Julie Mull.
[DNLM: 1. Critical Care—handbooks. 2. Emergencies—nursing—handbooks.   3. Patient Care Planning—handbooks.   4. Shock—nursing—handbooks.   5. Wounds and Injuries—nursing—handbooks. WY 39 S559]
RD93.S52   1987   617'.1026   87-9922
ISBN 0-87434-084-5

Dedication

To Elizabeth A. Scanlon, RN, MS
Director of Nursing
MIEMSS Shock Trauma Center

A pioneer who has dedicated her career to developing and strengthening the practice of trauma nursing. Her strong convictions and persistence are responsible for nursing autonomy and respect within the framework of collaborative practice. Her support, through guidance and challenges, provides a catalyst for our achievement of both personal and professional excellence.

CONTENTS

Contributors _____ ix

Foreword—Susan W. Veise-Berry, RN, MS _____ x

Preface—Julie Mull Strange, RN, CCRN _____ xi

Section I—Trauma Care: An Overview (Section Editor—Julie Mull Strange)

The Team Approach to Trauma—Julie Mull Strange _____ 2
The Nursing Process During Acute Resuscitation—Joyce E. Maslyk _____ 6
Prehospital Perspective—Patrick J. Canan, Julie Mull Strange _____ 8

Section II—Injuries—Acute Illnesses—Shock States

Shock states (Section Editor—Deana L. Holler)

Hemorrhagic Shock—Deana L. Holler _____ 14
Vasogenic Shock—Carolyn S. Childs _____ 19
Cardiogenic Shock—Deana L. Holler _____ 24

Neurologic (Section Editor—Carolyn S. Childs)

Cervical Spine Injury—Carolyn S. Childs _____ 28
Thoracic, Lumbar, and Sacral Spine Injury—Carolyn S. Childs _____ 36
Head Injury—Carolyn S. Childs _____ 42

Respiratory (Section Editor—Joyce E. Maslyk)

Upper Airway Obstruction—Julie Mull Strange _____ 51
Lower Airway Obstruction—Joyce E. Maslyk _____ 55
Laryngeal Fracture—Paula M. Kelly _____ 57
Tracheobronchial Tree Rupture—Joyce E. Maslyk _____ 60
Tension Pneumothorax—Joyce E. Maslyk _____ 62
Open Pneumothorax—Joyce E. Maslyk _____ 65
Pneumothorax—Joyce E. Maslyk _____ 67
Hemothorax—Joyce E. Maslyk _____ 69
Pulmonary Contusion—Joyce E. Maslyk _____ 73
Flail Chest—Joyce E. Maslyk _____ 76
Ruptured Diaphragm—Joyce E. Maslyk _____ 79
Penetrating Chest Trauma—Joyce E. Maslyk _____ 81

Cardiovascular (Section Editor—Deana L. Holler)

Traumatic Rupture of the Aorta or Great Vessels—Joyce E. Maslyk _____ 84
Acute Pericardial Tamponade—Joyce E. Maslyk _____ 87
Acute Myocardial Infarction—Michael J. Groves _____ 90
Myocardial Contusion—Joyce E. Maslyk _____ 93

Gastrointestinal (Section Editor—Julie Mull Strange)

Intraabdominal Trauma: Blunt and Penetrating—Julie Mull Strange _____ 95
Abdominal Trauma During Pregnancy: Blunt and Penetrating—Lynn Gerber Smith _____ 99
Acute Upper Gastrointestinal Bleeding—Julie Mull Strange _____ 107

Genitourinary (Section Editor—Julie Mull Strange)

Ruptured Ectopic Pregnancy—Julie Mull Strange _____ 113
Spontaneous Abortion—Julie Mull Strange _____ 116
Renal System Injury—Julie Mull Strange _____ 120
External Genitalia Injury—Carolyn S. Childs _____ 123

Musculoskeletal (Section Editor—Paula M. Kelly)

Traumatic Amputation—Paula M. Kelly _____ 125
Massive Pelvic Injury—Julie Mull Strange _____ 129
Fractures: Open/Closed—Paula M. Kelly _____ 134
Dislocations—Paula M. Kelly _____ 140
Soft Tissue Injuries—Paula M. Kelly _____ 142
Hand Injuries—Brenda R. Wright _____ 145

Section III—Additional Emergencies (Section Editor—Michael J. Groves)

Hypothermia—Julie Mull Strange _____ 156
Near Drowning: Freshwater/Saltwater—Paula M. Kelly _____ 160
Acute Whole-Body Radiation Exposure—Paula M. Kelly _____ 166
Burns
—General Burn Care Considerations—Deana L. Holler _____ 170
—Chemical Burns—Deana L. Holler, Joyce E. Maslyk _____ 173
—Caustic Chemical Ingestion—Deana L. Holler, Joyce E. Maslyk _____ 176
—Thermal Burns—Deana L. Holler _____ 179
—Electrical Burns—Deana L. Holler, Joyce E. Maslyk _____ 189
Inhalation Injuries: Smoke, Carbon Monoxide, Cyanide/Hydrogen Cyanide, Polyvinyl Chloride—
Julie Mull Strange _____ 193
Maxillofacial Injuries—Deana L. Holler _____ 199
Substance Abuse in the Trauma Patient—Michael J. Groves _____ 204
Venomous Snakebites—Michael J. Groves _____ 206
Eye Injuries—Brenda R. Wright _____ 211

Section IV—Complications (Section Editor—Julie Mull Strange)

Diabetes Insipidus—Michael J. Groves _____ 222
Pulmonary Thromboembolus—Michael J. Groves _____ 224
Pulmonary Edema—Michael J. Groves _____ 227
Adult Respiratory Distress Syndrome—Michael J. Groves _____ 229
Deep Vein Thrombosis—Michael J. Groves _____ 232
Use of Neuromuscular Blocking Agents—Michael J. Groves _____ 236
Malnutrition in the Trauma Patient—Michael J. Groves _____ 240
Peritonitis—Julie Mull Strange _____ 244
Acute Pancreatitis—Julie Mull Strange _____ 248
Paralytic Ileus—Julie Mull Strange _____ 252
Mechanical Bowel Obstruction—Julie Mull Strange _____ 256
Acute Renal Failure—Deana L. Holler _____ 259
Fat Embolism Syndrome—Julie Mull Strange _____ 264
Compartment Syndrome—Paula M. Kelly _____ 267
Gas Gangrene—Carolyn S. Childs _____ 270
Transfusion Reactions—Deana L. Holler _____ 272
Disseminated Intravascular Coagulation—Deana L. Holler _____ 278

Section V—Psychosocial Support of the Trauma Patient
(Section Editor—Michael J. Groves)

Introduction—Michael J. Groves _____ 286
Potential for Anxiety/Fear—Michael J. Groves _____ 286
Impaired Verbal Communication—Michael J. Groves _____ 288
Ineffective Individual Coping—Michael J. Groves _____ 289
Potential for Powerlessness—Michael J. Groves _____ 291
Disturbance in Self-Concept—Michael J. Groves _____ 293
Potential for Spiritual Distress—Michael J. Groves _____ 295
Potential for Alterations in Family Processes—Michael J. Groves _____ 296

Section VI—Pediatric Trauma (Section Editor—Julie Mull Strange)

Introduction—Martin R. Eichelberger, MD _____ 299
Pediatric Airway Obstruction—Julie Mull Strange _____ 300
Pediatric Hypovolemic Shock—Julie Mull Strange _____ 305
Pediatric Hypothermia—Julie Mull Strange _____ 310
Pediatric Gastric Distention—Julie Mull Strange _____ 312
General Pediatric Care Considerations—Julie Mull Strange _____ 313
Psychosocial Support of the Child—Julie Mull Strange _____ 317

Section VII—Studies and Procedures (Section Editor—Michael J. Groves)

Intrahospital Transport of the Shock Trauma Patient—Michael J. Groves _____ 322
Therapeutic Embolization—Paula M. Kelly _____ 324
Aortography—Paula M. Kelly _____ 325
Positive Contrast Study—Paula M. Kelly _____ 326
Nuclear Medicine Imaging—Paula M. Kelly _____ 327
Diagnostic Peritoneal Lavage—Julie Mull Strange _____ 328
Endoscopy—Julie Mull Strange _____ 329
Bronchoscopy (Fiberoptic)—Carolyn S. Childs _____ 330
Pulmonary Artery Catheterization—Michael J. Groves _____ 331
Intracranial Pressure Monitoring—Carolyn S. Childs _____ 332
Intracompartment Pressure Measurement—Paula M. Kelly _____ 333
Autotransfusion—Deana L. Holler _____ 334
Preparation for Surgery—Carolyn S. Childs _____ 336
Intraaortic Balloon Pump—Deana L. Holler _____ 337
Pacemaker Insertion, Temporary Transvenous Pacing—Carolyn S. Childs ____ 339
The Pneumatic Antishock Garment—Patrick J. Canan _____ 340
The Mechanical Chest Compression Device—Patrick J. Canan _____ 342
Closed-Tube Thoracostomy—Joyce E. Maslyk _____ 344
Organ Donation—Deana L. Holler, Michael J. Groves _____ 345
The Critically Ill or Injured Patient Requiring Special Care—Deana L. Holler ____ 347
Endotracheal Intubation—Julie Mull Strange, C. Russell Baker _____ 349
Needle Cricothyroidotomy—Julie Mull Strange _____ 353
Surgical Cricothyroidotomy—Julie Mull Strange _____ 354

Appendices

Appendix 1—Approved Nursing Diagnoses, April 1986 _____ 357
Appendix 2—Supplemental Nursing Diagnoses _____ 358
Appendix 3—Sample Trays and Specialty Carts Lists—Julie Mull Strange ____ 359
   —Multiuse Tray   —Isolation Trays   —Emergency Airway Tray
   —Instrument Set   —Emergency Transportation Cart   —Thoracoabdominal Tray
   —Peritoneal Lavage Tray   —Pediatric Admission Cart   —Halo Tray
   —Gardner-Wells Tong Tray   —Burn Cart   —Neuroarteriogram Tray
   —Plastics Tray
Appendix 4—Hospital Resources Document, Caring for the Injured Patient ____ 365
Appendix 5—Trauma Score _____ 370
Appendix 6—Tetanus Prophylaxis _____ 371
Appendix 7—Acid-Base Imbalances—Michael J. Groves _____ 372
Appendix 8—Fluid-Electrolyte Imbalances—Michael J. Groves _____ 374
Appendix 9—Triage Decision Scheme _____ 376

Index _____ 377

Contributors

Editor-in-Chief
Julie Mull Strange, RN, CCRN
Primary Admitting Nurse III
Acute Trauma Resuscitation Area
MIEMSS—Shock Trauma Center
Director—IMPACT

Section Editors & Authors

Carolyn S. Childs, RN, MSN
Clinical Nurse Specialist
General Operating Rooms
Johns Hopkins Hospital
Educational Consultant—IMPACT

Michael J. Groves, RN, BSN
Primary Admitting Nurse II
Acute Trauma Resuscitation Area
MIEMSS—Shock Trauma Center
Educational Consultant—IMPACT

Deana L. Holler, RN, BSN
Primary Admitting Nurse III
Acute Trauma Resuscitation Area
MIEMSS—Shock Trauma Center
Educational Consultant—IMPACT

Paula M. Kelly, RN
Primary Admitting Nurse III
Acute Trauma Resuscitation Area
MIEMSS—Shock Trauma Center
Educational Consultant—IMPACT

Joyce E. Maslyk, RN, BSN
Associate Nurse Supervisor
Acute Trauma Resuscitation Area
MIEMSS—Shock Trauma Center
Educational Consultant—IMPACT

Contributing Authors

C. Russell Baker, RN, BSN, CRNA
Anesthesia Department
Acute Trauma Resuscitation Area/Operating Room
MIEMSS—Shock Trauma Center

Patrick J. Canan, BS, EMT-A
Trauma Technician
Acute Trauma Resuscitation Area
MIEMSS—Shock Trauma Center

Lynn Gerber Smith, RN, MS
Primary Admitting Nurse II
Acute Trauma Resuscitation Area
MIEMSS—Shock Trauma Center

Brenda R. Wright, RN, BSN
Primary Admitting Nurse II
Acute Trauma Resuscitation Area
MIEMSS—Shock Trauma Center

Acknowledgment

To all those who influenced, supported, and challenged us.
JMS, CSC, MJG, DLH, PMK, JEM

FOREWORD

The emergency health care system in this country has made tremendous progress over the years by recognizing the elements essential to efficient and effective care of critically ill and injured shock trauma patients. The nursing profession, recognized as a key component in the delivery of quality care, has contributed significantly to this progression.

Now, another major contribution has been made with the publication of this book, which represents a valuable accumulation of knowledge by a group of highly skilled and experienced trauma nurses. The contributors have created a pragmatic resource by consolidating a vast amount of information and presenting it in a format not found in most standard references. This book is concise but comprehensive by design, thus providing a firm basis for a clear flow of thought processes so essential in the emergent phase of care. The pace at which the material is presented reflects the nature of the work.

This unique book offers vital information for effective nursing assessment, diagnosis, and management of disorders specific to critically ill or injured shock trauma patients during the initial phase of nursing care. Succinct and understandable, it is designed to expeditiously dispense clinical information that can be put into practice effectively. The aim of the book is to standardize the initial nursing management of the critically injured patient by presenting an early, systematic approach to patient problems.

As the most up-to-date reference manual on this topic available today, it will be valuable to all emergency/critical care trauma nurses, however experienced. Although clinical judgment itself is best learned at the patient's bedside, the basis for such decision making must originate from a well-constructed and educationally sound knowledge base. This book serves as an axis for the movement of nursing practice—allowing trauma nurses to expand capabilities and maximize their roles in assessment and intervention during the emergent phase of care.

Recognizing the importance of employing a systematic approach to the trauma patient's initial care, the authors present a framework that serves to bridge the gap between prehospital and postresuscitation care. This framework lends itself to the logical flow of nursing management priorities beyond the emergent phase of care, thus providing a firm basis for the continuity of nursing practices through the critical care phase of care. This text presents a source book that will allow practicing nurses to broaden their scope of knowledge while developing and refining essential skills.

A description of the book and its valuable contribution to the field of trauma/critical care nursing would be incomplete without acknowledging its creators. The cumulative years of clinical practice represented—and experience encountered—by these expert clinicians have obviously enhanced the content. The warmth and genuine care that these professionals have unselfishly extended to their patients is evident throughout. For despite the apparent task-oriented approach to the initial care of the trauma patient, the authors have provided the elements that make the trauma care experience human and real.

Congratulations to all those who have given of themselves to make this body of knowledge available. Your gift to nursing is ever so valuable.

Susan W. Veise-Berry, RN, MS
Clinical Nurse Supervisor
Acute Trauma Resuscitation Area
MIEMSS

PREFACE

Trauma continues to affect the lives and futures of over 70 million Americans each year. Swiftly and without warning, it inflicts physical and psychosocial crises on its victims and their families. The price trauma exacts on society exceeds $88 billion annually, reflecting health care costs, lost wages, and unrealized potential and productivity. Recovery from the physical, emotional, and economic scars of trauma is slow and may take a lifetime. Recognizing that current trauma prevention is inadequate, at best, health care providers must anticipate the complex needs of the multisystem-injured patient and prepare to meet the challenges of providing quality care.

Time is a precious, crucial factor in the care of the critically ill or injured patient, as it is in the first minutes to hours after injury that mortality from trauma is highest. The precarious resuscitation phase permits no time for speculation or vacillation; there is little margin for error. Decisions must be made quickly and confidently; actions must reflect knowledge and skill. Accurate assessment, appropriate interventions, and definitive diagnosis and therapy, performed with knowledge, precision, and speed with a collaborative team approach, most greatly influence the patient's immediate survival and final outcome.

The comprehensive care required by this patient and his family—not only at the scene of the accident and during resuscitation, but throughout the critical care, recovery, and rehabilitative phases—requires the expertise of specially trained professionals with advanced clinical skills. This team of experts includes prehospital care providers; nurses; physicians; social workers; family counselors; respiratory, physical, and occupational therapists; and countless others. Despite the tremendous need for trauma care specialists, current training programs fail to adequately prepare health care students to face the challenges of trauma care. In the clinical setting, the patient's critical and ever-changing condition often precludes students' direct involvement in care. In addition, as more hospitals strive for designation as qualified trauma centers, practicing clinicians in all areas are now expected to deliver high-quality care to this complex patient—a task that can overwhelm even the most experienced nurse or physician.

Currently available publications rarely provide substantial trauma nursing directives using a standardized approach regarding the comprehensive patient needs and necessary nursing interventions. Material specific to the initial resuscitation and stabilization phase of care that combined theory with direct clinical application was nonexistent. *Shock Trauma Care Plans* offers a unique approach to the spectrum of actual and potential health care needs of multisystem-injured/critically ill patients during resuscitation and acute care. It focuses primarily on traumatic injuries, acute illnesses, and major complications; however, sections on additional emergencies, pediatrics, psychosocial support, and studies and procedures commonly used provide the reader with a comprehensive look at shock trauma care.

This text is written in an easy-to-follow, standardized care plan format, which is based on the nursing process. Each topic is addressed in a similar fashion: Assessment (mechanism of injury/etiology and physical findings), Diagnostic Studies, Nursing Diagnosis (those accepted by the North American Nursing Diagnosis Association and supplemental diagnoses), Goals (telling the reader what must be done), Interventions and Rationale (which reflect the interdependent roles of health care providers during initial care), Additional Considerations, when applicable (a preview of future patient needs, such as transfer to regional centers, rehabilitation issues, or specific patient teaching), and Associated Care Plans and Associated Studies and Procedures (for comprehensive cross-referencing). The directive tone and the in-depth rationales make this text applicable to anyone who must make clinical decisions concerning the critically ill or injured patient—both practicing clinicians and health care providers new to trauma and critical care.

Shock Trauma Care Plans can serve as a ready reference during resuscitation and acute care when time is of the essence. Standard plans of care may also aid the development of standards of trauma nursing care and individualized plans of patient care, improve documentation of nursing therapy, and lend themselves to staff education and quality assurance audits. Regardless of how the reader chooses to use this text, we hope this contribution will promote and enhance the quality of care provided to the shock trauma patient and his family.

Many people, in a variety of roles, contribute to the development of a project such as *Shock Trauma Care Plans,* yet often those closest to the production go unrecognized despite their special efforts. Therefore, I wish to acknowledge several very special contributors: Susan Taddei, our Acquisitions Editor, whose belief and support made this a reality; Bernadette Glenn, our Acquisitions Assistant; David Moreau, our Editorial Services Manager; Greg Murowski, our first EMS consultant, who initially identified the value of *Shock Trauma Care Plans* for prehospital providers; our nursing, physician, and trauma technician colleagues in the Acute Resuscitation Area at MIEMSS, who offered expert advice and consultation; and our clinical reviewers, who helped solidify and polish selected care plans. My sincere appreciation to my coauthors for their professionalism and sense of humor, their belief in *Shock Trauma Care Plans,* and their perseverance. Finally, I thank the families and extended support systems of my coauthors and especially my husband Bill and my children Nick and Lauren. Ultimately it was all of your constant support, cooperation, and understanding that enabled all of us to accomplish this challenge.

Julie Mull Strange

TRAUMA CARE: AN OVERVIEW

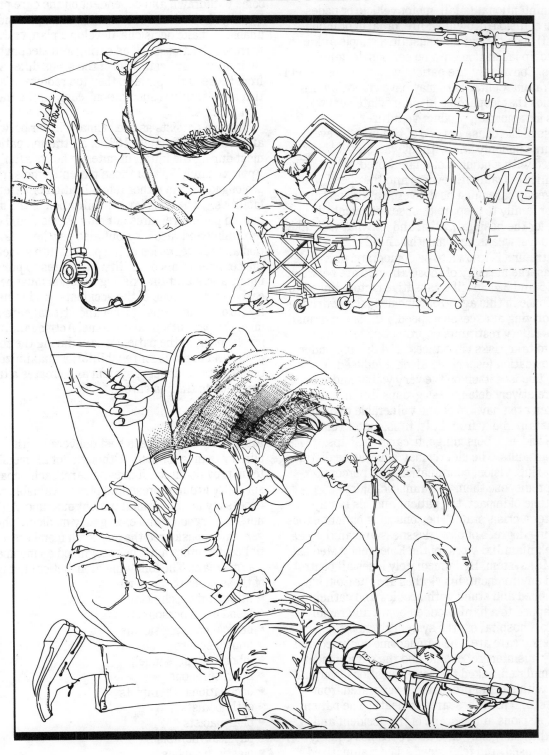

THE TEAM APPROACH TO TRAUMA

The patient

Trauma is a startling experience or a sudden force that disturbs the victim's physical, mental, psychosocial, and spiritual equilibrium and commonly produces lasting effects for the patient and his family.[8] The basis of the traumatic event may be intentional (assault, homicide, or suicide) or unintentional (a fall, motor vehicle or pedestrian/vehicle collision, drowning, fire, or farm or industrial accident). The patient may sustain a simple ankle fracture or scalp laceration with no serious, long-term ramifications. Conversely, the patient who requires Level I or Level II Trauma Center care may have critical multisystem injuries that jeopardize his immediate survival and chances for a normal, productive future.

Regardless of the cause or type of trauma, the event usually occurs suddenly and without warning, leaving those involved with a number of unanswered "whys." The unpredictability of traumatic events and the speed with which emergency care must be delivered afford no time for the patient or family to prepare themselves, mentally or emotionally, for the hospitalization and for what will take place in the days, weeks, and months ahead.

Although trauma is known to be democratic in its selection of victims, the majority of those affected are between the ages of 15 and 35. Specific causative factors linked to trauma incidence in this age group include lack of driving experience, driving at excessive speed, infrequent or inadequate use of safety restraints or protective headgear, willingness to take risks or chances, and driving under chemical intoxication (especially alcohol-induced).[1] Trauma also imposes itself on the very young and the elderly, two relatively defenseless groups. Infants and young children are unaware of and vulnerable to danger. They may sustain injury from falls, fires, motor vehicle and bicycle accidents, poisonings, firearm mishaps, abuses, and assaults. The elderly may experience disturbances in hearing, vision, coordination, and perception, all of which predispose them to traumatic injury.

From the time of impact, the patient and his family generally enter a crisis state. The conscious patient experiences varying degrees of powerlessness and anxiety as he enters the unfamiliar world of the Emergency Medical Services (EMS) system. He immediately loses all control of events and environment: his clothes are cut from his body; he is probed and stuck with needles and catheters; and he is strapped to a hard, wooden board and rapidly whisked off to a hospital of "the system's" choosing. Once in the emergency care area, he can become confused and therefore may misinterpret events and the environment. He is overstimulated, asked the same questions over and over, treated with painful procedures, separated from those he loves, and usually scared to death! The patient who was unconscious at the scene of the accident and wakes up in the emergency care area becomes equally powerless, confused, and frightened.[3] The traumatized family usually enters the health care system in a similar crisis state.[2] They are shocked and bewildered or possibly in denial of the whole situation. They may respond with exaggerated and uncontrolled emotion during this initial "impact" phase.[4,6] As families begin to think more clearly, they commonly experience anger or guilt. They may become withdrawn and dependent on the care providers. Usually their anxiety about the unknown renders them unable to make decisions, develop a plan, or even continue normal activities, such as eating and sleeping. Although their overt manifestations of the crisis differ somewhat from those of the patient, they too require crisis intervention and "family resuscitation" early in the trauma admission process.[7]

Trauma persists as the primary killer between ages 1 and 44. Approximately 16% of all trauma patients die, most during the initial minutes to hours after the injury. Approximately 36% of those patients who survive require prolonged care in either rehabilitation or extended care facilities.[11] The complex rehabilitation of the multisystem-injured patient requires not only physical and cognitive retraining and recovery, but also psychosocial readaptation and reintegration of the patient into society, within the confines of his disability. Measures to prevent further injury and maintain existing function must be initiated early—at the scene of the accident—and remain a priority throughout resuscitation and critical care to maximize the patient's final outcome. Active family involvement in the patient's care during the recovery phase and in plans for rehabilitation maximizes the patient's natural support system and creates a truly holistic approach to trauma care.

The team

Effective trauma care is best delivered with a multidisciplinary team approach. Although not all members of the team provide direct, hands-on care, each department and specialty group represented plays a valuable role that is necessary for an optimal patient outcome. Although the nurses, surgeons, and emergency medicine physicians are generally considered the key team members, other essential contributors must be recognized as members of the trauma team. The following alphabetical list is a sampling of these other team members:
- attendants/technicians
- blood bank personnel
- critical care physicians
- housekeepers
- laboratory personnel
- neurosurgeons
- occupational therapists
- orthopedists
- pharmacists
- physical therapists
- plastic surgeons

- prehospital care personnel
- radiographers/radiologists
- respiratory therapists
- social workers/pastoral counselors
- unit clerks/secretaries.

Although a facility's team size may vary (from 2 to 10 or more members at the bedside), all involved personnel or departments cited above must be acknowledged as members of the overall team. Fragmented or suboptimal care delivery can easily occur without the active involvement and participation of all team members.

The success of the multidisciplinary trauma team depends on six essential components:
- an identifiable leader
- a clear understanding of roles and responsibilities
- open lines of communication
- a collegial atmosphere
- collaborative practice (interdependence)
- a preestablished plan of action.

Leader. Although the emergency medicine physician may direct the immediate lifesaving procedures while awaiting the arrival of the designated trauma admitting team, the trauma surgeon usually is responsible for the coordination of all members' contributions. During resuscitation and critical care, the team leader works in close cooperation with the primary admitting nurse and the primary care nurse to develop an overall plan of care and to coordinate all proposed activities of the other team members.

Clear understanding of roles and responsibilities. Major team problems can occur with inadequate role definition or unclear delineation of areas of responsibility. The admitting team works most efficiently and effectively when afforded a preadmission conference. This brief meeting enables the team leader to delegate tasks and procedures before the patient's arrival, and it provides time for clarification of responsibilities. Throughout the entire hospitalization, team members should maintain an acute awareness of each other's responsibilities and treatment plans to avoid fragmentation of care.

Open lines of communication. A successful team approach truly depends on open, effective communication. An atmosphere of trust and respect will enable all members to feel free to contribute information and suggestions, ask questions, delegate responsibility, and ask for help. Communicating clearly and effectively is a skill that requires practice and that, even for the experienced, may suffer during the high stress of a critical trauma admission. Yet communication breakdowns will only increase stress and can potentially affect patient care.

Collegial atmosphere. All members of the trauma team, regardless of their specialty, serve a vital role in the care of the critically ill and injured patient. Each contribution is essential and must be recognized as such. Mutual trust and collegial respect among all members strengthen the team effort.

Collaborative practice. The complex nature of trauma care requires a multidisciplinary team approach for optimal patient outcome. Collaboration, important throughout the hospitalization, is most necessary during the acute resuscitation, intraoperative, and critical care phases. During these highly critical times, team members must work in concert to assess patient needs; diagnose, plan, and implement therapy; and constantly evaluate all aspects of patient care. Each team member, regardless of discipline, must work interdependently and in close cooperation with all others because in health care today, especially trauma care, there is little place for the independent approach. True collaborative team practice requires a clear understanding of your own role and responsibilities and those of the other members, open lines of communication, and a supportive, collegial atmosphere in which mutual respect of others' knowledge and skills is shared by all. Nurses in areas of highest patient acuity must use their advanced training, knowledge, and judgment to appropriately implement medical and nursing orders, thus practicing the true meaning of collaborative interventions.[9] Additionally, the bedside nurse serves as a care coordinator by her very position at the patient's side. Residents, physical therapists, radiographers, medical and surgical specialists, family members, and others come and go throughout the day. But the nurse maintains a continuing presence. She must anticipate, schedule, and plan the efficient coordination of all patient-related activities. She is commonly the one person who sees the patient from a truly holistic perspective and prevents fragmentation of care.

Plan of action. A preestablished, systematic action plan, whether for resuscitation procedure sequence or for future interventions, requires input from all disciplines. Preadmission conferences, which enable delegation of tasks or procedures, facilitate an efficient, effective resuscitation. Daily patient rounds attended by all members of the patient's direct care team not only provide patient progress updates but also afford collaborative clinical problem solving and development of short- and long-term care plans. Multidisciplinary patient rounds ensure that cooperative efforts are focused and directed in a coordinated manner: the right hand is aware of what the left hand is doing. This proves most essential for the multisystem-injured patient who requires the services of orthopedics, plastic surgery, neurosurgery, critical care, rehabilitation medicine, and, usually, numerous other specialties.

Finally, all members of the trauma team must strive toward the ultimate goal of optimal patient outcome—his return to society as a productive, contributing member. Incorporating these six components successfully facilitates the delivery of quality comprehensive care throughout the hospitalization.

The system

Anticipation. One of the key components of successful trauma care is anticipation. From the moment they hear of the injury through rehabilitation, all members of the trauma team must plan for and stay one step ahead of actual and potential patient needs. In the early phases of care, prehospital and acute resuscitation team members must foster a keen sense of suspicion, always expecting the worst. Injuries, especially from blunt traumatic mechanisms, are often subtle or hidden, and patient changes occur rapidly and generally without significant warning. Therefore, the team must be trained to anticipate and rapidly intervene in all the clinical events that could transpire. The system and the environment must be designed and prepared to facilitate the team's efforts. Patient care during each phase of the hospitalization must anticipate and plan for the patient's needs during the next phase. For example, anticipating and planning for the patient's progression to the recovery and rehabilitation phase must begin during critical care, with much of the care aimed at preventing or minimizing potential patient problems and secondary disabilities. In essence, the team and the system must always plan and work today for what the patient will need tomorrow.

Transportation. Rapid, safe transportation of the critically ill or injured trauma patient to the most appropriate health care facility is a priority. Personnel trained in trauma and emergency care should accompany the patient and continue therapy until their arrival at the facility. Factors affecting the mode of transport—helicopter or ambulance—may include availability, geographic accessibility, comparative travel time to the appropriate definitive care center, patient injuries, and the patient's overall stability and potential for deterioration. A preestablished system for obtaining either mode of transportation should be in effect, and any specific patient criteria or guidelines for use should be well known by all EMS providers.

Prehospital care. As the first to assess the trauma patient and intervene, prehospital care providers are valuable members of the trauma team. Prehospital interventions begin the resuscitative process, but prehospital care is often unstructured, and trauma knowledge, skill level, and permitted interventions may vary on county, regional, and statewide levels. Despite improvements in prehospital trauma care, continuing controversies include:
- philosophy for and institution of "swoop and scoop" ("scoop and run") or "stay and stabilize" policies
- appropriateness and necessity of field skills and procedures (including use of esophageal obturator airways versus endotracheal intubation, use of McSwain darts, performance of emergency cricothyroidotomy, central line insertion, and pneumatic antishock garment application)
- need for standardized and nationally recognized certification and recertification programs
- use of hospital-trained personnel (physicians, nurses) in the field.

Debate persists on many of these issues because of the lack of appropriate research data.[10] Continued efforts must be directed toward solidifying and improving the relationship and continuity of care between prehospital and hospital-based personnel. Prehospital care is explored further in "Prehospital Perspective." Quality prehospital care can and does save lives, yet optimal care is not universally available. Therefore, preventable deaths and disability continue to plague the trauma population.[5]

Communication systems. Preestablished, organized communication systems are an integral component of an effective trauma system. Patient-related information coming in from the field and patient care directives going out from the hospital must be clearly and accurately transmitted. Prehospital patient reports should be relayed in a systematic, succinct manner addressing patient priorities. Hospital-based direction should come from physicians or nurses trained and experienced in trauma care and field procedures who will adapt instructions to the skill level available at the scene and to the protocols and procedures governing the responding field unit (advanced life support versus basic life support).

Receiving facilities. Emergency care facilities that receive trauma patients should have the staff and equipment to meet the complex needs of this patient population. Appendix 4, "Level I, II, and III Trauma Center Guidelines," outlines the American College of Surgeons Committee on Trauma's recommendations on personnel and standardized equipment availability for Level I, II, and III trauma centers. Trauma care that includes anticipating the patient's needs requires a constantly available and ready team of physicians, nurses, and support personnel/services, as previously discussed. Although a hospital may have the basic personnel and equipment, all the necessary support services may not be available. The patient may arrive, undergo acute resuscitation (A [airway], B [breathing], C [circulation], D's [disability—gross neurologic examination]), and then require transfer to a more appropriate regional or specialty center. For example, the burn patient may initially receive emergency care at the closest health care facility and then be transferred to the regional burn center for definitive care. Transfer criteria and a preestablished system for such referrals should be easily accessible and readily initiated to facilitate rapid, efficient patient transfer to the tertiary care center.

Quality assurance. Formal and informal multidisciplinary quality assurance programs should be in effect. Nursing audits, peer review systems, chart reviews, patient case reviews, and morbidity/mortality conferences are all examples of quality assurance efforts. These activities, especially case reviews, should involve prehospital care providers whenever possible and appropriate. A mechanism to provide feedback to prehospital personnel also offers a means of follow-up and quality assurance evaluation. Feedback should include positive reflections as well as constructive criticism when necessary.

Protocols for care. The critical, complex, and usually urgent needs of the multisystem-injured trauma patient necessitate the development and use of care guideline protocols. Such protocols delineate resuscitative priorities and aid consistent quality care delivery. Medical management protocols have been used for some time by many institutions. The development of nursing management protocols is long overdue. Effective trauma patient care requires a truly collaborative approach with input from both medical and nursing disciplines. Medical diagnoses, protocols, and interventions should be integrated with nursing diagnoses, protocols, and interventions to improve planning, problem solving, and comprehensive interventions, enhancing each discipline's contributions to care.[9]

The continued search for excellence

Trauma care has improved since the 1966 publication of *Accidental Death and Disability: The Neglected Disease of Modern Society* by the National Research Council. However, many aspects of this significant public health problem—includng prevention, treatment, and rehabilitation—require continued research, testing, and development.[5] Although established associations, task forces, and government committees are dedicated to actively researching and implementing trauma prevention techniques, this area of trauma care deserves and must receive more attention and participation, especially from health care providers. Prehospital issues—such as improved techniques for stabilizing and transporting the spinal cord–injured patient; the efficacy of using more invasive modalities (such as endotracheal intubation, cricothyroidotomy, and central intravenous lines); and standardized training and recertification programs—demand continued evaluation and research. Knowledge of the mechanisms of injuries must be broadened to further intensify the development of injury prediction systems. The list of clinical topics and issues of particular importance to the trauma patient seems endless. The following is only a sample of the vital topics that must yet be explored: sepsis, immune response, wound healing, physiologic chain of events after a head injury, cerebral edema control, shock-response mediators, nerve cell regeneration, microvascular techniques, fracture healing, and pain control. Trauma patient rehabilitation is a clinical specialty that offers vast research potential, as does the psychosocial spectrum. Striving for excellence in future trauma care necessitates incorporating a heavy research emphasis into clinical practice. The tried and true protocols and standards of care that have enabled improved trauma patient care must continually undergo close examination, reevaluation, and possibly alteration to take advantage of the latest findings and recommendations of trauma research.

THE NURSING PROCESS DURING ACUTE RESUSCITATION

Shock Trauma Care Plans focuses on one of the most complex and challenging nursing roles: rapid, appropriate nursing care of the critically ill and multiply injured trauma patient during initial resuscitation and stabilization. To meet this challenge, guidelines in the form of standardized care plans were devised for professional nurses caring for these patients. This chapter introduces and explains the entry format and possible methods of using the information contained in the care plans.

During the initial resuscitation and stabilization phase, the focus is on rapid diagnosis and treatment. These two steps commonly occur simultaneously. Given the rapidity of events and the need for decisiveness, standardized medical protocols have been developed to facilitate well-planned and orderly medical care of trauma patients.

For the same reasons, standardized shock trauma nursing care plans facilitate the logical intermeshing of medical and nursing care. A highly trained nurse, knowledgeable in the trauma/critical care area, should recognize signs and symptoms of potentially life-threatening or disabling injuries and complications. This nurse must use rapid, expert judgment and decision making in initiating standardized medical orders and nursing therapies. Thus, standardized nursing care plans can provide a baseline for developing the individualized care required by the critically ill or multiply injured patient.

The Nursing Process—the systematic approach developed to promote comprehensive nursing care—was used as the basis for developing the format and structuring the care plans. Using the Nursing Process enables a nurse to identify and prioritize patient problems; develop a plan of care to prevent, minimize, or resolve the problems; and evaluate the effects of nursing interventions. The steps of this continuous process include: 1) assessment, 2) nursing diagnosis, 3) planning, 4) implementation, and 5) evaluation.

Medical diagnosis—The care plans are presented according to specific injuries, illnesses, or complications for easy reference. The care plans are organized in the following sections: Shock, Neurologic, Respiratory, Cardiovascular, Gastrointestinal, Genitourinary, Musculoskeletal, Psychosocial Support, Pediatrics, Additional Emergencies, and Complications.

Assessment—During this phase, information is gathered concerning the type, severity, and urgency of the illness or injury. Mechanism of injury and etiology provide important information required by the trauma team. Traumatic injuries are produced by outside energy forces exerted on the body. These forces are divided into two categories: blunt trauma and penetrating trauma. An understanding of the physical forces causing injury alerts the trauma team to suspect potential life-threatening injuries that may not be initially obvious. Physical assessment of the patient includes an initial rapid, primary evaluation of *A*irway maintenance and cervical spine control, *B*reathing, *C*irculation, *D*isability (gross neurologic examination), and complete *E*xposure of the patient. Life-threatening conditions are diagnosed immediately and treated rapidly. After the primary survey and the initial resuscitation, a more detailed head-to-toe secondary assessment is completed and definitive care is initiated. The probable Physical Findings are listed according to system. Associated injuries are not uncommon in the critically ill and multiply injured trauma patient and are listed in the assessment section when appropriate.

Diagnostic studies—Diagnostic Studies are a major component of patient evaluation. These studies, such as laboratory data, diagnostic peritoneal lavage, and radiographs, assist with differential diagnosis, guide treatment, and confirm clinical impressions.

Nursing diagnosis—Nursing diagnoses are clinical diagnoses made by professional nurses describing actual or potential patient problems that nurses, by virtue of their education and experience, are capable and licensed to treat.[3] Nursing diagnoses are formulated based on the information gathered during the assessment phase of the nursing process. The majority of the nursing diagnoses describing actual and potential health problems of the critically ill and injured trauma patient are physiologically oriented. A physiologic nursing diagnosis is defined as an inferential statement made by a professional nurse describing physiologic disturbances that impede optimal function and direct the nurse to specific interventions, both independent and interdependent. The list of nursing diagnoses accepted by the North American Nursing Diagnosis Association (NANDA) was the primary basis for developing the nursing diagnoses in this book. Several supplemental nursing diagnoses were developed to describe patient problems not included in the NANDA list. These supplemental diagnoses are marked with an asterisk before the diagnosis and are listed in Appendix 2, "Supplemental Nursing Diagnoses." Several diagnostic statements combine a NANDA-approved and a supplemental diagnosis. To acknowledge this combination of diagnoses, these statements are also marked with an asterisk. The diagnostic statements are written in two parts connected by the phrase "related to." The statements describe the actual or potential health problems in relation to their etiology.

Goals—Each nursing diagnosis describes an actual or potential health problem. The goals are statements of desired, projected outcomes of nursing therapies prescribed to prevent, minimize, or resolve those problems. Goals provide the criteria by which nursing care is evaluated.

Nursing interventions—Nursing interventions are actions directed toward preventing, minimizing, or resolving the patient's actual or potential health problem. These interventions directly affect the factors causing the problem. The interventions can be interdependent, independent, or dependent nursing actions, decisions, and judgments and must be planned in collaboration with prescribed medical protocol and therapies.

Rationale—Each nursing intervention is explained and justified, and the pathophysiology of the illness or injury is further described in the rationale. Understanding the mechanisms of injury/etiology and the pathophysiology of specific patient problems increases the nurse's expertise and her ability to interrelate isolated signs and symptoms and anticipate sequelae, thus improving the quality of nursing practice.

Additional considerations—This section presents pertinent and essential information that does not easily fit into the care plan format. Such information may include transfer of patients to specialty referral centers, rehabilitation issues, or collaborative efforts made by various specialists to provide optimal care to the patient.

Associated care plans—These are listed at the end of each individual care plan. It is not uncommon for the traumatized patient to have sustained multiple-system injuries and complications. Generally, these patients will require multiple care plans for completion of comprehensive nursing care.

Associated procedures/studies—Specific procedures and studies referred to in the care plans are described in this section. This section was designed to aid the nurse in anticipating the need for specific diagnostic and therapeutic procedures/studies.

References—At the end of each section a complete Reference List is provided. Much of the information in this text is based on the experience of the authors as trauma nurses working in the Acute Trauma Resuscitation Area of a major Level I trauma center.

PREHOSPITAL PERSPECTIVE

In "The Team Approach to Trauma," major trauma team members were introduced and their roles discussed. This chapter will expand on one part of this team, prehospital providers, as this group is perhaps the least understood by in-hospital personnel. An overview of the development of Emergency Medical Services (EMS) systems in the United States will be provided in order for the reader to better understand the current state of EMS development. We feel this is essential because this development has led to the various levels of EMS providers with differing skills and training. After a discussion of the past and present, we will look to the future of EMS and the hope for a research-based continuation of system development. This chapter should stimulate a greater understanding of the role of the prehospital provider in trauma care—an understanding that will result in a more unified team effort.

Many factors contributed to the development of today's prehospital care systems. These systems originally developed on a local or, at best, regional level and served primarily as transport mechanisms to take patients to hospitals. Modern EMS development began with the extrapolation of lessons learned during military conflict to the general peacetime population. Military engagements of the 20th century (World Wars I and II and the Korean and Vietnam Wars) demonstrated the effectiveness of a systems approach to the management of battlefield casualties. As technology improved (for example, as helicopters came into use), a system developed to rapidly move the wounded soldier from the battlefield to a definitive care area. With the advent of this system, shortened transport time was discovered to be a major factor contributing to decreased mortality. Figure 1.1 demonstrates the relationship between evacuation time and mortality rate during 20th-century wars.

The systems created on battlefields abroad were slow coming to communities and cities in the United States. National attention was drawn to EMS development during the 1960 presidential campaign when John F. Kennedy declared that possibly the nation's greatest public health problem was traffic accidents.[9] In 1966 the National Academy of Science, in a white paper on trauma, reported that accidental death and disability had become the "neglected disease" of modern society. Ten years later, in the 1970s, it was said that the life expectancy of the American public was better after an injury in the fields of Vietnam than on our streets and highways at home.[1] Automobile accident–related injuries continued to occur at a rate of 10,000 per day in the United States. The need for changes in the community's response to the increasing numbers of trauma deaths was evident; however, major changes in our health care systems would take time.

A parallel, nonmilitary influence on EMS system development was field treatment of sudden death due to myocardial infarction. Prehospital care systems served as extensions of the hospital's coronary care unit. This led to the creation of mobile intensive care units staffed by emergency technicians trained in airway management, intravenous catheter placement, and dysrhythmia management. These systems, although primarily designed for the treatment of medical emergencies, were perceived by the general public as capable of handling any call for help. Although many of the calls were for accidents and related problems, the first rescue units received little trauma-related training.[10] The "stabilization and transport" philosophy, appropriate and effective for cardiac patients, was also used in the treatment of the trauma patient.

These varied influences on current EMS systems have led to a number of controversies in prehospital care delivery, all of which are closely intertwined. Debate focuses on the following:
- time/benefit ratio of field interventions
- appropriate field interventions/skill levels
- medical control of EMS operations
- use of predefined field protocols.

Essential to a discussion of these controversies is an understanding of the difference between supportive and restorative care.[4] Supportive measures—for example, antidysrhythmic drugs for the cardiac patient and use of a pneumatic antishock garment (PASG) and intravenous therapy for the shock trauma patient—buy the patient time until his arrival at the definitive care facility. Restorative measures are those interventions required for patient survival and generally are performed in the hospital setting. Obviously, administration of certain emergency cardiac drugs and defibrillation for dysrhythmias are restorative measures that can be accomplished during the prehospital phase. These measures reverse the critical situation and enable patient survival. However, restorative measures for the critically ill trauma patient usually are more complex surgical measures that are neither appropriate nor possible at the scene or en route to the hospital. For example, a common restorative measure necessary for surviving a penetrating chest injury is emergency thoracotomy; the patient with intraabdominal injuries requires emergency exploratory laparotomy; and the patient with a severe pelvic injury usually needs massive blood replacement, external fixation, and possibly therapeutic embolization.

With these differences in types of care measures in mind, it is possible to present patient scenarios and examine the above-mentioned controversies in light of potential, realistic situations.

Patient #1 is a 24-year-old male sustaining a gunshot wound to the left leg, resulting in an open femur fracture. This incident occurs during a robbery attempt at a store 20 minutes from a hospital. Supportive measures for this patient include the establishment of I.V. therapy, application of an immobilization/traction device, administration of oxygen, and application of a sterile dressing. Restorative measures would consist of irrigation and debridement of the open wound, surgical fixation of the fracture, and antibiotic therapy. In light of the above controversies, is the time required for supportive care measures justified by the benefit to the patient? Application of traction or immobilization of the fracture will reduce the patient's pain; help to prevent further nerve, blood vessel, and tissue damage; reduce the possibility of fat embolism; and minimize blood loss from the fracture site. This immobilization initially stabilizes the fracture and helps to prevent potential complications of this injury. I.V. establishment provides ready access in the event of continued or occult blood loss resulting in hemorrhagic shock. Administration of oxygen compensates for decreased oxygenation capability caused by blood loss and the release of fat globules to the pulmonary circulation. A sterile dressing decreases the potential for further bacterial contamination. It is clear from this explanation that the patient benefits greatly from these interventions with little additional risk. Additionally, these are all generally routine procedures in which the field provider should be well versed, thus decreasing the time needed for performance and the patient's risk from incorrect performance.

Patient #2 is a 25-year-old motorcycle driver not wearing a helmet at the time of her accident. Upon arrival the patient is unconscious and bleeding from the mouth and right ear, with obvious fractures of the right arm and left femur. No breath sounds are audible on the right side and her trachea is deviated to the left. Her pulse is weak at 124 and her blood pressure is palpable at 80.

Specific controversies surrounding the care of this patient include the decompression of the tension pneumothorax, the establishment of I.V. therapy, PASG application, and airway control. Matters for concern include medical authority to perform procedures, individual competency in each procedure, risk to the patient with incorrect performance, time used to perform procedures, and the effectiveness of the procedures. Another factor requiring serious consideration is the distance to a definitive care facility. This patient, if 10 minutes from a Level I trauma facility, would probably be treated much differently than if 1½ hours from the nearest hospital.

Despite recent trends toward extended field stabilization, one fundamental principle must be kept in mind: the purpose of field care is to prevent further patient deterioration and to expedite transport to a definitive care facility.[3] Cowley's "Golden Hour" concept for shock reversal cannot be forgotten. Patient survival is greatly enhanced by the initiation of restorative, definitive interventions within a maximum of 60 minutes from the time of injury.[5] The above patients demonstrate the basic current debate in field care—differentiation of situations where it is appropriate to "stay and stabilize" or "swoop and scoop." From this central controversy come

additional questions of which procedures are appropriate for the field, methods of training and certification, and assurance of continued competency.

EMS systems have made significant advances in prehospital patient care. The efforts that were originally directed toward improving prehospital cardiac care must now focus on optimizing prehospital trauma care. The continuing cost to society from trauma deaths and disabilities demands further development of prehospital trauma care. To provide for orderly, effective change, developments need to be research-based, with input from physicians, nurses, and field providers involved in the care of the trauma patient.[10]

Trunkey identifies several major issues currently facing prehospital care providers: 1) medical control, 2) determination of which procedures are useful in the field, and 3) the time:benefit ratio of these procedures (the time spent performing interventions in the field compared to the actual patient benefit).[11] These issues can serve as the basis for many research programs. Research concerning medical control could include comparisons of the use of field protocols and direct medical intervention (by radio/telemetry) in the field, flexibility of field protocols, and education and training of medical field advisors. Time:benefit ratio issues could lead to research in the areas of stabilization time, percentage of failed procedural attempts (possibly related to frequency of performance), and patient benefit from various interventions. Another potential research topic is comparisons of the effectiveness of multitiered EMS systems (systems composed of both basic and advanced life support units).

The ongoing growth of prehospital systems and the improved effectiveness and quality of prehospital trauma care depend on the development of trauma-related education, nationally standardized and recognized training programs, and continued efforts in progressive prehospital research programs. Collaborative efforts between prehospital and in-hospital care providers to address and resolve the issues previously discussed can stimulate growth, strengthen clinical expertise, and promote realization of our common goal—optimal trauma patient care.

A discussion of prehospital systems must include examination of the relationship that has developed between the prehospital and hospital-based care providers. Both groups share a common goal: the provision of optimal, effective trauma care. Prehospital care personnel are the first members of the trauma team to provide patient care. The decisions made and the actions initiated in the field provide the foundation for trauma resuscitation and are then expanded upon in the hospital facility. The valuable contributions of prehospital personnel, however, often go unrecognized and unappreciated. Despite the shared goal of both groups, a gap exists between the prehospital and in-hospital care providers. Closer evaluation of this relationship, which is essential for consistent, quality patient care, reveals a major deficit in the area of communication. Most problems occurring between these two components of the team revolve around ineffective or nonexistent communication.

Open, two-way communication is an integral element of any successful relationship. Three currently weak aspects of the prehospital-hospital relationship could be strengthened by improved communication: patient information, feedback, and mutual education.

Patient information

Patient information relayed from the field is the most vital communication link within this prehospital-hospital relationship. The dynamic nature of traumatic injuries often causes drastic changes in the patient's condition from the time of the initial report until his arrival in the emergency care area. Therefore, this initial patient report must be accurately relayed, since it serves as the baseline to which all future assessments are compared. The communication and consultation from the field should be formulated and presented in a systematic or priority format that not only promotes accuracy and objectivity but also reflects the urgency and priority of the patient's needs. Prehospital reports must contain the following information:

Patient data
- sex and approximate age
- weight (especially important for children)
- mechanism of injury†
- obvious or suspected injuries
- vital signs (including trends reflecting improvement or deterioration)
- level of consciousness (Glasgow Coma Scale)
- therapy initiated at the scene (oxygen and drug administration, I.V. catheter insertion, PASG application, immobilization)
- available medical history
- estimated time of arrival (to definitive care facility).

Other pertinent data
- time—**Note:** *Maintain an awareness of the overall time frame from the initial time of the accident or injury until the patient's arrival at the definitive care facility to estimate how much of the "Golden Hour" is spent in the field.*
  - ☐ estimated time of the accident or injury
  - ☐ extrication time and how long the patient was trapped
  - ☐ on-scene time after extrication
  - ☐ loading time
  - ☐ transport time to the definitive care facility.
- on-scene contributing factors
  - ☐ use of safety restraints (seat belt, child safety seat)
  - ☐ approximate speed of the vehicle(s) involved
  - ☐ chemicals found at the scene (alcohol, drugs).
- special patient considerations—**Note:** *This advance information concerning specific patient situations enables the admitting team to anticipate potential patient needs, plan for specific procedures, notify specialized personnel, and prepare equipment accordingly.*

☐ patient under arrest (especially if handcuffs or leg shackles are in place)
☐ patient with a psychiatric history
☐ patient who is violent, homicidal, or suicidal
☐ pregnant patient
☐ infant or young child being transported to an adult center
☐ extremely obese patient
☐ patient with a known infectious disease
☐ non-English-speaking patient
☐ patient contaminated with toxic material.

When presented in a concise, standardized format, this information reflects the patient's overall status and stability. The initial data should be appropriately relayed to all members of the admitting team prior to the patient's arrival when possible. Upon arrival in the emergency care area, the prehospital care provider should update the team with a concise report of any changes or trends, additional findings, and therapies instituted en route.

Mutual education/feedback

The daily interaction of prehospital and in-hospital team members provides significant opportunities for mutual education. This educational process occurs on both informal and formal levels. The informal level consists primarily of feedback and discussions concerning specific situations and cases. The formal level involves joint participation in multidisciplinary educational programs.

Informal education. Both the prehospital and in-hospital care providers can benefit from a critical examination of the patient care delivered in specific situations. It is important that a system exist for the regular exchange of both positive and negative feedback between the two components of the team. This feedback, whether in written or verbal form, promotes consistent care by monitoring the quality of care and the effectiveness of protocols in the field. Whenever possible, feedback mechanisms should permit one-on-one communication concerning the patient care provided. This communication should not occur during the critical phase of trauma resuscitation but instead shortly thereafter, while events are still fresh in everyone's minds. Although sometimes difficult, this process must be conducted without judgmental or defensive attitudes, which can rapidly halt effective communication. Repeated unsatisfying communication may decrease participation in the feedback program. Planning communication in advance and keeping the goal of improved patient care clearly in mind will promote an open, mutual exchange of information.

Formal education. Formal educational programs, such as case presentations, symposia, disaster exercises, and procedure inservices, provide opportunities for enhancing knowledge levels. The prehospital-hospital relationship is

---

†The mechanism of injury and any details concerning the accident are extremely valuable data that assist the team in predicting potential associated injuries. In combination with patient survey findings, the mechanism of injury triggers the team's index of suspicion for injuries commonly seen as a result of the specific type of accident.

improved by the social interaction and the development of a common knowledge base inherent in joint multidisciplinary educational programs. Each component is afforded the opportunity to share valuable information that provides insight into the specialized care required and provided in the respective areas. Developing a wider trauma knowledge base and gaining insight into other phases of trauma care often eliminate or minimize future communication or care-related problems.

Collaboration must exist between all members of the trauma team, especially prehospital and in-hospital care providers. Continued cooperative efforts between these two facets of the trauma team will result in a more unified approach to trauma care. This chapter should have led to a greater understanding of the various pressures upon prehospital systems and their relationship with in-hospital providers.

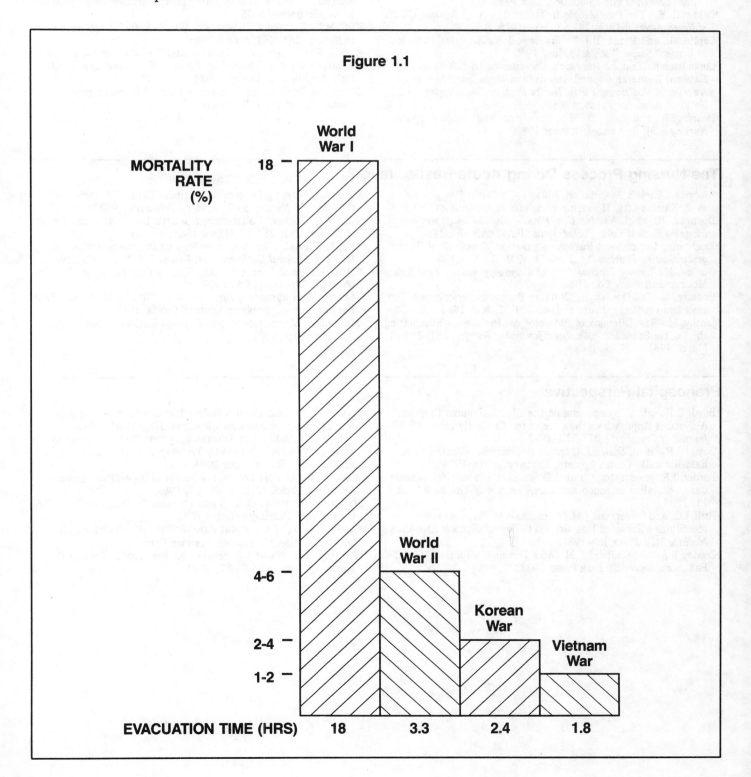

Figure 1.1

REFERENCES

TRAUMA CARE: AN OVERVIEW

The Team Approach to Trauma

[1] Baker, S.P., et al. *The Injury Fact Book.* Lexington, Mass.: Lexington Books, 1984.

[2] Braulin, J.L.D., et al. "Families in Crisis: The Impact of Trauma," *Critical Care Quarterly* 38-46, December 1980.

[3] Caldwell, E. "The Psychologic Impact of Trauma," *Nursing Clinics of North America* 13(2):247-53, June 1978.

[4] Caplin, G., and Parad, H.J. "A Framework for Studying Families in Crisis," *Social Work* 3-15, July 1960.

[5] Committee on Trauma Research, Commission on Life Sciences, National Research Council, Institute of Medicine. *Injury in America: A Continuing Public Health Problem.* Washington, D.C.: National Academy Press, 1985.

[6] Dearing, B., and Dang, D. "The Family in Crisis," *Life Support Nursing* 3(5), September/October 1980.

[7] Eichelberger, M.R. *Pediatric Trauma.* Baltimore: Presented before the National Trauma Symposium, 1985.

[8] Groves, M.J. "Initial Communication with Trauma Patients," in *Trauma Nursing.* Edited by Cardona, V.D. Oradell, N.J.: Medical Economic Books, 1985.

[9] Kim, M.J. "Without Collaboration, What's Left?" *American Journal of Nursing* 281, 284, March 1985.

[10] Lewis, F.R. "Prehospital Trauma Care," in *Current Therapy of Trauma 1984-1985.* Edited by Trunkey, D.D., and Lewis, F.R. Philadelphia: B.C. Decker, 1984.

[11] Maryland Institute for Emergency Medical Services Systems. *Annual Report-1983.* Baltimore.

The Nursing Process During Acute Resuscitation

[1] American Nurse's Association. *Nursing—A Social Policy Statement.* Kansas City, Mo.: American Nurse's Association, 1980.

[2] Doenges, M., et al. *Nursing Care Plans—Nursing Diagnoses in Planning Patient Care.* Philadelphia: F.A. Davis Co., 1984.

[3] Emergency Department Nurses Association. *Standards of Emergency Nursing Practice.* St. Louis: C.V. Mosby Co., 1983.

[4] Gordon, M. *Nursing Diagnosis: Process and Application.* New York: McGraw-Hill Book Co., 1982.

[5] Guzetta, C., and Dossey, B. "Nursing Diagnosis: Framework, Process and Problem," *Heart & Lung* 281-91, May 1983.

[6] Jacoby, M. "The Dilemma of Physiological Problems—Eliminating the Double Standard," *American Journal of Nursing* 281, 284-85, March 1985.

[7] Kim, M.J. "Nursing Diagnosis in Critical Care," *Dimensions of Critical Care Nursing* 5-67, January/February 1983.

[8] Kim, M.J. "Without Collaboration, What's Left?" *American Journal of Nursing* 281, 284-85, March 1985.

[9] Kim, M.J., et al. *Classification of Nursing Diagnoses: Proceedings of the Fifth National Conference.* St. Louis: C.V. Mosby Co., 1984.

[10] Little, D.E., and Carnevali, D.L. *Nursing Care Planning.* Philadelphia: J.B. Lippincott Co., 1969.

[11] Mayers, M. *A Systematic Approach to the Nursing Care Plan.* East Norwalk, Conn.: Appleton-Century-Crofts, 1972.

[12] Mundinger, Mary. *Autonomy in Nursing.* Rockville, Md.: Aspen Systems Corp., 1980.

Prehospital Perspective

[1] Boyd, D.R., ed. "A Symposium on the Illinois Trauma Program: A Systems Approach to the Care of the Critically Injured," *Journal of Trauma* 13:275-320, 1973.

[2] Boyd, D.R., et al. *Systems Approach to Emergency Medical Care.* East Norwalk, Conn.: Appleton-Century-Crofts, 1983.

[3] Border, J.R. (moderator). "Panel Discussion: Prehospital Trauma Care—Stabilize or Scoop and Run," *Journal of Trauma* 23:708-11, 1983.

[4] Brill, J.C., and Geiderman, J.M. "A Rationale for Scoop and Run: Identifying a Subset of Time-Critical Patients," *Topics in Emergency Medicine* 3(2): 37-43, July 1981.

[5] Cowley, R.A., and Dunham, C.M. *Shock Trauma/Critical Care Manual.* Baltimore: University Park Press, 1982.

[6] Franaszek, J. "Stabilization Before Transportation—But How Much?" *Topics in Emergency Medicine* 3(2): 31-35, 1981.

[7] Lewis, F.R. "Prehospital Trauma Care," in *Current Therapy of Trauma 1984-1985.* Edited by Trunkey, D.D., and Lewis, F.R. Philadelphia: B.C. Decker, 1984.

[8] McSwain, N. "Another Look at the Technical Imperative," *Topics in Emergency Medicine* 3(2): 87-90, July 1981.

[9] Statistical Abstracts of the United States. Washington, D.C.: U.S. Government Printing Office, 1979.

[10] Stewart, R.D., "Prehospital Care of Trauma," in *Trauma Quarterly.* Rockville, Md.: Aspen Systems Corp., 1985.

[11] Trunkey, D.D. "Is ALS Necessary for Prehospital Trauma Care?" *Journal of Trauma* 24:86-87, 1984.

INJURIES—ACUTE ILLNESSES—
SHOCK STATES

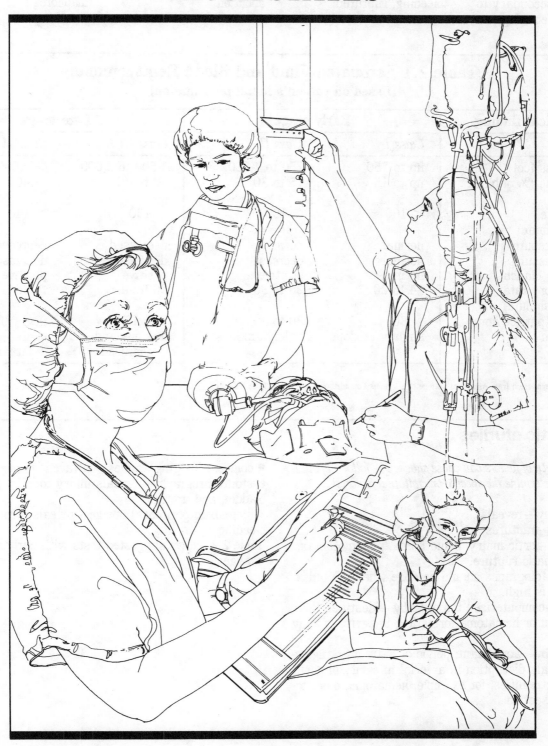

Medical diagnosis

HEMORRHAGIC SHOCK

Assessment

Mechanism of injury/etiology:
• bleeding secondary to blunt or penetrating

trauma
• association with GI bleeding, ruptured

ectopic pregnancy, spontaneous or induced abortion

Physical findings:
• skin—pallor, coolness, diaphoresis

Table 2.1 Estimated Fluid and Blood Requirements[1]
(Based on patient's initial presentation)

Physical finding	Early stage		Late stage	
	Class I	*Class II*	*Class III*	*Class IV*
Blood loss (cc)	up to 750	750 to 1,500	1,500 to 2,000	> 2,000
Blood loss (% of blood volume)	up to 15	15 to 30	30 to 40	> 40
Pulse rate (beats/minute)	< 100	> 100	> 120	> 140
Blood pressure	normal	normal	decreased	decreased
Pulse pressure	normal	decreased	decreased	decreased
Capillary blanch	normal	positive	positive	positive
Respiratory rate (breaths/minute)	14 to 20	20 to 30	30 to 40	> 35
Urine output (cc/hour)	≥ 30	20 to 30	5 to 15	negligible
Mentation	slightly anxious	mildly anxious	anxious and confused	confused and lethargic

[1]For a 70-kg male.
Reprinted with permission from American College of Surgeons Committee on Trauma (ATLS) Manual.

Diagnostic studies

Note: *A variety of factors can cause shock. The following studies can help determine the specific precipitating factor(s).*

• radiography—reveals:
☐ pelvis—fractures
☐ chest—aortic injury, hemothorax, pneumothorax, diaphragmatic rupture.
Additional radiographs should be done when the index of suspicion is high.
• imaging—computerized tomography—identifies fluid accumulation or hematoma formation; integrity of bony structures
• angiography—aortogram; pelvic or extremity angiography—reveals disruption in arterial integrity of aorta, pelvis, or extremities, for example, hematoma, obstruction, or transection

• contrast imaging studies—intravenous pyelography, cystourethrography—reveals injury to kidneys, ureters, bladder, and urethra
• diagnostic peritoneal lavage—reveals intraabdominal bleeding
Table 2.2 shows suggested tests with early and late changes:

Table 2.2 Changes in Laboratory Values During Shock

Blood study	Early	Late
Hemoglobin/hematocrit	WNL (within normal limits)	↓
WBC	WNL	↑
Prothrombin time	WNL	may be extremely prolonged
Partial thromboplastin time	WNL	may be extremely prolonged
Platelets	WNL	↓
Sodium	↑	↑ or ↓
Potassium	↓	↑
Glucose	↑	↓
Blood urea nitrogen	WNL	↑
Creatinine	WNL	↑
Chloride	↓	↑
Lactate[1]	WNL or ↑	↑
pH	↑	↓
PaO$_2$	remains WNL or ↓	↓
PaCO$_2$	↓	↑
HCO$_3$	WNL	↓
Oxygen saturation	WNL or ↓	↓

[1]Lactate, although not absolutely required, reflects anaerobic metabolism at the cellular level.
Note: *Sending a blood sample for hepatitis-associated antigen (HAA) determination is not necessary in the assessment, planning, or evaluation of the trauma patient; however, it is advantageous for patient and staff safety to know if the patient is HAA⁺.*

• invasive monitoring—reflects and aids management of the patient's hemodynamic status
☐ pulmonary artery catheter—measures pulmonary arterial pressure, pulmonary capillary wedge pressure, carbon dioxide, and mixed venous gases
☐ arterial pressure catheter—permits accurate, continuous arterial pressure monitoring, waveform assessment, and blood sampling
☐ central venous catheter—measures the right heart's ability to accept a fluid load.

Nursing diagnosis

Potential for decreased tissue perfusion related to fluid volume deficit secondary to hemorrhage.

GOAL: Optimize tissue perfusion.

Note: *A systematic approach using the A, B, C sequence promotes rapid resuscitation and stabilization of the hemorrhagic shock patient. Early, aggressive airway management, including oxygenation and ventilation in combination with rapid volume expansion, helps prevent postshock complications.*

SHOCK

Interventions

1. Assess the patient's respiratory status:
- evaluate his airway
- auscultate breath sounds
- administer supplemental oxygen as ordered

- integrate ABG and chest radiograph results to prepare for intubation and chest-tube insertion.

2. Assess the patient's cardiovascular (CV) status and establish baseline data:
- assess bleeding source and volume lost
- monitor and document the patient's vital signs (blood pressure, heart rate, and pulse pressure) and perfusion parameters (capillary refill time, skin color, and temperature) every 5 to 15 minutes
- monitor continuous ECG rhythm
- obtain baseline and serial blood samples, and monitor results frequently for changes
- include blood typing and cross matching in initial sampling.

3. Assess the patient's neurologic status:
- monitor his level of consciousness.

4. Assess the patient's renal status:
- insert an indwelling urinary catheter unless contraindicated.
Note: *Contraindications include blood at the urinary meatus, scrotal or perineal hematoma, and a high-riding prostate as detected on rectal examination.*
- monitor intake/output trends
- hematest urine samples
- send urine samples for analysis.

5. Control bleeding by:
- applying direct pressure
- elevating an extremity
- putting the patient in Trendelenburg position
- applying a pneumatic antishock garment (PASG).

Rationale

Early shock
This assessment establishes a baseline for trend analysis. Supplemental oxygen augments oxygen saturation of RBCs. Prompt, aggressive oxygen therapy can relieve hypoxemia and its potential complications, including adult respiratory distress syndrome, renal failure, and coagulopathy. Clinical signs may not correlate with ABG findings. The chest radiograph determines a mechanical as opposed to physiologic cause of further respiratory deterioration.
Late shock
An uncompensated physiologic state requires aggressive oxygen therapy to support the already stressed respiratory system.

Early shock
The bleeding source may be obscured, and in early shock vital signs and laboratory data may not accurately reflect the condition's potential severity.
Late shock
The ongoing CV assessment reflects the class and progression of shock. These parameters are indicators of compensation and decompensation (see Table 2.2). Dysrhythmias may develop from hypoxemia, electrolyte imbalance, cardiac contusion, central venous pressure or pulmonary artery line insertion, and any preexisting cardiac condition. Baseline laboratory values are necessary for accurate trend analysis. Typing and cross matching ensure readily available blood for transfusion.

Early shock
Slight or mild anxiety may be an early sign of shock.
Late shock
Deterioration in neurologic status, except from a central nervous system injury, indicates Class III or IV shock.

Intake/output trends reflect tissue perfusion and the adequacy of volume replacement therapy (50 ml/hour in adults; see chart for early/late shock). Gross or microscopic hematuria indicates the need for intravenous pyelography and/or cystourethrography. The specific gravity value reflects hydration. Glycosuria and ketonuria may underscore the need for further metabolic investigation. The patient's urine sample must accompany his serum sample for toxicologic evaluation.

Direct pressure promotes clotting. Elevation and Trendelenburg position increase venous return, which increases core circulation. A PASG increases peripheral vascular resistance and myocardial afterload. Additional benefits of a PASG include splinting, hemorrhage control, and tamponade for lower extremity and pelvic fractures.

6. Replace fluid volume:
• ensure venous access by starting two large-bore 14 to 16g peripheral I.V.s
• administer I.V. fluids, blood, and blood products as ordered
• anticipate the use of autotransfusion.

Multiple large-bore peripheral I.V. lines ensure venous access for rapid volume infusion and I.V. drug administration. Ringer's lactate is typically the fluid of choice, with normal saline solution being the second choice. RBC transfusions increase oxygen-carrying capacity and decrease the amount of anaerobic metabolism. Blood should not be infused with dextrose or Ringer's lactate solution. Blood component therapy ensures replacement of clotting factors. Prompt, aggressive volume replacement with colloid, crystalloid, and component therapy aids reduction of potential complications. Autotransfusion provides safe, warm, and readily available blood.

7. Monitor the patient's hemodynamic status:
• prepare for the use of invasive monitoring lines, including arterial, central venous pressure, and pulmonary artery catheters.

Vasoconstriction and increased arterial constriction in hypotensive states make Korotkoff sounds less audible. An arterial pressure catheter provides waveform assessment, access for frequent arterial blood sampling, and accurate blood pressure readings. Central venous pressure lines serve as a guide to the right heart's ability to accept fluid load. Pulmonary capillary wedge pressure (PCWP) measures left ventricular function. Right atrial, pulmonary artery, and PCWP pressures may be monitored. Cardiac output and mixed venous sampling may be obtained, and the intrapulmonary shunt can be calculated from the above measurements.

8. Anticipate the need for inotropic agents.

Inotropic agents enhance cardiac output by increasing renal, coronary, mesenteric, and cerebral blood flow.

Nursing diagnosis

Potential for continued fluid volume deficit related to hemorrhage secondary to coagulopathy.

GOAL: Prevent, minimize, or correct clotting disorders.

Interventions

1. Obtain baseline coagulation studies (prothrombin time, partial thromboplastin time, platelets, fibrinogen).

2. Transfuse RBCs, platelets, fresh-frozen plasma, and cryoprecipitate as ordered through micropore tubing.

3. Warm all blood before infusing (especially when giving massive transfusions).

4. Anticipate the need for calcium.

5. Monitor the patient's serum pH; anticipate the need for sodium bicarbonate.

Rationale

In later stages of shock, large volume replacement is required. Blood component therapy replaces clotting factors lost from hemorrhage. Laboratory data trend analysis accurately reflects the patient's coagulation profile.

Filtration via tubing removes microscopic clots and debris.

Cold, banked blood lowers the patient's core temperature, thereby increasing the risk of myocardial dysrhythmias and paradoxical hypotension. Hypothermia can compound microvascular bleeding.

Calcium supplements are usually not required but may be necessary for a patient requiring massive transfusions. Banked blood contains calcium-binding citrate.

Acidosis aggravates microvascular bleeding.

SHOCK

6. Use autotransfusion to retrieve shed blood for infusion, unless contraindicated. (See "Autotransfusion" in Section VII.)

Autologous blood is safe, warm, readily available, less costly than banked blood, and usually acceptable to patients with religious objections to homologous transfusions.

Nursing diagnosis

Potential for hypothermia related to decreased tissue perfusion and rapid infusion of I.V. fluids.

GOAL: Maintain a normothermic state.

Interventions

1. Continuously monitor trends in the patient's core temperature.

2. Warm the patient with:
• hemocoil or blood warmer
• blood infusions with warmed normal saline solution (if blood is required for shock)
• oxygen warmed with a heated humidity device
• warm solution for diagnostic peritoneal lavage
• warm sheets
• hyperthermia blanket
• warming lights.

Rationale

Core temperature monitoring is needed to evaluate therapy properly. The following, in descending order, provide the most accurate measurement of core body temperature:
• pulmonary artery catheter
• continuous esophageal probe
• continuous bladder probe
• continuous rectal probe
• rectal temperature taken every 30 minutes to 1 hour.

Hypothermia can precipitate paradoxical hypotension, cardiac dysrhythmias, and cardiac arrest. As the core temperature decreases, the sinoatrial node is cooled, causing myocardial electrical dysfunction. Hypothermia and acidosis promote increased microvascular bleeding.

Associated care plans

Hypothermia
Psychosocial Support of the Trauma Patient
Disseminated Intravascular Coagulation
Adult Respiratory Distress Syndrome
Acute Renal Failure

Associated procedures

Pulmonary Artery Catheterization
Autotransfusion
Preparation for Surgery
Endotracheal Intubation

SHOCK

Medical diagnosis

VASOGENIC SHOCK (Septic, Neurogenic, and Anaphylactic)

Assessment

Mechanism of injury/etiology:
- spinal cord injury (disruption, edema, contusion, or hemorrhage)
- allergies
- infection (usually gram-negative bacteria but can be gram-positive or fungal)
- neurologic injury or disorder
- substance abuse

Physical findings:

Septic shock
- See Table 2.3 below.

Neurogenic shock
- bradycardia (slow-bounding pulse)
- hypotension
- warm, dry skin
- poikilothermy (assuming the environmental temperature)
- loss of strength or motor ability below the level of the lesion
- respiratory distress
- decreased cardiac output

Anaphylactic shock
- generalized urticaria
- cool, pale skin
- nausea, vomiting
- progressive respiratory failure, including choking sensation ("I can't breathe"); wheezing, dyspnea, swelling of uvula and tongue; laryngeal edema (causes barking or high-pitched cough); bronchospasms; respiratory arrest
- hypotension

Note: *A rapid course characterizes anaphylactic shock, with symptoms developing rapidly from vasodilation caused by histamine release. Treatment must be started immediately to prevent death.*

Table 2.3 Septic Shock	
Warm or hyperdynamic (early) stage	**Cold or hypodynamic (late) stage**
• tachycardia • tachypnea • warm, pink skin • hyperthermia • polyuria • restlessness • respiratory alkalosis	• tachycardia • tachypnea • pallor • hypothermia • oliguria • unresponsiveness • disseminated intravascular coagulation • hypotension • decreased cardiac output

Diagnostic studies

Septic shock
- cultures—of fluids from I.V. puncture sites, sinuses, and surgical or nonsurgical wounds, and of sputum, urine, blood, spinal fluid (if indicated)
- computed tomography (CT) scan—identifies areas of potential abscesses
- radiography—chest or abdominal films may reveal fluid accumulation, free air, abscesses
- WBC—reveals indication of infectious process

Neurogenic shock
- fluid challenge—rules out hypovolemia as shock cause
- radiography—spinal films
- CT scan—may reveal cord edema, contusion, hemorrhage
- myelography—may reveal cord obstruction

Anaphylactic shock
- bronchoscopy—evaluates laryngeal and upper airway edema

Nursing diagnosis

Potential for fluid volume deficit related to peripheral vasodilation.

GOAL: Restore and maintain normovolemia.

Interventions

1. Assess the cardiovascular baseline:
- skin color
- pulse
- blood pressure
- capillary refill time (CRT)
- edema.

2. Ensure I.V. access with a minimum of two large-bore catheters.

3. Place the patient in Trendelenburg position and apply a pneumatic antishock garment, unless contraindicated.

4. Assemble equipment and assist in insertion of a pulmonary artery or central venous pressure line. (See "Pulmonary Artery Catheterization" in Section VII.)

5. Insert an indwelling urinary catheter; monitor intake and output closely.

6. Monitor, document, and report hemodynamic trends.

7. Validate monitor readings through clinical findings.

8. Monitor laboratory data and report abnormal or changing trends in:
- hemoglobin/hematocrit level
- coagulation profile.

Rationale

Septic shock—depending on the shock phase, the patient may initially have an increased cardiac output, causing a flushed or pink appearance, elevated blood pressure, and a full-bounding pulse. As the hypodynamic phase develops, the cardinal signs of shock become evident. This low-flow state is characterized by tachycardia, a decreasing blood pressure, prolonged CRT, and pallor. (See Physical Findings: Septic Shock.)

Neurogenic shock—the loss of vascular neural tone causes peripheral pooling, resulting in systemic hypotension.

Anaphylactic shock—histamine release causes:
- vasodilation, resulting in hypotension and thready pulse
- increased capillary permeability with third-space shifting of fluids, especially notable in face (eyelids), tongue, hands, and genitalia.

Fluid volume loss secondary to redistribution requires replacement with blood, blood products, and crystalloids.

These measures facilitate venous return from the lower extremities.

Ideally, left ventricular function should be evaluated continuously through pulmonary arterial monitoring. However, if this is not possible, central venous pressure monitoring will provide general indications of cardiac function by monitoring right ventricular status. Cardiac status serves as a guide for fluid replacement and drug therapy.

Fluid replacement can be judged effective if urine output is adequate: a minimum of 50 cc/hour in the adult.

Trend analysis indicating stability, improvement, or deterioration is used to adjust therapy.

Errors in treatment can occur if monitor readings are taken as the sole indication of physiologic conditions without validating the patient's clinical picture. High-technology equipment places responsibility on the caregiver to understand, troubleshoot, and correct technical problems.

Peripheral pooling caused by vasodilation results in a relative hypovolemia. Initially, endotoxin activity indirectly affects cardiac function. As the shock state progresses, the endotoxins (bradykinin, histamine, lactic acid, carbon dioxide, kallikrein, and myocardial depressant factor) cause peripheral vasodilation, reflected by a lower hemoglobin/hematocrit level. Microcirculation pooling makes blood unavailable to the central circulatory system. Disseminated intravascular coagulation may develop with increasing cellular permeability.

9. Administer and evaluate inotropic drug therapy to maintain a mean arterial pressure of > 80 to 110 mm Hg:
- dopamine
- dobutamine.

Inotropic agents enhance cardiac output to increase renal, mesenteric, coronary, and cerebral blood flow.

10. Monitor core body temperature and provide appropriate care.

In septic shock, infection elevates temperature, requiring corrective measures. Care may range from antipyretic suppositories to cool packs to thermia blankets. In neurogenic shock, thermoregulation mechanisms are altered or lost secondary to loss of the sympathetic response. Care is directed toward correcting hypothermia or hyperthermia. Spinal cord-injured patients with elevated temperatures should be evaluated for sources of infections.

Nursing diagnosis

Potential for impaired gas exchange related to accumulation of fluid in alveoli and pulmonary interstitium.

GOAL: Maintain or restore optimal pulmonary function.

Interventions

Rationale

1. Assess the patient's respiratory status; evaluate:
- respiratory rate, rhythm
- chest expansion or abdominal movement
- breath sounds
- ABG results
- signs of bronchospasms.

Increasing cardiovascular demands increase oxygen consumption regardless of the underlying cause of the shock state. In septic shock's hyperdynamic phase, a patient may be in respiratory distress despite relatively normal ABG results. Initially, a decreasing PaO_2 level may be an early indication of atrioventricular shunting at the arteriole level. Adventitious breath sounds suggest altered capillary permeability and beginning pulmonary edema. In the hypodynamic state, ABG results reflect hypoxia or metabolic acidosis.

  In anaphylactic shock, histamine release causes increased capillary permeability; therefore, third-space shifting of fluids may occur. Histamine also causes smooth muscle contraction; therefore, bronchospasms may occur.

2. Optimize respiratory function through such measures as:
- breathing exercises
- chest physiotherapy
- incentive spirometry
- progressively supportive oxygen therapy, such as intubation or tracheostomy with mechanical ventilation. (See "Endotracheal Intubation" in Section VII.)

In spine-injured patients, lost neural innervation of respiratory muscles can impair respiratory function. This predisposes the patient to retained secretions and, if untreated, to pneumonia; the cough mechanism is altered or completely absent. Identifying the deficit level proves essential. Lesions at C_4, which provides diaphragm innervation, or above produce total loss of spontaneous respiration. Lesions at T_{6-7} and above paralyze intercostal muscle function, rendering the patient unable to deep-breathe or cough. Major abdominal muscles essential to expiration receive innervation from T_{6-12}. Position changes and chest physiotherapy aid mobilization and drainage of secretions.

3. Interpret and report untoward trends in ABG results.

Decreasing PaO_2 and increasing $PaCO_2$ values indicate a deteriorating respiratory status. The cause must be determined and more aggressive ventilatory therapy instituted.

4. Administer bronchodilators, as ordered.

Bronchodilators act on beta$_2$ receptor sites to produce airway dilation.

Nursing diagnosis

(Neurogenic shock) Potential for ineffective breathing patterns related to fatigue of remaining respiratory muscles secondary to neurologic injury.

GOAL: Promote and maintain maximum respiratory function.

Interventions

1. Assess and monitor the patient's respiratory status every hour or more frequently, as his condition warrants:
- observe respiratory rate and rhythm
- observe quality of chest expansion, abdominal movement
- auscultate breath sounds
- monitor ABG results and report trends.

2. Optimize respiratory function through such measures as:
- breathing exercises
- chest physiotherapy
- incentive spirometry
- progressively supportive oxygen therapy, such as intubation or tracheostomy with mechanical ventilation.

3. Report increasing respiratory distress and anticipate use of supplemental oxygen. Ensure availability of equipment needed for intubation and mechanical ventilation.

Rationale

In neurogenic shock, dependent on the level and extent of spinal cord damage, respiratory status must be assessed continually in all patients. The onset of respiratory distress can be slow and insidious, necessitating continual awareness of the patient's respiratory status. Respiratory status may be affected by:
- the level and extent of cord damage
- increasing neurologic deficit (up to 72 hours after the trauma, resulting from further cord edema or hemorrhage)
- excessive fatigue from the extra work load placed on the remaining functional respiratory muscles
- pulmonary complications following trauma or associated injuries.

See rationale #2 (for pulmonary hygiene) in the preceding nursing diagnosis.

Nursing diagnosis

(Septic shock) Potential for systemic infection related to bacterial or fungal invasion.

GOAL: Reduce or eliminate the risk of infection.

Interventions

1. Prevent or minimize the introduction of pathogenic or potentially pathogenic organisms:
- use frequent handwashing
- maintain aseptic technique for all invasive procedures
- initiate or maintain isolation measures, if indicated
- schedule laboratory tests collectively to reduce the number of venipunctures.

Rationale

Many patients survive trauma only to succumb to overwhelming septicemia in the posttraumatic phase. Reasons for increased post-trauma risk for infection include the following:
- shock states alter the immune response so that normally non-pathogenic organisms may have a pathogenic effect
- hospital-acquired organisms may be of a highly resistant nature
- invasive procedures provide ports of entry
- antibiotic therapy, while treating one organism, may allow another to proliferate
- bloody or serous wound drainage provides an excellent medium for pathogenic growth.

Conscientious and diligent measures, such as handwashing and maintaining aseptic technique, can minimize the risk of infection.

2. Assemble equipment for and assist in bedside procedures (such as irrigation and drainage of small abscesses or sinus drainage). Label and send culture specimens to the laboratory. Dispose of exudate and contaminated equipment and linens according to institutional policy.

As signs of infection develop or advancing infection occurs, measures are directed toward identification of the organism and removal or drainage of the infectious source.

3. Administer antibiotics, as ordered. Monitor drug levels. Observe and report signs of ineffectiveness, toxicity, or side effects of medications.

Organism-specific antibiotics are chosen according to culture and sensitivity results.

4. Prepare the patient for surgery, if needed. (See "Preparation for Surgery" in Section VII.)

Associated care plans	**Associated procedures and study**
Cardiogenic Shock	Bronchoscopy
Hemorrhagic Shock	Pulmonary Artery Catheterization
Cervical Spine Injury	Preparation for Surgery
Thoracic, Lumbar, and Sacral Spine Injury	The Critically Ill or Injured Patient Requiring Special Care
Head Injury	The Pneumatic Antishock Garment
Psychosocial Support of the Trauma Patient	Intraaortic Balloon Pump
Disseminated Intravascular Coagulation	Endotracheal Intubation

SHOCK

CARDIOGENIC SHOCK

Assessment

Mechanism of injury/ etiology:
- history of acute myocardial infarction (AMI)
- severe triple-vessel disease and distal coronary artery occlusion
- papillary muscle rupture
- septal perforation
- cardiac tamponade
- ventricular wall rupture
- end-stage cardiomyopathy
- severe valve disease
- severe dysrhythmias
- tension pneumothorax
- massive pulmonary embolism
- final stage of other shock states

Physical findings:
Respiratory
- sudden onset of respiratory distress
- shortness of breath
- dyspnea
- orthopnea
- tachypnea
- moist rales deteriorating to pulmonary edema

Cardiovascular
- severe chest pain
- hypotension
- cool, clammy skin
- pallor
- absent or weak peripheral pulses
- hypothermia
- dysrhythmias
- ECG changes (elevated ST in V1–V3, ST depression in V4–V6, Q waves in V2–V4, ST elevations and T-wave inversion in V2–V6)
- abnormal heart sounds—murmur, click, friction rub, gallop rhythms (ventricular diastolic, atrial, summation)
- signs of right ventricular failure, including:
  - ☐ jugular vein distention
  - ☐ peripheral edema
  - ☐ hepatomegaly

Neurologic/Psychological
- anxiety, fear
- irritability
- restlessness
- confusion
- decreased mentation

Genitourinary
- urine output < 20 to 25 cc/hour

Diagnostic studies

- laboratory data
  - ☐ ABG analysis—commonly reflects hypoxemia and accompanying acidosis (metabolic and respiratory)
  - ☐ enzymes—elevated creatine phosphokinase-MB, lactate dehydrogenase, and serum glutamic-oxaloacetic transaminase levels (elevation may not occur for 48 hours after AMI) reflects myocardial tissue damage
  - ☐ serum lactic acid level >1.4 mEq/liter reflects anaerobic metabolism
  - ☐ elevated serum blood urea nitrogen/creatinine level—reflects inadequate renal perfusion
  - ☐ urine electrolytes—reflects elevated sodium concentrations.
- radiography
  - ☐ chest film—may show cardiomegaly and alveolar interstitial changes indicating pulmonary edema

- invasive monitoring
  - ☐ arterial pressure catheter—provides continuous arterial pressure monitoring, aortic balloon pump synchronization, and blood-sampling access
  - ☐ pulmonary artery catheter—permits pulmonary arterial pressure and pulmonary capillary wedge pressure (PCWP) measurement, cardiac output and cardiac index (CI) calculation (PCWP > 18 mm Hg; CI < 2.1 liters/minute/m²), access for mixed venous blood sampling
  - ☐ central venous pressure (CVP) catheter—measures right ventricular function, reflects patient's overall systemic volume status

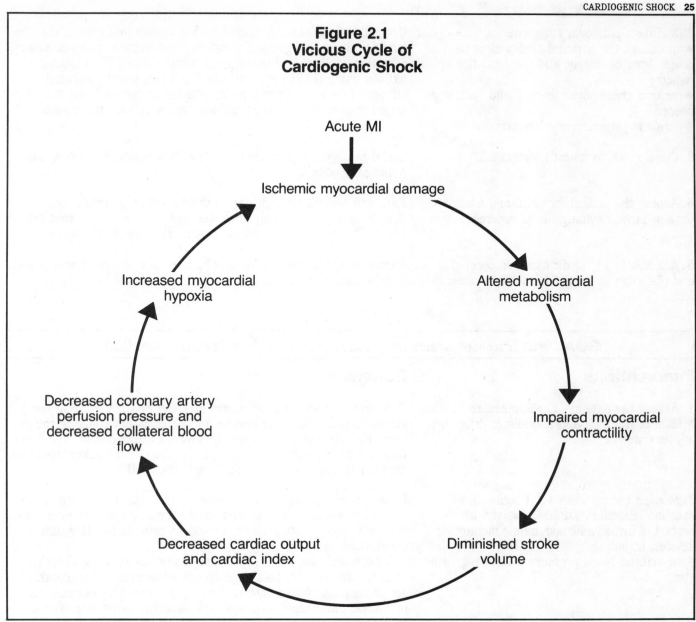

**Figure 2.1
Vicious Cycle of
Cardiogenic Shock**

Acute MI

Ischemic myocardial damage

Altered myocardial metabolism

Impaired myocardial contractility

Diminished stroke volume

Decreased cardiac output and cardiac index

Decreased coronary artery perfusion pressure and decreased collateral blood flow

Increased myocardial hypoxia

Nursing diagnosis

Potential for decreased tissue perfusion related to inadequate cardiac output secondary to left ventricular failure.

GOAL #1: Optimize pulmonary tissue perfusion and oxygen availability.

Interventions

1. Assess the patient's respiratory status:
● evaluate his airway
● auscultate breath sounds
● apply supplemental oxygen as ordered
● integrate ABG and chest radiograph results
● prepare for intubation, mechanical ventilation, and positive end-expiratory pressure (PEEP).

Rationale

Rales and rhonchi are typical in the patient with pulmonary edema. Administering supplemental oxygen helps correct acidemia caused by poor perfusion, ventilatory insufficiency, and pulmonary edema. Increasing myocardial oxygen supply and decreasing myocardial oxygen demand reduce the work of respiration in an already stressed myocardium. PEEP treats pulmonary edema by maintaining positive pressure and keeping alveoli open.

2. Maintain pulmonary hygiene:
• encourage the nonintubated patient to cough, breathe deeply, and use incentive spirometry
• perform chest physiotherapy and suction as needed
• turn the patient every 2 hours.

Optimal lung expansion minimizes atelectasis and pneumonia. Frequent position changes and chest physiotherapy reduce pulmonary secretion pooling. Full turning is contraindicated if an intraaortic balloon pump (IABP) is in use. In this case, slight positional changes may be preferred. Suctioning helps maintain a patent airway; however, it may be contraindicated in pulmonary edema.

3. Closely monitor chest radiographs.

Serial radiographs help identify atelectatic spots, infiltrates, and pulmonary edema.

4. Assess the patient for pain, and administer a sedative or analgesic as ordered.

Pain and associated tachycardia impede optimal ventilation. Breathing asynchronously with the ventilator increases respiratory effort. These problems increase myocardial oxygen demands.

5. Administer I.V. medications as ordered, and observe the patient for hemodynamic effects.

Narcotics administered I.M. may be unevenly absorbed as a result of poor tissue perfusion.

GOAL #2: Increase cardiac output and decrease left ventricular work load.

Interventions

Rationale

1. Assess the patient's cardiovascular status:
• Monitor his ECG and administer drug therapy as ordered.

Dysrhythmias weaken left ventricular contractility, putting more stress on ischemic heart muscle and potentially extending the infarct. Correcting dysrhythmias improves cardiac output. The insertion of a pacemaker may be necessary. (See "Pacemaker Insertion, Temporary Transvenous Pacing" in Section VII.)

2. Monitor the patient's vital signs. Draw baseline laboratory studies. Assist with insertion of invasive hemodynamic monitoring devices, including:
• an arterial blood pressure monitoring catheter

Hemodynamic pressure measurements and vital signs reflect the shock's progression and severity and provide a guide to effectiveness of therapy. Initial laboratory values provide baseline data for trend analysis.
   Vasoconstriction and hypotension make auscultating Korotkoff sounds difficult. Cuff pressures do not accurately reflect central aortic pressure. Mean arterial blood pressures aid determination of cardiac output and total systemic vascular resistance. The intraarterial waveform also acts as a check on IABP.

• a pulmonary artery (PA) catheter with CVP port.

The PA catheter can measure left ventricular, right atrial, pulmonary artery, and pulmonary capillary wedge pressures. These measurements assist with diagnosis and with determination and evaluation of the treatment regimen (drugs, ventilation, and IABP). They also enable calculation of cardiac output, cardiac index, and intrapulmonary shunt. Mixed venous blood samples can be drawn from the PA line.

3. Administer diuretics as prescribed.

Diuretics reduce circulating fluid volume, which decreases left ventricular work load, tachypnea, and orthopnea.

4. Administer vasodilators and vasopressors as prescribed:
• assess the patient for hypovolemia before administering drugs
• closely monitor the patient's blood pressure
• keep the head of the bed flat
• administer a fluid challenge if necessary.

Vasodilators reduce left ventricular work load and afterload by improving systolic emptying. This decreases preload and myocardial oxygen requirements. Vasopressors produce vasoconstriction, raising blood pressure and increasing cardiac output, and may increase myocardial oxygen requirements. Both vasodilators and vasopressors must be titrated to achieve maximum cardiac performance. Hypovolemia can exacerbate hypotension in the patient receiving vasodilators and can decrease vasopressor efficacy.

5. Administer inotropic agents as ordered.

Inotropic agents increase cardiac output by causing the heart's beta-receptors to improve myocardial contractility. These drugs enhance cardiac output and increase renal, mesenteric, coronary, and cerebral blood flow.

6. Assist with insertion of the IABP. (See "Intraaortic Balloon Pump" in Section VII.)

The IABP provides counterpulsation to:
- increase coronary artery blood flow
- increase cardiac output
- increase oxygen supply
- decrease myocardial work and oxygen consumption.

7. Assess the patient's neurologic status.

Changes in mentation may reflect the degree of cerebral perfusion.

8. Assess the patient's renal status:
- insert an indwelling catheter
- monitor urine output.

Urine output reflects renal perfusion.

Associated care plans

Myocardial Contusion
Acute Pericardial Tamponade
Acute Myocardial Infarction
Pulmonary Thromboembolus
Tension Pneumothorax
Pulmonary Edema

Associated procedures

Pulmonary Artery Catheterization
Intraaortic Balloon Pump
Pacemaker Insertion, Temporary Transvenous Pacing

CERVICAL SPINE INJURY

Assessment

Note: *For the purposes of this care plan, cervical spine injury is defined as spinal cord deficit with or without bony or ligamentous injury. However, immobilization and stabilization techniques will be the same for the patient with bony or ligamentous injury without neurologic deficit.*

Mechanism of injury/ etiology:
- blunt trauma—rapid acceleration/deceleration causing flexion or hyper-extension of the neck
- vertical compression and subluxation—as in diving accidents (falls landing on head)
- penetrating trauma—as from missiles, such as in gunshot wounds or stab wounds; impaling injuries

Physical findings:
Neurologic
- highly variable level of consciousness, from awake and alert to unre-sponsive, depending on associated injuries
- cervical pain
- altered motor function, from weakness to paraly-sis
- altered sensation, from paresthesia or hyperes-thesia to insensateness
- bony or ligamentous in-jury without neurologic deficit
- forearms flexed over chest (indicative of C_5 in-jury from loss of triceps innervation)

Respiratory
- shortness of breath
- diaphragmatic breath-ing
- respiratory distress
- respiratory arrest

Cardiovascular
- bradycardia
- warm, dry skin
- labile blood pressure
- poikilothermy (assum-ing the environmental temperature)
- vasogenic (neurogenic) shock state

Gastrointestinal
- absent bowel sounds
- gastric distention

Genitourinary
- urinary retention
- priapism

Associated injuries:
- head: fractures, epidural/subdural hema-tomas
- facial: fractures, lacer-ations
- chest: pneumothorax, hemothorax, rib and ster-nal fractures
- abdominal: intraab-dominal injuries
- musculoskeletal: pelvic and long-bone fractures

Diagnostic studies

- radiography
  - ☐ lateral cervical spine radiography (most important radiograph)—to evaluate all seven cervical vertebrae
  - ☐ computed tomography scan—to rule out associated head injury; provides further visualization of cervical spine; done in conjunction with myelography
  - ☐ tomography—to reveal more extensive, poorly visu-alized, or hidden fractures that may be overshadowed by other structures
  - ☐ myelography—to locate evidence of pressure or im-pingement on the spinal cord or a nerve root
- laboratory studies
  - ☐ ABGs—may reveal hypoxemia
  - ☐ hemoglobin/hematocrit—may reflect hypovolemia from associated injuries

Potential for motor and sensory deficit related to potential spinal cord injury.

> **GOAL:** Maintain an increased index of suspicion and protect the patient from spinal cord injury.

Note: *Every unevaluated trauma patient must be treated as having a cervical spine injury until proven otherwise.*

*Supplemental nursing diagnosis

NEUROLOGIC

Interventions

1. Maintain proper spinal alignment via:
- stabilization with sandbags
- manual in-line traction
- rigid cervical collar
- backboard or breakaway orthopedic stretcher
- logroll techniques.

2. Instruct the patient concerning proper head/neck position and the need to avoid turning his head (depending on his level of consciousness and cooperation).

3. Continually reassess spine alignment and immobilization techniques; adjust as necessary.

Rationale

An acute awareness of the potential for spinal cord injury must begin from the time of injury. Any motion of the cervical spine or head may cause further damage to the spinal cord or nerve roots.

The awake, oriented patient can maintain immobilization of the head and neck independently. Explicit instructions and stressing of the need for immobilization may elicit his cooperation.

Constant monitoring of immobilization techniques ensures proper spine alignment.

Nursing diagnosis

Potential for motor and sensory deficit related to spinal cord injury.

> **GOAL:** Maintain alignment and stabilize the cervical spine.

Interventions

1. Maintaining cervical immobility, move the patient to a turning frame.

2. Assemble equipment and assist with application of cervical traction devices (see "Sample Trays and Specialty Carts Lists" in Appendix 3 for information on Halo and Gardner-Wells trays).

3. Prepare the patient for surgery. (See "Preparation for Surgery" in Section VII.)

Rationale

The turning frame—equipped with features that assist in maintaining body alignment—provides ease and safety in turning the patient from the supine to prone position. These features include safety straps, a semicircular bar, armboards, and continuous traction for cervical traction via Halo or Gardner Wells tongs.

Cervical spine alignment, initially accomplished with Halo or Gardner-Wells tongs, may require early surgical intervention, including cervical spine plating or cervical fusion and wiring.

Nursing diagnosis

Potential for impaired gas exchange related to decreased mechanical ventilatory control secondary to cervical cord injury.

> **GOAL #1:** Promote optimal respiratory function.

Interventions

1. Obtain a baseline respiratory assessment; monitor the patient closely for signs of respiratory distress or deterioration; determine the need for urgent therapy as evidenced by:
● apnea
● respiratory distress
● shallow, diaphragmatic breathing.

2. Evaluate and document breath sounds, ABGs, chest radiographs.

3. Ensure early administration of supplemental oxygen; anticipate the need for intubation and mechanical ventilation. (See "Endotracheal Intubation" in Section VII.)

4. Prepare equipment for fiberoptic bronchoscopy; assist as needed. (See "Bronchoscopy" in Section VII.)

Rationale

C_1-C_2 injuries produce immediate respiratory arrest because of severed neural innervation. Injury at or above C_4 leads to respiratory arrest from paralysis of the major respiratory muscles, including the diaphragm. The cervical spine-injured patient risks developing respiratory dysfunction as cord level injury increases from edema or expanding contusions or as fatigue of breathing increases.

Respiratory insufficiency poses the most serious threat, making constant assessment of respiratory status essential. The onset may be slow and insidious and may develop up to 3 to 7 days after injury. Trend analysis of breath sounds, ABG results, and chest radiographs aids identification of respiratory complications and monitors ventilatory effectiveness.

If emergency intubation is required before confirmation of a cervical spine injury, nasal intubation is the preferred route to avoid neck hyperextension. While blind nasal intubation can be performed by an experienced practitioner, the use of a fiberoptic bronchoscope facilitates tube placement.

GOAL #2: Prevent or minimize retained secretions.

Interventions

1. Auscultate breath sounds frequently; provide optimal pulmonary hygiene:
● suction frequently
● perform tracheal lavage (if secretions are thick and difficult to suction)
● turn on turning frame every 2 hours or as condition warrants
● perform chest physiotherapy every 2 to 4 hours.

Rationale

A cervical spine-injured patient may lose nerve innervation to respiratory muscles, impairing function. This predisposes the patient to retained secretions and, if untreated, to pneumonia. The cough mechanism is altered or completely absent. Knowledge of the deficit level is essential. Lesions at C_4 or above produce total loss of spontaneous respiration (C_4 innervates the diaphragm). Lesions at T_6 to T_7 and above paralyze intercostal muscle function. This patient will be unable to deep-breathe or cough. Major abdominal muscles for expiration receive innervation from T_6 to T_{12}.

Position changes and chest physiotherapy aid mobilization and secretion drainage. The prone position is necessary but may not be tolerated for long periods initially. **Caution:** *A sudden position change in the spine-injured patient may trigger the vasovagal response, in turn triggering cardiac arrest.*

Nursing diagnosis

Potential for fluid volume deficit related to loss of sympathetic vasomotor tone secondary to spinal cord injury.

GOAL: Restore and maintain normovolemia.

Interventions

1. Monitor the patient's cardiovascular status for signs of neurogenic shock state (See "Vasogenic Shock" in Section II):
● monitor the patient closely for hypotension with bradycardia
● monitor and document vital signs, as indicated by stability of the cardiovascular system.

2. Ensure placement of large-bore peripheral I.V. catheters. Administer I.V. fluids, as ordered. Monitor and document fluid intake closely.

3. Assist with the insertion of hemodynamic monitoring equipment:
● pulmonary artery catheter
● arterial line.
Monitor blood pressure and pulmonary pressures. Monitor or assist with cardiac output measurements.

4. Administer and evaluate vasopressor therapy, as ordered, to maintain a mean arterial pressure > 80 to 110 mm Hg.

5. Place the patient in Trendelenburg position and apply a pneumatic antishock garment, unless contraindicated.

Rationale

Severe instability of the cardiovascular system, especially with high paraplegic and quadriplegic patients, occurs immediately after injury and lasts several days. Just as neural loss to the muscle function necessary for respiration creates instability or inadequacy, so loss of neural innervation to the cardiovascular system creates instability or altered functioning. Loss of neural regulatory control may produce changes or fluctuations in blood pressure and heart rate. Generally, the body achieves homeostasis within 1 year. Lesions at T_6 or above interfere with maintenance of vasomotor tone. Classic signs of a spine injury are hypotension with bradycardia. If hypotension with tachycardia occurs, associated injuries should be sought.

The placement of I.V. lines and hemodynamic monitors permits provision and evaluation of fluid and drug therapy. Stimulation, such as rapid position changes or deep tracheal suctioning, may trigger the vasovagal response. This rare but dangerous phenomenon occurs because the parasympathetic system is unchecked by the usual antagonistic sympathetic system; thus, sufficient stimulation not only slows the heart but stops it. These lines also permit continual monitoring of the patient's condition and rapid intervention for vasovagal responses.

Vasopressors increase cardiac output by acting on the heart's beta-receptors, improving myocardial contractility and causing peripheral vasoconstriction.

These measures facilitate venous return from the lower extremities.

NEUROLOGIC

Nursing diagnosis

Alteration in urinary elimination related to neurogenic bladder.

GOAL #1: Prevent bladder distention.

Interventions

1. Assemble equipment and insert an indwelling urinary catheter, using sterile technique.

Rationale

Injuries at T_{11} to T_{12} and S_1 cause urinary dysfunction. Loss of neural innervation to the bladder may be partial or complete, temporary or permanent. Spinal shock causes a flaccid bladder immediately after injury. Recovery of bladder function depends on the level or completeness of the lesion. Level of function is determined after the spinal shock phase.

An indwelling catheter is used during the acute phase of spinal cord injury. Thereafter, a bladder retraining program of intermittent catheterizations is started.

GOAL #2: Prevent or minimize the risk of urinary tract infections.

Interventions

1. Observe the fluid intake pattern and monitor urine output.

2. Observe characteristics of urine:
- color and clarity
- odor
- presence of sedimentation.

3. Report signs of infection to the physician.

4. Obtain urine for analysis and culture and sensitivity tests.

5. Administer antibiotics as ordered.

Rationale

Complications from urinary catheterization can be prevented or minimized by meticulous catheter care. The adequacy of fluid intake is evaluated by correlating output. Spine-injured patients are at increased risk for developing urinary tract infections. Therefore, closely observe and monitor possible infection sites. Recognizing early signs of developing infection permits prompt antibiotic treatment, minimizing the risk of developing septicemia. Specific antibiotic therapy will be based on culture and sensitivity tests.

Nursing diagnosis

Potential for ineffective breathing patterns related to diaphragmatic elevation secondary to gastric distention from a paralytic ileus.

GOAL: Recognize signs of a paralytic ileus; prevent aspiration of vomitus.

Interventions

1. Monitor and document the patient's bowel sounds.

2. Insert a gastric decompression tube.

3. Confirm proper positioning of the gastric tube. Maintain tube patency; irrigate and aspirate the air vent and the drainage port at least every 2 hours.

4. Maintain gastric decompression with 80 to 120 mm Hg (intermittent) or 30 to 40 mm Hg (continuous) suction.

5. Assess and document the amount and characteristics of gastric secretions; document initial pH and test every 2 to 4 hours.

6. Assess gastric secretions for blood. Monitor abdominal girth measurements.

7. Give antacids, as ordered.

Rationale

Paralytic ileus is common with all levels of spine injuries. Temporary disruption of the autonomic nervous system is thought to be the cause; however, many other stimuli may precipitate a paralytic ileus, such as shock and anesthetic agents. Complete quadriplegia increases the risk of paralytic ileus. Coupled with the loss of the cough mechanism, quadriplegic patients may vomit and aspirate gastric contents, which may result in respiratory arrest. This is the most common cause of sudden death in quadriplegic patients during the first 48 hours after injury.

Peptic ulcers may develop as a result of increased hydrochloric acid production. Secretion analysis, including pH and hematest, aids prevention by allowing early institution of ulcer therapy. Loss of pain sensation further necessitates testing of secretions for early detection of occult bleeding. Antacids combat gastric hyperacidity (pH < 5).

Nursing diagnosis

Potential for ineffective thermoregulation related to loss of autonomic nervous system secondary to cord damage.

GOAL: Maintain normothermia.

Interventions

1. Obtain a baseline and closely monitor trends in the patient's core temperature.

2. Warm the patient by using:
- warmed oxygen via heated humidity or ventilator cascade
- hemocoil or blood warmer
- warmed blankets
- closely monitored hyperthermia blanket
- warming lights around the bed or stretcher.

3. Cool the patient by using:
- hypothermia blanket
- light blanket or sheet.

Rationale

Loss of autonomic control of the sweat glands causes altered regulation of the body temperature. Messages normally sent to the hypothalamus, or "thermostat," are disrupted in the spine at the lesion level. Quadriplegic patients are most severely affected. Monitoring body temperature allows early initiation of appropriate thermia interventions. The most common contributing factors to hypothermia include exposure at the scene of the accident, air conditioning in the emergency department, and shock states.

Nursing diagnosis

Potential for impaired skin integrity related to immobility secondary to paralysis.

GOAL: Protect and maintain patient's skin integrity.

Interventions

1. Maintain spinal immobilization and place the patient on a turning frame. Turn every 2 hours.

2. Inspect the skin for areas of redness, pressure, or breakdown; begin patient teaching when appropriate.

3. Maintain correct body alignment and pad all pressure areas.

4. Move the patient carefully to avoid shearing or friction forces. Use lifting rather than dragging movements.

5. Avoid extremes of temperature in bathwater.

Rationale

Immobility, trauma, compromised defense mechanisms, and malnutrition all contribute to the development of poor skin integrity. The patient who has lost sensation will be unaware of the need to move because of interrupted pressure or pain signals normally relayed to the brain. Nursing interventions are directed at protection and prevention of skin breakdown, early detection and treatment of reddened areas, and patient/family instruction about inspection and care of the patient's skin.

Padding of common pressure points and proper body alignment help protect the skin. Friction from dragging over sheets increases the risk for breakdown.

Temperature extremes increase the risk of thermal burns.

Nursing diagnosis

Potential for alteration in tissue perfusion related to sluggish venous return secondary to loss of vasomotor control, loss of muscle tone, and immobility.

GOAL #1: Prevent the development of deep vein thrombosis (DVT).

Interventions

1. Apply pneumatic compression devices to the legs, if ordered.

2. Apply graduated elastic stockings.

3. Instruct in and assist with active and passive range-of-motion (ROM) exercises.

4. Turn and position the patient every 2 hours.

5. Observe for signs of DVT:
- low-grade temperature
- localized warm skin area on legs
- asymmetry of calves
- phlebitis.

6. Administer prophylactic anticoagulant therapy, as ordered (usually low-dose heparin, 5,000 to 7,500 units every 12 hours).

7. Monitor clotting and prothrombin times and platelet count, as ordered.

Rationale

Spine injuries produce cardiovascular dysfunction. All spine-injured patients are at risk for DVT development. The main causative factor is sluggish venous return produced when vasomotor tone is lost. Loss of muscle tone and temporary or permanent immobility contribute to poor circulating return, thus setting up ideal conditions for thrombus formation. Various interventions help promote venous return. Pneumatic compression devices provide alternate compression and release of pressure to the lower extremities. This simulates the "milking action" on the veins normally provided by muscle activity. Elastic stockings provide a similar action.

ROM exercises promote muscle activity, which in turn increases venous return.

Frequent turning and positioning help prevent compression, which slows circulation and impedes venous return.

Spine-injured patients will not exhibit Homans' sign—pain in the calf when the foot is dorsiflexed—because of loss of sensation. (See "Deep Vein Thrombosis" in Section IV.)

Heparin acts to prevent the conversion of fibrinogen to fibrin in the clotting chain and impairs the activation of several other clotting factors. Heparin's action is rapid, has a low incidence of side effects, and is reversible with the antagonist protamine. To prevent excessive anticoagulation, clotting profiles are monitored. Prior to administration of heparin, the laboratory results are checked and, if necessary, the dosage is regulated.

GOAL #2: Detect early signs of and institute prompt therapy for pulmonary thromboembolism (PTE).

Interventions

1. Observe for signs of pulmonary thromboembolism:
- sudden onset of hypoxia
- tachypnea
- dyspnea
- tachycardia
- elevated temperature.

2. Initiate nursing measures as described in "Pulmonary Thromboembolus" in Section IV.

Rationale

Pulmonary thromboemboli are a major complication during the acute phase following spine injury and may lead to a fatal outcome. Spinal shock, prolonged bed rest, immobility, and loss of muscle tone contribute to the development of DVT and subsequent PTE. Most patients (90%) with PTE have thrombi that originate in the deep veins of the legs.

Additional considerations

Psychological and physical rehabilitation begin at the time of injury. This devastating injury changes the structure of the entire family. Allow the patient and family time to make adjustments. Provide a team approach to help the patient and family develop coping strategies that will be productive. Every aspect of the patient's and family's lives, including their roles, will be affected and will require continuous psychosocial and physical assessment.

NEUROLOGIC

Associated care plans

Head Injury
Vasogenic Shock
Maxillofacial Injuries
Penetrating Chest Trauma
Intraabdominal Trauma: Blunt and
  Penetrating
Massive Pelvic Injury
Psychosocial Support of the Trauma Patient
Malnutrition in the Trauma Patient
Pulmonary Thromboembolus
Deep Vein Thrombosis

Associated procedures and studies

Positive Contrast Study
Intrahospital Transport of the Shock Trauma Patient
Bronchoscopy
Preparation for Surgery
Endotracheal Intubation
The Pneumatic Antishock Garment

Medical diagnosis

THORACIC, LUMBAR, AND SACRAL SPINE INJURY

Assessment

Mechanism of injury/ etiology:
• blunt trauma—as from automobile, motorcycle, diving, and especially industrial accidents; falls onto buttocks; and cave-ins
• penetrating trauma— such as from gunshot and stab wounds

Physical findings:
Neurologic
• altered level of consciousness varying from awake to unresponsive, depending on associated injuries (the patient is usually awake and alert)
• motor and sensory loss below the level of cord injury

Complete syndrome
• complete paraplegia (T_2 or below) or quadriplegia or tetraplegia (T_1 or above)

Incomplete syndromes
• Central cord syndrome—damage to the center of the cord only; extreme weakness or loss of arm movement but intact leg movement
• anterior artery syndrome—loss of motor function and pain and temperature sensation below the level of the lesion with preservation of proprioception, vibration, and touch sensation
• Brown-Séquard syndrome—damage to one side of the cord only; loss of motor function on the injured side, loss of pain and temperature sensation on the opposite side of the body
• conus and cauda equina injuries—loss of motor function only; sensory function intact,

variable pattern of involvement, possible recovery potential; loss of bowel, bladder, and sexual function
• sacral sparing—radicular arteries of the outer circumference of the cord are spared; sensation in the sacral area is spared despite an otherwise paralyzed patient

Cardiovascular
• warm, dry skin
• regular, full pulse
• bradycardia
• neurogenic shock state
• poikilothermy (assuming the temperature of the environment)

Respiratory
• chest wall abrasions, contusions, wounds
• decreased breath sounds
• tachypnea

Gastrointestinal
• decreased or absent bowel sounds
• abdominal wall abrasions, contusions, wounds
• gastric distention

Genitourinary
• hematuria
• bladder distention
• priapism

Associated injuries:
Chest
• lung contusion
• pneumothorax
• myocardial contusion
• ruptured aorta

Abdominal
• ruptured spleen or liver
• kidney injuries

Musculoskeletal
• pelvic or long-bone fractures

Diagnostic studies

• radiography—thoracic, lumbar, sacral radiographs
  ☐ computed tomography scan, for fracture identification
  ☐ tomography, for more extensive, poorly visualized, or hidden fractures that may be overshadowed by other structures
  ☐ myelography, for evaluation of pressure or impingement on the spinal cord or on a nerve root

• laboratory studies
  ☐ hemoglobin/hematocrit—may reflect hypovolemia from associated injuries
  ☐ ABGs—may reveal hypoxemia

NEUROLOGIC

Nursing diagnosis

Potential for motor and sensory deficit related to potential spinal cord injury.

> **GOAL:** Maintain alignment and stabilize the spine.

Note: *Every unevaluated trauma patient must be treated as having a cervical spine injury until proven otherwise.*

Interventions

1. Initiate or maintain proper spine alignment by:
- maintaining the patient on a spine board until spinal injuries are ruled out
- placing the patient on a turning frame
- placing the patient on a scoop or break-away stretcher for ease in transferring to other beds
- utilizing the logroll technique
- minimizing patient movement
- educating the patient concerning spine alignment, if he is cooperative
- preparing for surgery.

Rationale

Spine injury must be ruled out in all trauma patients. C_5 to C_6 and T_{12} to L_1 are the weakest and thus most common locations for spine injuries because of the natural curves in the spine. Injury at T_2 or below causes complete paraplegia. Maintaining immobilization of the spine until injury has been ruled out will prevent cord injury in a fracture without spinal cord disruption. In a fracture with cord disruption, immobilization minimizes further cord damage. Early surgical intervention may be needed for spine stabilization.

Nursing diagnosis

Potential for impaired gas exchange related to decreased mechanical ventilatory control secondary to cervical cord injury.

> **GOAL:** Promote optimal respiratory function.

Interventions

1. Obtain a baseline respiratory assessment; monitor the patient closely for signs of respiratory distress or deterioration; determine the need for urgent therapy as evidenced by:
- apnea
- respiratory distress
- shallow, diaphragmatic breathing.

2. Evaluate and document breath sounds, ABGs, chest radiographs.

3. Ensure early administration of supplemental oxygen; anticipate the need for intubation and mechanical ventilation. (See "Endotracheal Intubation" in Section VII.)

4. Auscultate breath sounds frequently; provide optimal pulmonary hygiene:
- suction frequently
- perform tracheal lavage (if secretions are thick and difficult to suction)
- turn on turning frame every 2 hours or as condition warrants
- perform chest physiotherapy every 2 to 4 hours.

Rationale

Thoracic spine-injured patients may lose neural innervation to some respiratory muscles, altering respiratory function. Depending on the lesion level, compromise may or may not be as great as with cervical spine injuries. Associated injuries or fatigue of remaining muscles may compound this problem and place these spine-injured patients at high risk for pulmonary complications. The onset of complications may be slow and insidious. Because of the risk of respiratory deterioration, patients need monitoring for 3 to 7 days after injury. Any complaints of respiratory difficulty require immediate investigation. Lesions at T_6 to T_7 and above paralyze intercostal muscle function. This patient will be unable to deep-breathe or cough. Major abdominal muscles for expiration receive innervation from T_6 to T_{12}.

Position changes and chest physiotherapy aid mobilization and drainage of secretions.

*Supplemental nursing diagnosis

NEUROLOGIC

Nursing diagnosis

Potential for fluid volume deficit related to loss of sympathetic vasomotor tone secondary to spinal cord injury.

> **GOAL:** Restore and maintain normovolemia.

Interventions

1. Ensure placement of two large-bore peripheral catheters. Administer I.V. fluids, as ordered. Monitor and document fluid intake closely.

2. Monitor cardiovascular status, including:
• blood pressure
• heart rate and rhythm.

3. Assemble equipment and assist with placement of hemodynamic monitoring lines:
• pulmonary artery catheter
• arterial catheter.
Monitor pulmonary artery and blood pressures. Document and report trends.

4. Administer inotropic agents as ordered.

5. Assemble equipment and insert an indwelling urinary catheter using sterile technique. Monitor output. (See "Alteration in urinary elimination related to neurogenic bladder" nursing diagnosis in "Cervical Spine Injury," in Section II.)

Rationale

Loss or partial loss of vasomotor tone produces instability in the cardiovascular system. In general, the higher the lesion, the more profound the effect.

Injury below T_6 allows partial sympathetic function to continue. The sympathetic nervous system remains intact with lower lumbar or sacral cord injuries. However, vasomotor tone to the lower limbs is lost. The extent of invasive hemodynamic monitoring will depend on the level of injury, concomitant cardiovascular instability, and associated injuries.

Inotropic agents increase cardiac output by acting on the heart's beta-receptors to improve myocardial contractility.

The purpose of bladder catheterization is twofold. Adequate urine output is an indicator of adequate fluid replacement and hydration. Additionally, spine-injured patients have a flaccid bladder during the spinal shock phase. Recovery prognosis is determined by the lesion level and neurologic function after resolution of the spinal shock phase.

Nursing diagnosis

Potential for alteration in thermoregulation related to loss of autonomic nervous system control secondary to spinal cord damage.

> **GOAL:** Maintain normothermic state.

Interventions

1. Obtain a baseline core temperature and closely monitor trends.

2. Warm the patient by using:
• warmed oxygen via heated nebulizer or ventilator cascade
• hemocoil or blood warmer
• warmed blankets
• hyperthermia blanket
• warming lights around bed or stretcher.

3. Cool the patient by using:
• hypothermia blanket
• light blanket or sheet.

Rationale

As stated, the higher the lesion, the more profound the effect. High thoracic spine injuries pose more difficulty with thermal regulation than low thoracic or lumbar/sacral injuries. Quadriplegia produces the most severe effects. Hypothermia occurs most commonly.

Nursing diagnosis

Potential for ineffective breathing patterns related to diaphragmatic elevation secondary to gastric distention from a paralytic ileus.

> **GOAL:** Recognize paralytic ileus and prevent aspiration of vomitus.

Interventions

1. Assess, monitor, and document the quality of bowel sounds.

2. Insert a gastric decompression tube.

3. Assess proper placement of the gastric tube. Maintain tube patency; irrigate and aspirate both the air vent and the drainage port at least every 2 hours.

4. Maintain gastric decompression with 80 to 120 mm Hg (intermittent) or 30 to 40 mm Hg (continuous) suction.

5. Assess and document the amount and characteristics of gastric secretion; document the initial pH and test every 2 to 4 hours.

6. Assess gastric secretions for blood. Monitor abdominal girth measurements.

7. Administer antacids as ordered.

Rationale

Paralytic ileus is common to all levels of spine injuries. Temporary disruption of the autonomic nervous system is thought to be the cause, but associated injuries may also be responsible. Complete quadriplegia increases the risk for paralytic ileus. Coupled with the loss of the cough mechanism, it may lead to aspirated stomach contents, possibly resulting in respiratory arrest. This is the most common cause of sudden death in quadriplegic patients during the first 48 hours after injury. Gastric ulcers may develop as a result of steroid release in reaction to trauma. Loss of pain sensation increases the chance of a silent bleed.

Antacids are given to combat gastric hyperacidity. The pH should be maintained at ≥ 5.

Nursing diagnosis

Potential for impaired skin integrity related to immobility secondary to paralysis.

> **GOAL:** Protect and maintain the patient's skin integrity.

Interventions

1. Maintain spinal immobilization and place the patient on a turning frame. Turn every 2 hours.

2. Inspect the skin for areas of redness, pressure, or breakdown; begin patient teaching when appropriate.

Rationale

Immobility, trauma, compromised defense mechanisms, and malnutrition all contribute to the development of poor skin integrity. The patient who has lost sensation will be unaware of the need to move because of interrupted pressure or pain signals normally relayed to the brain. Nursing interventions are directed at protection and prevention of skin breakdown, early detection and treatment of reddened areas, and patient/family instruction about inspection and care of the patient's skin.

3. Maintain correct body alignment and pad all pressure areas.

4. Move the patient carefully to avoid shearing or friction forces. Use lifting rather than dragging movements.

Padding of common pressure points and proper body alignment help protect the skin. Friction from dragging over sheets increases the risk for breakdown.

5. Avoid extremes of temperature in bathwater.

Temperature extremes increase the risk of thermal burns.

Nursing diagnosis

Potential for alteration in tissue perfusion related to sluggish venous return secondary to loss of vasomotor control, loss of muscle tone, and immobility.

GOAL #1: Prevent the development of deep vein thrombosis (DVT).

Interventions

Rationale

1. Apply pneumatic compression devices to the legs, if ordered.

2. Apply graduated elastic stockings.

Spine injuries produce cardiovascular dysfunction. All spine-injured patients are at risk for DVT development. The main causative factor is sluggish venous return produced when vasomotor tone is lost. Loss of muscle tone and temporary or permanent immobility contribute to poor circulating return, thus setting up ideal conditions for thrombus formation. Various interventions help promote venous return. Pneumatic compression devices provide an alternate compression and release of pressure to the lower extremities. This simulates the "milking action" on the veins normally provided by muscle activity. Elastic stockings provide a similar action.

3. Instruct in and assist with active and passive range-of-motion (ROM) exercises.

ROM exercises promote muscle activity, which in turn increases venous return.

4. Turn and position the patient every 2 hours.

Frequent turning and positioning help prevent compression, which slows circulation and impedes venous return.

5. Observe for signs of DVT:
- low-grade temperature
- localized warm skin area on legs
- asymmetry of calves
- phlebitis.

Spine-injured patients will not exhibit Homans' sign—pain in the calf when the foot is dorsiflexed—because of their loss of sensation. (See "Deep Vein Thrombosis" in Section IV.)

6. Administer prophylactic anticoagulant therapy, as ordered (usually low-dose heparin, 5,000 to 7,500 units every 12 hours).

7. Monitor clotting and prothrombin times and platelet count, as ordered.

Heparin acts to prevent the conversion of fibrinogen to fibrin in the clotting chain and impairs the activation of several other clotting factors. Heparin's action is rapid, has a low incidence of side effects, and is reversible with the antagonist protamine. To prevent excessive anticoagulation, clotting profiles are monitored. Prior to administration of heparin, the laboratory results are checked and, if necessary, dosage is regulated.

GOAL #2: Detect early signs of and initiate prompt therapy for pulmonary thromboembolus (PTE).

Interventions

1. Observe for signs of PTE:
- sudden onset of hypoxia
- tachypnea
- dyspnea
- tachycardia
- elevated temperature.

2. Initiate nursing measures as described in "Pulmonary Thromboembolus" in Section IV.

Rationale

Pulmonary thromboemboli are a major complication during the acute phase following spine injury and may lead to a fatal outcome. Spinal shock, prolonged bed rest, immobility, and loss of muscle tone contribute to the development of DVT and subsequent PTE. Most patients (90%) with PTE have thrombi that originate in the deep veins of the legs.

NEUROLOGIC

Associated care plans

Cervical Spine Injury
Vasogenic Shock
Penetrating Chest Trauma
Intraabdominal Trauma: Blunt and
    Penetrating
Massive Pelvic Injury
Psychosocial Support of the Trauma Patient
Deep Vein Thrombosis
Pulmonary Thromboembolus

Associated procedures and study

Positive Contrast Study
Intrahospital Transport of the Shock Trauma Patient
Preparation for Surgery
Endotracheal Intubation

HEAD INJURY

Assessment

Mechanism of injury/ etiology:
• penetrating trauma, as from bullets and stab wounds or open head injuries
• blunt trauma, as from motor vehicle accidents, falls, or assaults
• skull fractures
• anticoagulant ther-apy—may precipitate or worsen a cerebral bleed

Physical findings:
See Table 2.4 below.

Note: *The head-injured patient can exhibit an extremely wide range of clinical manifestations. Although the patient may be awake and alert and neuro-logically intact initially, he may deteriorate rapidly. The trauma patient who has sustained force sufficient to cause injury, no matter where that injury is located, requires a thorough history taking, examination, and testing to rule out a neurologic problem or establish baseline neurologic criteria. This care plan presupposes that the patient has a significant head injury on arrival at the emergency department. Because this patient commonly has associated injuries, associated care plans are referenced.*

Table 2.4	
Skull fractures	**Findings**
Linear	• Edematous, tender, ecchymotic, or lacerated scalp
Depressed	• Bruised or lacerated scalp • Neurologic changes relative to the degree of brain involvement
Basilar anterior fossa	• Subconjunctival hemorrhage • Periorbital ecchymosis (raccoon eyes) • Epistaxis • Anosmia (Cranial Nerve I) • Visual defect (Cranial Nerve II) • Rhinorrhea
middle fossa	• Otorrhea • Deafness (Cranial Nerve III) • Tinnitus • Peripheral facial palsy • Hemotympanum
posterior fossa	• Ecchymosis posterior to ear, overlying mastoid (Battle's sign)
Brain/Brain stem injury	**Findings**
Concussion	• Temporary disturbance of consciousness and memory with restoration within a variable period of time; duration of both disturbances is index of severity of injury • Possible transient confusion; disturbances of vision, equilibrium, and hearing during recovery • Retrograde or antegrade memory loss • No residual neurologic deficit
Contusion and laceration	• Variable; altered level of consciousness to coma with decorticate or decerebrate posturing • Deficit depending on area of brain involved and severity of the insult; brain involvement may be the area directly under the impact (coup injury) or the area opposite the impact (contrecoup) • Possible disorganized, confused behavior

NEUROLOGIC

Hemorrhage/Hematomas	Findings
Epidural hematoma	• Early finding in patients presenting with head injury • Signs of brain stem compression, usually within 24 hours • Short period of unconsciousness followed by a lucid interval (only 20% of cases) • Lucid interval followed by progressive depression of consciousness • Focal signs: ipsilateral pupil dilation, weakness of contralateral extremities

Subdural hematoma
  acute: symptomatic within 24 hours
 	
  subacute: symptomatic in 2 to 10 days
	• Depressed consciousness level, usually from the time of injury
	• Ipsilateral pupil dilation and contralateral weakness
	
	• Headaches
	• Altered level of consciousness and focal signs of compression
	• Failure to show improvement

Posterior fossa hematoma	• Headache and vomiting • Nystagmus • Cerebellar ataxia • Respiratory depression
Intracerebral hematoma	• Single or multiple, subcortical or deep hematomas; symptoms frequently indistinguishable from contusion of the cortex • Lucid interval followed by decreased consciousness level • Focal signs based on location • Possible clinical silence (frontal or nondominant temporal lobes)
Subarachnoid hemorrhage	• Severe headache and restlessness • Nuchal rigidity, elevated temperature, photophobia, and a positive Kernig's sign • Extensor plantar reflexes bilaterally

Associated injuries:
- facial fractures, lacerations, contusions
- cervical spine injuries
- chest injuries
- abdominal injuries
- musculoskeletal injuries

Diagnostic studies

- radiography
  - ☐ computerized tomography (CT) scan of the head
  - ☐ skull radiographs for fractures
  - ☐ angiography (has been replaced by CT scan for evaluation of intracranial mass lesions but remains essential to demonstrate vascular injuries).
- laboratory data

☐ ABG—usually reflects hypoxemia
☐ hematocrit/hemoglobin—detects bleeding (unusual but possible in head injuries).
☐ coagulation profile—is altered by development of disseminated intravascular coagulation
☐ toxicology screen—may reveal chemical substances that alter or confuse neurologic findings.

Note: *Lumbar puncture is contraindicated as brain stem herniation can occur in the presence of increased intracranial pressure. Electroencephalography has little usefulness in the emergency setting because the test's validity depends on drug-free, normothermic conditions. These factors may not be present or known early in the resuscitation phase.*

Nursing diagnosis

Potential for impaired gas exchange related to ineffective breathing patterns and upper airway obstruction secondary to head injury.

GOAL: Establish and maintain an adequate airway.

Interventions

1. Assess the patient's respiratory status, evaluate his airway, and auscultate breath sounds.

2. Prepare for intubation, mechanical ventilation, and positive end-expiratory pressure. (See "Endotracheal Intubation" in Section VII.)

Rationale

As for all trauma patients, airway patency and maintenance are paramount. In the head injury patient, upper airway obstruction is the most common cause of impaired ventilation. If cervical spine injury has not been ruled out, hyperextending the neck is contraindicated, necessitating a fiberoptic bronchoscope for oral intubation. Unless a cerebral spinal fluid leak has been ruled out, nasal intubation is avoided. Medullary and pontine lesions commonly cause irregular breathing. The lesion site and specific breathing patterns cannot be correlated, and several breathing patterns may be seen in the same patient.

Nursing diagnosis

Potential for impaired gas exchange and infection related to lower airway obstruction secondary to retained secretions, atelectasis, and possible aspiration.

GOAL #1: Prevent or minimize retained secretions.

Interventions

1. Ensure the availability and anticipate the use of supplemental oxygen.

2. Auscultate breath sounds frequently. Provide optimal pulmonary hygiene, including:
• frequent suctioning
• turning every 2 hours
• positioning in semi-Fowler's position (unless contraindicated)
• performing chest physiotherapy
• providing incentive spirometry.
(See "Lower Airway Obstruction" in Section II.)

Rationale

The patient in any degree of respiratory distress requires supplemental oxygen before, during, and after airway establishment to promote optimal gas exchange.

Lower airway obstruction produced by retained secretions or atelectasis decreases alveolar function and impairs gas exchange. Auscultation of rales and wheezes indicates probable lower airway obstruction. Pulmonary hygiene must be initiated early during the resuscitation phase to optimize aeration and reduce the risk of complications from aspirated and retained secretions. These measures mobilize secretions, prevent pooling, and promote full lung expansion. Prompt and consistent removal of pulmonary secretions reduces the risk of infection, pneumonia, and other pulmonary complications.

GOAL #2: Restore and maintain effective cerebral oxygenation.

Interventions

1. Obtain blood for ABG analysis.

2. If hyperventilation therapy is ordered, obtain an ABG sample for analysis at least every 4 hours and monitor results for $PaCO_2$ between 25 and 30 mm Hg. Collaborate with the physician and respiratory therapist if ventilator adjustments are needed to maintain hyperventilation.

Rationale

Ventilation adequacy can be determined from ABG results. Hypoxemia usually occurs secondary to head injury (50% of patients exhibit $PaO_2 < 80$ mm Hg; 20% to 30%, $PaO_2 < 65$ mm Hg). Obstructed airways, upper or lower, may be the usual cause. Also, concussion alone may produce hypoventilation. Hyperventilation, with $PaCO_2$ levels maintained between 25 and 30 mm Hg, is an effective means of decreasing cerebral blood volume, which is a major cause of intracranial hypertension in the early phases of head injury.

Nursing diagnosis

Potential for fluid volume deficit related to blood loss secondary to uncontrolled hemorrhage from large scalp wound.

> **GOAL:** Restore and maintain normovolemia.

Note: *The primary cause of decreased blood pressure in head-injured patients is blood loss from associated injuries. These must be aggressively sought and managed.*

Interventions

1. Assist with I.V. line placement of at least two large-bore peripheral catheters.

2. Assess the patient's cardiovascular status, including:
- blood pressure
- pulse
- skin color
- capillary refill time
- hemoglobin/hematocrit results.

3. Anticipate and assist with insertion of hemodynamic monitoring devices:
- arterial blood pressure catheter
- pulmonary artery catheter.

Rationale

Large scalp lacerations with uncontrolled bleeding can cause hypovolemia. Adequate venous access provides the fluid replacement route.

Careful monitoring of cardiovascular parameters aids planning of proper replacement with crystalloid, colloid, or blood/blood products without overhydration. Cerebral edema may result from overhydration, worsening the patient's neurologic status.

These catheters allow more precise monitoring of hemodynamic parameters, such as mean arterial, central venous, and pulmonary artery and wedge pressures.

Nursing diagnosis

Potential for decreased cardiac output related to possible dysrhythmias secondary to heightened sympathetic vasomotor activity in the medulla resulting from head injury.

> **GOAL:** Recognize, prevent, or minimize dysrhythmias; rule out associated myocardial injury.

Interventions

1. Monitor cardiac activity, including:
- continual ECG monitoring
- a 12-lead ECG
- serial ECGs.

2. Obtain blood for creatine phosphokinase (CPK) and CPK-MB measurement.

3. Administer antidysrhythmics, as ordered.

Rationale

Mechanisms causing cardiac dysrhythmias remain unclear but may result from overactive sympathetic vasomotor mechanisms in the medulla. Patients with a subarachnoid hemorrhage following aneurysm rupture have shown elevated levels of epinephrine and norepinephrine. Continuous ECG monitoring permits rapid detection of and intervention for dysrhythmias. A 12-lead ECG provides a baseline for detection of myocardial electrical changes. CPK and CPK-MB levels and ECGs rule out myocardial infarction or myocardial contusion. Cardiac changes associated with head injuries are usually not severe, but if myocardial failure develops, antidysrhythmics are given.

Nursing diagnosis

Potential for fluid volume deficit related to blood loss secondary to coagulopathy caused by release of thromboplastin from damaged brain tissue.

GOAL: Restore normal clotting time.

Interventions

1. Obtain blood for a coagulation profile. Monitor this profile every 12 hours or more frequently, if indicated.

2. Administer fresh-frozen plasma, platelets, or whole blood as ordered.

Rationale

Brain tissue contains the highest level of thromboplastin in the body. Cerebral tissue destruction or blood-brain barrier disruption can release large quantities of thromboplastin, creating a consumptive coagulopathy. Of all head-injured patients, 40% to 70% have decreased clotting factors. Fresh-frozen plasma or whole blood administration will correct low fibrinogen levels. Continued severe bleeding may require platelet replacement. (See "Disseminated Intravascular Coagulation" in Section IV.)

Nursing diagnosis

*Potential for fluid and electrolyte imbalance related to increased urine output secondary to disruption in antidiuretic hormone (ADH) secretion.

GOAL: Restore normal fluid and electrolyte balance.

Interventions

1. Monitor and report urine and serum osmolality and electrolyte (Na^+, K^+, Cl^-) levels.

2. Insert an indwelling urinary catheter using aseptic technique. Monitor intake and output.

3. Weigh the patient daily.

4. Administer vasopressin, as ordered.

Rationale

Trauma, stress, and surgery may elevate glucocorticoid levels. Corticosteroids act in several ways to regulate the body's salt and water content. Disturbance of the posterior lobe of the pituitary gland may produce diabetes insipidus. Inappropriate ADH secretion usually accompanies trauma of any type. Normally, ADH markedly increases permeability of the distal renal tubule to water and urea, which promotes free water retention and leads to systemic hyponatremia. However, disturbance of ADH secretion produces large amounts of urine of low specific gravity. A fluid and electrolyte imbalance with dehydration may develop. Hyponatremia is treated by restricting fluid to 10 to 22 cc/kg of body weight of normal saline solution per day. Vasopressin may be used to increase the reabsorption rate of water from the distal renal tubules. (See "Diabetes Insipidus" in Section IV.)

Nursing diagnosis

*Potential for further neurologic deterioration related to increased intracranial pressure (ICP) secondary to expanding space-occupying lesions and cerebral edema.

GOAL #1: Establish neurologic baseline.

*Supplemental nursing diagnosis

Interventions

1. Assess and monitor the patient's neurologic status, including:
- level of consciousness
- pupils (reaction, size, and position)
- sensory and motor function (using the Glasgow Coma Scale or your institution's modified form of the scale).

Rationale

Baseline findings provide a reference to evaluate improvement or deterioration of the neurologic state. Level of consciousness is the most sensitive indicator of neurologic status. The most frequently injured cranial nerve, Cranial Nerve III controls pupil constriction and dilation.

GOAL #2: Detect early signs of increasing ICP.

Interventions

1. Prepare equipment for and assist with insertion of ICP monitoring device, or, if institutional policy requires surgical suite for this procedure, prepare the patient for surgery. (See "Preparation for Surgery" and "Intracranial Pressure Monitoring" in Section VII.)

2. Monitor and report an ICP remaining above 15 mm Hg for 5 minutes while the patient is at rest.

Rationale

Intracranial hypertension commonly develops before clinical deterioration becomes apparent. ICP monitoring is required for comatose patients and those patients who need rapid surgical intervention and have the potential for developing increased ICP. Any life-threatening injury may necessitate immediate resuscitative surgery before all diagnostic tests have been completed. If surgery occurs before completion of neurologic tests, intraoperative ICP monitoring is indicated.

Similar to blood pressure readings, ICP varies with activity. In the head-injured patient, however, alert the neurosurgeon to prolonged elevation or pressures that remain elevated after activity or procedures such as suctioning.

GOAL #3: Maintain ICP within normal range.

Interventions

1. Elevate the head of the bed 30 degrees, or place the patient in reverse Trendelenburg position if elevating the head of the bed is contraindicated (as with concomitant cervical spine injury); maintain the neck in neutral position.

2. Drain specific amounts of cerebral spinal fluid, as ordered, through an intraventricular catheter.

3. Check $PaCO_2$ levels to evaluate for range of 25 to 30 mm Hg.

4. Administer osmotic agents, as ordered.

Rationale

Under normal physiologic conditions, ICP should be below 15 mm Hg mean pressure in a flat position. An upright position will reduce the pressure to zero. With increased ICP, elevating the head of the bed usually provides a quick and effective measure to reduce the ICP to an acceptable range. Maintaining the neck in a neutral position promotes venous return from the head, thereby reducing cerebral blood volume.

Reducing cerebral mass can be accomplished by reducing brain mass proper or cerebral spinal fluid volume. Reducing cerebral mass in order to reduce ICP can be accomplished by surgical removal of damaged brain mass or by withdrawal of specific amounts of cerebral spinal fluid.

Maintaining $PaCO_2$ levels of 25 to 30 mm Hg reduces ICP by decreasing cerebral blood volume.

Osmotic agents reduce ICP by creating hyperosmotic serum, which draws water from the tissues, producing a diuretic effect. Mannitol is the osmotic agent of choice because it has little, if any, rebound effect (a phenomenon in which, several hours after osmotic use, ICP "rebounds," or returns, to a level higher than the initial reading).

5. Administer high-dose barbiturate therapy, as ordered.

This treatment seeks to reduce ICP by reducing the cerebral metabolic rate. Patients who are refractory to other treatments may respond to barbiturate therapy. The cardiac depressant effect of barbiturates makes pulmonary artery monitoring essential.

6. Obtain serial CT scans, if ordered. Prepare the patient for surgery, if indicated.

Serial CT scans identify an expanding intracranial lesion. Alerting the operating room staff as soon as surgery is indicated facilitates quick transport and adequate preparation.

Nursing diagnosis

Potential for alteration in neurologic function related to seizure activity secondary to head injury.

GOAL #1: Prevent seizure activity.

Interventions

1. Administer anticonvulsants, as ordered.

Rationale

Of all patients with an open head injury, 30% to 60% develop posttraumatic seizures; only 5% of those with a closed head injury develop this complication. Seizures increase metabolic needs of the brain, thereby increasing cerebral blood flow and ICP. Anticonvulsants may be administered either prophylactically following head injury or in response to seizure activity.

GOAL #2: Recognize seizure activity, maintain a patent airway, and optimize the patient's safety.

Interventions

1. Assess and report seizure characteristics, such as:
- patient reporting an aura
- length of seizure
- tonic/clonic activity
- incontinence
- postictal condition (altered mental status)
- seizure-related injuries, especially intraoral lacerations.

Rationale

Description of the seizure aids diagnosis and treatment. Suspicion of an unwitnessed seizure may evolve from recognition of postictal conditions, such as altered mental status, intraoral lacerations, and incontinence. Currently, seizure precautions no longer include use of a padded tongue blade because it increases the risk of patient injury.

2. Establish or maintain a patent airway. (See "Upper Airway Obstruction" in Section II.)

The recommended interventions include:
- performing the jaw-thrust maneuver
- inserting a nasal airway
- positioning the patient on his side while maintaining proper body alignment.

3. Pad the bed side rails.

4. Remove physical obstructions.

No attempts should be made to control or limit the patient's movement during a seizure because they may result in injury. Rather, the environment should be cleared of obstructions to the patient's movement.

Nursing diagnosis

Potential for alteration in thermoregulation related to hypothalamic malfunction secondary to head injury.

GOAL: Restore and maintain normothermia.

*Supplemental nursing diagnosis

NEUROLOGIC

Interventions

1. Monitor the patient's core body temperature.

2. Observe for other signs of increased temperature:
- hot, dry skin
- diaphoresis
- flushed skin.

3. Initiate antihyperthermic measures, such as use of a cooling blanket and antipyretic drugs, as ordered.

Rationale

Damage to the hypothalamus causes hyperthermia. This increases the brain's metabolic demands, increasing cerebral blood flow and ICP. These interventions detect and treat hyperthermia.

Nursing diagnosis

Potential for infection related to multiple invasive procedures or mechanism of injury.

GOAL: Detect early signs of septic shock.

Interventions

1. Observe for changes in level of consciousness or vital signs. (See "Vasogenic Shock" in Section II.)

2. Observe potential infection sites, including:
- venous line (peripheral and central)
- pulmonary artery or arterial line
- indwelling urinary catheter
- associated injury sites
- facial sinuses
- ICP monitoring sites.

3. Use strict aseptic technique for all invasive procedures and dressing changes.

4. Administer antibiotics, as ordered.

Rationale

Patients who survive the initial major trauma may succumb to an infection or multiple-system organ failure. Certain mechanisms of injury, such as those producing an open head wound or a cerebral spinal fluid leak, also predispose the patient to meningitis or brain abscesses. Septic shock may manifest itself early as a change in neurologic or cardiovascular status.

Care of the head-injured patient involves many invasive monitoring devices, any of which may serve as a source of infection.

Meticulous care of dressing sites and urinary catheters minimizes their potential as ports of entry.

Antibiotic selection will depend on the type of infection.

Nursing diagnosis

Potential for alteration in nutrition related to catabolic state secondary to traumatic injury.

GOAL: Provide adequate nutrition.

Interventions

1. Assess proper placement of the feeding tube. Administer tube feedings or parenteral hyperalimentation, as ordered.

Rationale

Trauma increases nutritional demands. A brief initial hypermetabolic state is tolerated by most patients, but establishment of good nutrition is important to reduce the likelihood and severity of sepsis. Most comatose head-injured patients tolerate tube feedings well, although hyperalimentation through a central venous line offers another route when enteral feeding is contraindicated. (See "Malnutrition in the Trauma Patient" in Section IV.)

Additional considerations

Approximately 200,000 adults sustain and are hospitalized for head injuries each year in the United States. Conservative estimates on lost income alone from these individuals is $22 billion a year. Long-term costs to the patient, family, and society are too astronomical to calculate. Multiple, complex problems in the rehabilitation phase require a coordinated team effort by all health care members. Rehabilitation for recovery of cognitive deficits may require from 3 to 24 months. A persistent vegetative state or brain death may ensue from severe head injuries. In these circumstances, nursing care will be directed toward family support, and if all attempts at treatment of the head-injured patient fail, consideration should be given to requesting organ donation from the next of kin, as appropriate.

Associated care plans

Vasogenic Shock
Hemorrhagic Shock
Diabetes Insipidus
Disseminated Intravascular Coagulation
Cervical Spine Injury
Lower Airway Obstruction
Upper Airway Obstruction
Use of Neuromuscular Blocking Agents
Malnutrition in the Trauma Patient
Maxillofacial Injuries
Psychosocial Support of the Trauma
  Patient

Associated procedures

Pulmonary Artery Catheterization
Preparation for Surgery
Intrahospital Transport of the Shock Trauma Patient
Endotracheal Intubation
Intracranial Pressure Monitoring
Organ Donation

Medical diagnosis

UPPER AIRWAY OBSTRUCTION

Assessment

Note: *Assume every trauma patient has a cervical spine injury—until proven otherwise. To prevent further injury to the spinal cord during airway management, ensure proper cervical spine alignment. Use one person to apply manual in-line traction to the head and cervical spine, and as soon as possible, apply a hard cervical collar to immobilize the head and cervical spine in proper alignment. Remember: Immobilize the chest before immobilizing the head and neck, so the body cannot act as a lever. Do not turn the head or hyperextend the neck, even in the rush to clear an obstruction; use the jaw-thrust or chin-lift method without the head-tilt.*

Mechanism of injury/ etiology:
- blunt or penetrating trauma to the upper airway
- burns of the face, head, neck
- smoke inhalation within the past 12 to 24 hours
- aspiration of foreign objects

Physical findings:
Respiratory
- cyanosis
- anxious facial expression, suggesting respiratory distress
- restlessness or unresponsiveness
- inability to talk
- complaints of inability to "get enough air"
- nasal flaring
- use of accessory muscles

- supraclavicular and/or intercostal retractions
- stridor (noisy, crowing respirations)
- gasping breaths
- extreme respiratory distress
- airway blocked by edema, tongue, or foreign object(s), such as dentures, broken teeth, blood, mucus, gum, tobacco, food, bone fragments

Maxillofacial
- malocclusion

Associated injuries:
- maxillofacial fractures/ wounds
- burns
- laryngeal/tracheal injury
- head/cervical spine injury

Diagnostic studies

(Physical examination usually confirms diagnosis immediately)
- radiographs of neck and chest—may locate objects lodged in or blocking the lower airway
- bronchoscopy—helps evaluate the lower airway for aspirated material

Nursing diagnosis

Ineffective airway clearance related to obstruction by the tongue, foreign matter, or edema.

GOAL #1: Restore a patent airway; avoid stimulating the gag reflex.

Interventions

1. Assess the patient rapidly for:
- air flow from the nose and mouth
- chest movement
- bilateral breath sounds.

2. Manually remove any obvious obstructing matter from the nose or mouth; gently suction the oropharynx with a tonsillar tip catheter.

Rationale

This rapid assessment helps determine whether the obstruction is complete or partial.

If the upper airway is obstructed by foreign matter or accumulated blood or mucus, simply suctioning the oropharynx or manually removing the debris may open the airway. Perform these maneuvers gently and carefully to avoid pushing debris farther into the airway.

RESPIRATORY

Note: *Assume that all trauma patients have a full stomach prior to admission. Avoid stimulating the gag reflex, as it may trigger vomiting, thus increasing the risk of aspiration. Should vomiting occur, rapidly suction the patient's oropharynx and coordinate logrolling onto one side while maintaining manual cervical alignment.*

3. Perform the jaw-thrust or chin-lift maneuver.

These maneuvers physically open the airway—by elevating the mandible, which in turn lifts the tongue away from the posterior pharyngeal wall—while maintaining proper spinal alignment. *Do not tilt or turn the patient's head to either side or hyperextend the head/neck.*

4. Insert an artificial oral or nasal airway.

Soft tissue relaxation allows the tongue to rest against the posterior pharyngeal wall, the most common cause of upper airway obstruction. Artificial airways reposition the tongue and may temporarily relieve the obstruction by allowing air to pass around or through the airway.

5. Ensure the availability of oral and nasal intubation equipment; assist with intubation as necessary. (See "Endotracheal Intubation" in Section VII.)

The patient who is unresponsive or has maxillofacial injuries usually requires emergency intubation because he is unable to maintain a patent airway. This inability results from loss of the gag reflex, excessive edema, and/or the inability to swallow.

6. Ensure the availability of properly functioning manual or mechanical ventilation devices.

Usually, the patient who requires intubation for airway management also requires assisted ventilation. Expect long-term management.

7. Ensure the availability of emergency cricothyroidotomy equipment (including surgical instruments and tracheostomy tubes in various sizes). Assist as necessary. (See "Needle Cricothyroidotomy" and "Surgical Cricothyroidotomy" in Section VII and "Emergency Airway Tray" in Appendix 3.)

Upper airway obstruction is a life-threatening situation! Extensive maxillofacial injuries or tracheobronchial tree trauma may make intubation physically impossible. Advanced preparation, by maintaining a ready-to-use airway tray, saves valuable time during this emergency.

GOAL #2: Maintain a patent airway.

Interventions

Rationale

1. Monitor the patient closely for signs of respiratory distress, including:
- air hunger
- retractions
- tachypnea
- stridor.

Ensure the availability of intubation equipment.

Although the patient's airway may be patent initially, he may develop respiratory difficulties resulting from neurologic deterioration, progressive soft tissue swelling, or laryngeal spasms (as with inhalation injury).

2. Ensure the availability and proper functioning of suction apparatus. Suction the patient as needed and document secretion characteristics. (See "Lower Airway Obstruction" in Section II.)

Accumulations from continued bleeding and mucus formation may obstruct the artificial airway. Retained secretions may obstruct the lower airway and cause complications, such as pneumonia or atelectasis. Pooled secretions also promote bacterial growth. Evaluating the quantity and characteristics of the tracheal secretions helps detect additional respiratory problems, such as pulmonary contusion.

Nursing diagnosis

Potential for impaired gas exchange related to aspiration of foreign objects into the lungs.

GOAL: Restore and maintain adequate gas exchange.

Interventions

1. Ensure the availability and proper functioning of equipment for supplemental humidified oxygen administration and mechanical ventilation.

2. Monitor the patient closely for indications of respiratory deterioration; obtain a baseline chest radiograph and ABG analysis.

3. Auscultate breath sounds frequently; provide optimal pulmonary hygiene, including:
• frequent suctioning
• turning and positioning in semi-Fowler's, unless contraindicated
• chest physiotherapy
• incentive spirometry.

4. Ensure the availability of bronchoscopy equipment. (See "Bronchoscopy" in Section VII.)

Rationale

The patient in any degree of respiratory distress requires supplemental oxygen before, during, and after airway establishment to promote optimal gas exchange. Upper airway obstruction may lead to lower airway obstruction: aspirated foreign objects decrease alveolar function and impair adequate gas exchange.

Signs of pulmonary insult or complications may not become evident for several hours. Baseline studies and trend analysis assist early detection of lower airway complications.

Auscultation of wheezes suggests lower airway obstruction. Pulmonary hygiene must be initiated early in the resuscitation phase to optimize aeration and prevent complications from aspirated and retained secretions. Hygiene measures mobilize secretions, prevent pooling, and promote full lung expansion.

Bronchoscopy helps detect pulmonary aspirates and affords deep pulmonary suctioning.

Nursing diagnosis

Potential for infection related to bacterial growth in lungs or cricothyroidotomy site secondary to aspiration of foreign objects or wound contamination.

GOAL #1: Reduce the risk of bacterial growth in the lungs.

Interventions

1. Provide optimal pulmonary hygiene, as described above.

Rationale

Prompt and consistent removal of pulmonary secretions reduces the risk of pneumonia and other pulmonary complications.

GOAL #2: Reduce the risk of bacterial growth in the cricothyroidotomy site.

Interventions

1. Promote sterile technique during emergency procedures, including the use of:
• masks and gloves
• masks for bedside staff
• sterile tray/instruments.

Rationale

Sterile technique decreases the risk of contaminates entering the wound and, ultimately, the respiratory tract.

RESPIRATORY

2. Perform aseptic wound care every 8 hours and as needed for excessive wound drainage.

Frequent aseptic wound care reduces the opportunity for bacterial growth. Monitoring the wound site, surrounding tissue, and drainage aids early detection of inflammation or infection.

Associated care plan	**Associated procedures and study**
Lower Airway Obstruction	Bronchoscopy
	Endotracheal Intubation
	Needle Cricothyroidotomy
	Surgical Cricothyroidotomy

Medical diagnosis

LOWER AIRWAY OBSTRUCTION

Assessment

Mechanism of injury/ etiology:
- commonly seen in varying degrees in patients with severe blunt and penetrating chest trauma

- associated with:
  - ☐ aspiration
  - ☐ smoke inhalation
  - ☐ near drowning
  - ☐ shock (all types)
  - ☐ pulmonary or fat embolism

- ☐ chemical ingestion
- ☐ immobility

Physical findings:
Respiratory
- decreased breath sounds

- rales, wheezes
- tachypnea

Cardiovascular
- cyanosis

Diagnostic studies

- ABGs—may indicate hypoxia, hypercapnia
- chest radiograph—may reveal atelectasis, infiltrates

Nursing diagnosis

Potential for impaired gas exchange and infection related to retained secretions and atelectasis.

> **GOAL #1:** Recognize early signs of lower airway obstruction. Optimize gas exchange.

Interventions

1. Assess the patient's respiratory status, checking particularly for:
- wheezes and rales
- increased respiratory effort
- alterations in ventilatory pattern
- tracheal secretions, amount and characteristics.

Monitor serial ABGs and chest radiographs.

2. Ensure the availability and proper functioning of equipment for humidified oxygenation, intubation, and mechanical ventilation. (See "Endotracheal Intubation" in Section VII.)

Rationale

Signs of obstruction at the alveolar level may not become evident for hours to days after the initial insult. Therefore, frequent reassessment and trend analysis are essential to prompt recognition. Serial ABGs (for example, every 12 hours) and daily chest radiographs aid early detection of pulmonary complications, such as pulmonary edema or adult respiratory distress syndrome.

The patient in any degree of respiratory distress requires supplemental oxygen before, during, and after the establishment of an airway to promote optimal gas exchange.

> **GOAL #2:** Prevent or minimize retained secretions. Minimize risk of infection.

Interventions

1. Auscultate breath sounds frequently. Provide optimal pulmonary hygiene, including:
- frequent suctioning
- turning the patient every 2 hours
- positioning in semi-Fowler's, unless contraindicated
- performing chest physiotherapy
- supervising incentive spirometry.

Evaluate and document characteristics and amount of tracheal secretions.

2. Obtain a specimen for sputum culture and administer antibiotics, as ordered.

3. Prepare the patient for bronchoscopy, as indicated. (See "Bronchoscopy" in Section VII.)

Rationale

Retained secretions are the most common form of lower airway obstruction in the seriously injured multiple trauma patient. Obstruction of the lower airways by secretions takes time to develop: hours, days, or even weeks. The lungs constantly secrete mucus, which the healthy person can easily clear. However, the traumatized patient has a decreased energy reserve and may be immobilized, contributing to his inability to clear secretions. Secretion accumulation in the alveoli limits or prohibits air from entering, resulting in localized atelectasis. Initiating an optimal pulmonary hygiene routine early in the resuscitation phase optimizes aeration and may prevent further complications.

Retained secretions provide a rich medium for growth of microorganisms and infection, which can lead to permanent lung damage. Antibiotic therapy is based on positive culture results.

Inability to clear lower airway obstructions with the above measures is an indication for bronchoscopy.

Associated care plans

Pulmonary Edema
Pulmonary Contusion
Adult Respiratory Distress Syndrome

Associated procedure and study

Bronchoscopy
Endotracheal Intubation

Medical diagnosis

LARYNGEAL FRACTURE

Assessment

Mechanism of injury/ etiology:
- high- or low-energy blunt trauma to the neck (often deceleration-type force): collision with interior structures of an automobile during an accident, clothesline accident, sporting injuries, strangulation, throttling
- penetrating neck injury

Physical findings:
Respiratory
- slight or progressive dysphonia
- aphonia
- hemoptysis
- painful swallowing
- dyspnea
- stridor
- tachypnea
- cyanosis
- use of accessory muscles of respiration

- anxiety, restlessness secondary to hypoxemia
- inability to make high-pitched "e" sound

Soft tissue
- contusions and abrasions of the anterior or anterolateral neck
- laceration or puncture wound of the neck
- swelling and tenderness

- subcutaneous emphysema, crepitus

Associated injuries:
- fracture/dislocation of cervical vertebra
- intralaryngeal laceration
- fractured trachea
- perforated pharynx
- ruptured esophagus

Diagnostic studies

- laryngoscopy, direct and indirect, flexible or rigid
- computerized tomography scan of the neck
- lateral cervical spine radiograph, including anterior portion of the neck, to rule out associated cervical

spine injury
- radiographic contrast study of the pharynx and esophagus—helps rule out associated injury

Nursing diagnosis

Potential for ineffective airway clearance related to soft tissue edema and displacement of fractured cartilage into the airway.

GOAL #1: Recognize patients at risk for laryngeal fractures.

Interventions

1. Question the patient, prehospital care providers, and family members about the mechanism of injury.

2. Question the patient and family members about dysphonia.

3. Ask the patient to make a high-pitched "e" sound.

4. Palpate the patient's neck for subcutaneous emphysema.

5. Note the presence of hemoptysis.

Rationale

Knowledge of the mechanism of injury will raise the clinician's index of suspicion.

Patients and family will often attribute a change in voice quality to causes other than trauma, such as dry throat or nervousness.

Vocal cord movement depends on mobile arytenoid cartilage, and proper vocal cord tension requires an intact, recurrent laryngeal nerve. Injury to either of these structures will prevent formation of this sound.

The presence of subcutaneous air indicates an airway disruption that allows air to escape into surrounding soft tissue.

Intralaryngeal lacerations commonly occur with laryngeal fractures.

GOAL #2: Restore a patent airway.

Interventions

1. Ensure the availability of endotracheal intubation equipment; assist with intubation as necessary. (See "Endotracheal Intubation" in Section VII.)

2. Ensure the availability of emergency cricothyroidotomy or tracheostomy equipment; assist as necessary. (See "Needle Cricothyroidotomy" and "Surgical Cricothyroidotomy" in Section VII.)

Rationale

Excessive soft tissue swelling and/or displacement of a fractured cartilage segment may obstruct the airway, necessitating endotracheal intubation.

Segments of displaced cartilage in the airway may prevent passage of an endotracheal tube, necessitating establishment of an airway below the site of injury.

GOAL #3: Maintain a patent airway.

Interventions

1. Monitor nonintubated patients closely for signs of dyspnea, accessory muscle use, and stridor; ensure the availability of emergency intubation, cricothyroidotomy, and tracheostomy equipment.

2. Ensure the availability of necessary equipment, supplies, and personnel to establish a patent airway whenever the patient must be transported for diagnostic studies.

3. Keep suctioning equipment at the bedside.

4. Keep the patient NPO.

5. Provide humidified oxygen as ordered.

Rationale

Continued swelling 48 hours postinjury may obstruct the airway, necessitating emergency intubation.

Frequent pharyngeal suctioning may be necessary if intralaryngeal lacerations are associated with laryngeal fracture.

Development of laryngeal spasms may cause aspiration.

Humidified oxygen helps keep the injured airway moist and reduces the patient's tidal volume.

Nursing diagnosis

Potential for fear related to difficulty in breathing secondary to laryngeal injury.

GOAL: Decrease the patient's fear.

Interventions

1. Explain all procedures to the patient using comprehensible terms; repeat explanations as necessary.

2. Monitor bedside conversations by other health care personnel.

Rationale

Fear may alter the patient's ability to comprehend events, and it may impair short-term memory; clear, careful explanations, repeated as necessary, can help reduce fears.

Increased patient fear may result from misinterpretation of conversations.

Nursing diagnosis

Potential for impaired verbal communication related to dysfunction of vocal cords or placement of artificial airway.

> **GOAL:** Establish and maintain effective methods of communication.

Interventions

1. Assess the patient's ability to communicate in ways other than verbally.

2. Provide the patient with an appropriate alternative to verbal communication.

Rationale

The patient will not be able to speak while an artificial airway is in place.

Associated care plans

Upper Airway Obstruction
Lower Airway Obstruction
Psychosocial Support of the Trauma
    Patient

Associated procedures and study

Bronchoscopy
Intrahospital Transport of the Shock Trauma Patient
Endotracheal Intubation
Needle Cricothyroidotomy
Surgical Cricothyroidotomy

RESPIRATORY

Medical diagnosis

TRACHEOBRONCHIAL TREE RUPTURE

Assessment

Mechanism of injury/ etiology:
- penetrating chest trauma
- blunt chest trauma— chest compression, rapid deceleration

Physical findings:
Respiratory
- dyspnea
- hemoptysis
- subcutaneous emphysema—especially of the head and neck
- signs and symptoms of a pneumothorax or tension pneumothorax

- large, continuous air leak from a chest tube

Common sites of injury:
- distal trachea
- proximal main stem bronchi

Note: *Tracheobronchial tree injuries from blunt*

trauma usually occur within 2.5 cm of the carina.

Associated injuries:
- pneumothorax or tension pneumothorax
- upper rib fractures

Diagnostic studies

- chest radiography—may reveal pneumomediastinum
- bronchoscopy—to verify the tear

Nursing diagnosis

Potential for impaired gas exchange related to decreased inspired air, lung collapse and compression secondary to air leakage from tracheobronchial tree rupture.

GOAL #1: Maintain a high index of suspicion.

Interventions

1. Suspect tracheobronchial injury in a patient with:
- pneumothorax or tension pneumothorax
- subcutaneous emphysema
- hemoptysis
- large, continuous air leak after closed-tube thoracostomy
- mediastinal emphysema on chest radiograph.

Rationale

Tracheobronchial tree rupture is a rare injury caused primarily by blunt trauma. If the peribronchial tissue is disrupted and communicates with the chest cavity, the patient usually has signs and symptoms of a pneumothorax or possibly tension pneumothorax. The pneumothorax is treated by closed-tube thoracostomy to evacuate air and blood and reexpand the lung. Suspect a tracheobronchial rupture if there is a large, persistent air leak after chest tube insertion.

GOAL #2: Establish and maintain an adequate airway and optimize gas exchange.

Interventions

1. Ensure the availability and proper functioning of equipment for administration of humidified oxygen, intubation, and mechanical ventilation. (See "Endotracheal Intubation" in Section VII.)

Rationale

A patient with any degree of respiratory distress needs supplemental oxygen and prompt airway management.

2. Assist with chest radiography as necessary.

The chest radiograph is very valuable in confirming the findings that arouse suspicion of a tracheobronchial tree rupture, such as:
- pneumothorax
- subcutaneous emphysema
- mediastinal emphysema
- upper rib fractures
- deep cervical emphysema.

These findings indicate the need for more definitive diagnostic procedures.

3. Prepare the patient for bronchoscopy. (See "Bronchoscopy" in Section VII.)

Bronchoscopy verifies a tracheobronchial tree rupture.

4. Prepare the patient for surgery. (See "Preparation for Surgery" in Section VII.) Notify operating room personnel.

Surgical reconstruction is performed if the tracheobronchial tear is greater than one third the airway's circumference. The patient may not need surgical intervention, however, if the tear, visualized by bronchoscopy, is less than one third the airway's circumference and if chest tube insertion and an underwater seal drainage system result in complete lung reexpansion and air leak cessation.

Nursing diagnosis

Potential for impaired gas exchange and infection related to lower airway obstruction secondary to possible blood aspiration, retained secretions, and atelectasis.

GOAL: Prevent or minimize retained secretions; minimize the risk of infection.

Interventions

Rationale

1. Ensure the availability and anticipate the use of supplemental humidified oxygen.

A patient with any degree of respiratory distress needs supplemental oxygen before, during, and after establishing an airway to promote optimal gas exchange. Lower airway obstruction from retained secretions, aspiration, or atelectasis impairs alveolar function and gas exchange.

2. Auscultate breath sounds frequently. Provide the patient with optimal pulmonary hygiene, including:
- frequent suctioning
- tracheal lavage if secretions are thick and difficult to suction
- turning every 2 hours
- positioning in semi-Fowler's (unless contraindicated)
- chest physiotherapy every 2 to 4 hours.

Rales and wheezes indicate lower airway obstruction. Pulmonary hygiene, initiated early during resuscitation, optimizes aeration and minimizes complications from retained secretions, aspiration, and atelectasis. These measures help mobilize secretions, prevent pooling, and promote full lung expansion. Also, prompt and consistent removal of pulmonary secretions lowers the risk of bacterial infection, such as pneumonia, and other pulmonary complications.

Associated care plans	Associated procedures and study
Pneumothorax	Bronchoscopy
Tension Pneumothorax	Preparation for Surgery
Lower Airway Obstruction	Endotracheal Intubation
Laryngeal Fracture	

Medical diagnosis

TENSION PNEUMOTHORAX

Assessment

Mechanism of injury/ etiology:
- blunt or penetrating chest trauma, including fractured ribs, tracheobronchial tree rupture, an occluded open pneumothorax
- a complication associated with the use of positive end-expiratory pressure on mechanically ventilated patients, especially those with preexisting lung disease

†Classic sign of a tension pneumothorax

Physical findings:
Respiratory
- rapidly progressing restlessness
- extreme agitation
- dyspnea
- tachypnea
- nasal flaring
- intercostal retraction
- rapidly progressing respiratory failure and cyanosis
- deviation of the cervical trachea toward the unaffected side†
- apical pulse displacement toward the unaffected side†
- possible neck vein distention—if blood loss is significant, neck vein distention is usually not evident
- absent breath sounds on the affected side
- hyperinflation and minimal chest wall expansion on the affected side
- hyperresonance to percussion on the affected side

- abrasions, lacerations, or ecchymosis

Cardiovascular
- hypotension
- tachycardia

Associated injuries:
- tracheobronchial tree rupture or laceration
- esophageal rupture or laceration
- lung laceration or perforation
- open pneumothorax
- hemopneumothorax
- rib fractures

Diagnostic study

- chest radiography—confirms clinical impressions

Nursing diagnoses

1. *Potential for decreased cardiac output, tissue perfusion, and hypoxia related to:*
   - *vena cava compression, resulting in decreased diastolic filling of the heart*
   - *mediastinal shift toward the unaffected side, resulting in cavoatrial junction compression and angulation, further decreasing diastolic filling secondary to progressive air accumulation within the chest cavity, causing increased positive intrapleural pressure.*

2. *Potential for decreased gas exchange related to ventilatory interference secondary to lung collapse on the affected side and contralateral lung compression produced by increased positive intrapleural pressure and mediastinal shift.*

GOAL #1: Recognize early signs of a tension pneumothorax and maintain a patent airway.

Interventions

1. Monitor the patient for signs of a tension pneumothorax, especially if he is in severe respiratory distress. Assess for:
- severe air hunger
- rapidly progressing restlessness and agitation

Rationale

A tension pneumothorax is a life-threatening emergency. It develops as air leaks into the chest cavity through a "one-way valve" from a lung, tracheobronchial tree, or chest wall injury. The progressive air accumulation rapidly increases the positive pressure within the chest cavity. As a result, the venae cavae are compressed and diastolic filling is decreased, thus lowering cardiac

*Supplemental nursing diagnosis

- nasal flaring and intercostal retraction
- deviation of the cervical trachea toward the unaffected side
- apical pulse displacement toward the unaffected side
- possible neck vein distention
- absent breath sounds, hyperinflation, minimal chest wall expansion, and hyperresonance to percussion on the affected side
- hypotension and tachycardia.

2. Ensure the availability and proper functioning of equipment for administration of humidified oxygen, intubation, and mechanical ventilation. (See "Endotracheal Intubation" in Section VII.)

output. The mediastinum also shifts toward the unaffected side, causing cavoatrial junction angulation that reduces venous return to the heart and further lowers cardiac output. Decreased cardiac output leads to peripheral hypoxia and acidosis. The increasing intrapleural pressure also causes the affected lung to collapse. As the pressure increases and the mediastinum shifts toward the unaffected side, contralateral lung compression interferes with that lung's ventilation. Gas exchange in both lungs is severely impaired because of parenchymal collapse. Pulmonary blood shunted through nonventilated or hypoventilated alveoli leads to severe hypoxia. The combination of hypoxia and acidosis can be fatal if intrapleural pressures are not immediately restored to atmospheric or subatmospheric levels.

GOAL #2: Relieve increased intrapleural pressure and return pressures to atmospheric or subatmospheric levels.

Interventions

1. Immediately remove any dressing occluding an open pneumothorax.

2. Ensure the availability of equipment for a needle thoracentesis; assist as necessary.

3. Ensure the availability of equipment for a closed-tube thoracostomy; assist as necessary. (See "Closed-Tube Thoracostomy" in Section VII.)

4. Assist with chest radiography as necessary.

5. Monitor and report trends in ABG levels. Administer sodium bicarbonate as ordered.

Rationale

A tension pneumothorax is life threatening and demands immediate treatment. Initial management is focused on returning the intrapleural pressure to atmospheric or subatmospheric levels. This goal can be achieved simply by removing an occlusive dressing covering an open pneumothorax or by inserting a 14G to 18G over-the-needle catheter anteriorly into the second or third intercostal space in the midclavicular line. The catheter is inserted over the rib to avoid injuring intercostal vessels and nerves lying below the rib. As the needle enters the chest cavity, a large quantity of air under pressure is released, converting the tension pneumothorax to a pneumothorax. The lung usually completely reexpands after a chest tube is inserted.

A chest radiograph confirms diagnosis of a tension pneumothorax. It usually shows collapse of the affected lung, compression of the unaffected lung, ipsilateral diaphragm depression, and a mediastinal shift toward the uninvolved side. Despite the fact that a chest radiograph confirms the diagnosis, a tension pneumothorax is a *life-threatening emergency.* Never delay treatment while awaiting definitive diagnosis by radiography.

Sodium bicarbonate neutralizes the acidosis resulting from decreased tissue perfusion and hypoxia.

Nursing diagnosis

Potential for impaired gas exchange and infection related to lower airway obstruction secondary to retained secretions and atelectasis.

GOAL: Prevent or minimize retained secretions.

Interventions

1. Ensure the availability and anticipate the use of supplemental humidified oxygen.

2. Auscultate breath sounds frequently. Provide optimal pulmonary hygiene, including:
- frequent suctioning
- turning the patient every 2 hours
- positioning in semi-Fowler's (unless contra-indicated)
- chest physiotherapy
- incentive spirometry.

Rationale

A patient in any degree of respiratory distress needs supplemental oxygen before, during, and after airway establishment to promote optimal gas exchange. Lower airway obstruction from retained secretions or atelectasis impairs alveolar function and gas exchange.

Rales and wheezes reflect probable lower airway obstruction. Pulmonary hygiene must be initiated early in resuscitation to optimize aeration and prevent aspirated and retained secretion complications. These measures mobilize secretions, prevent pooling, and promote full lung expansion. Promptly and consistently removing pulmonary secretions reduces the risk of infection, pneumonia, and other pulmonary complications.

Associated care plans

Open Pneumothorax
Pneumothorax
Pulmonary Contusion
Hemothorax
Lower Airway Obstruction
Tracheobronchial Tree Rupture

Associated procedures

Closed-Tube Thoracostomy
Endotracheal Intubation

Medical diagnosis

OPEN PNEUMOTHORAX ("Sucking" Chest Wound)

Assessment

**Mechanism of injury/
etiology:**
• blunt chest trauma,
usually associated with
large chest wall defects
• penetrating chest
trauma, usually associ-
ated with smaller chest
wall defects

Physical findings:
Respiratory
• dyspnea
• tachypnea
• cyanosis
• restlessness
• sucking sound from
the chest wound

• subcutaneous emphy-
sema
• decreased or absent
breath sounds

Associated injuries:
• tension pneumothorax
• pneumothorax

• hemothorax
• pulmonary contusion
• cardiac tamponade
• tracheobronchial tree
rupture

Diagnostic study

• chest radiography—confirms presence of air in the
pleural space and reexpansion of lung; may identify associated injuries

Nursing diagnosis

*Potential for ineffective breathing patterns and impaired gas exchange related to lung collapse and loss of
thoracic bellows needed to produce a pressure gradient for air exchange.*

GOAL: Restore normal breathing patterns and improve gas exchange.

Interventions

1. Apply a sterile, nonocclusive dressing at
the end of exhalation. The dressing must extend beyond the edges of the wound. Tape
the dressing on three sides. Monitor the patient for early signs of a tension pneumothorax. Immediately remove the dressing if
the patient shows signs of a tension pneumothorax.

2. Ensure the availability and proper functioning of equipment for humidified oxygen
administration, intubation, and mechanical
ventilation.

Rationale

Generally, penetrating chest wounds from projectiles or stabbings
have a smaller diameter and self-seal. If the defect is large and
cannot self-seal, a "sucking" chest wound develops. If the wound
diameter is two thirds the tracheal diameter, air passes by the
route of least resistance: through the defect. During inspiration,
air enters the chest wound, collapsing the lung on the injured
side. Normal lung ventilation is impaired because the bellows effect is lost and an adequate amount of air is not drawn into the
lung via the trachea. The result is oxygen depletion, hypoxia, and
carbon dioxide retention. Applying a nonocclusive dressing prevents more air from entering the thoracic cavity. Apply the dressing at the end of exhalation because intrathoracic pressure is most
negative then. Create a flutter valve by taping the dressing on
three sides. When the patient inhales, the dressing is sucked over
the wound, preventing air entry. When the patient exhales, the
open end of the dressing lets air escape. A nonocclusive dressing
lowers the risk of a tension pneumothorax.

Generally, a patient with an open pneumothorax is intubated
promptly and placed on a mechanical ventilator to improve his ventilatory status.

3. Ensure the availability of equipment for a closed-tube thoracostomy; assist as needed. Apply an occlusive petrolatum gauze dressing after chest tube insertion. Assist with chest radiography, as needed.

A chest tube is inserted at a site away from the open chest wound. It is connected to an underwater seal suction device to reexpand the involved lung. Monitor the chest tube closely for continuous air leaks or massive bleeding. Either condition reflects possible associated injuries. A chest radiograph confirms lung reexpansion and may show associated injuries. An occlusive dressing can now be applied because the chest tube minimizes the risk of a tension pneumothorax.

4. Prepare the patient for surgical intervention. (See "Preparation for Surgery" in Section VII.)

Depending on the location and extent of the open, "sucking" chest wound, surgical debridement is usually required, and thoracic exploration may be required.

Nursing diagnosis

Potential for infection related to wound contamination.

GOAL: Prevent or minimize further wound contamination and reduce the risk of infection.

Interventions

1. Apply all wound dressings using sterile technique.

2. Obtain the patient's history of medication allergies and tetanus immunization; administer antibiotics and tetanus vaccine, as ordered.

Rationale

Dressings provide a mechanical barrier to environmental contaminants, reducing the introduction of additional organisms.

Antibiotics rarely are ordered prophylactically; more commonly, they are started after a positive culture has been obtained. Typically, the wound is surgically debrided and irrigated. All patients with open wounds require immunization against tetanus.

Associated care plans

Tension Pneumothorax
Pneumothorax
Hemothorax
Acute Pericardial Tamponade
Tracheobronchial Tree Rupture
Pulmonary Contusion

Associated procedures

Closed-Tube Thoracostomy
Preparation for Surgery

RESPIRATORY

Medical diagnosis

PNEUMOTHORAX

Assessment

Mechanism of injury/ etiology:
- penetrating chest trauma
- blunt chest trauma
- iatrogenic injury

Physical findings:

Respiratory
- chest pain
- dyspnea (may be worse in patients with preexisting lung disease)
- tachypnea
- decreased or absent breath sounds on affected side
- hyperresonance
- subcutaneous emphysema (may not be present)
- unequal chest expansion

Classification of pneumothoraces:
- small—15% of pleural cavity
- moderate—15% to 60% of pleural cavity
- large—greater than 60% of pleural cavity

Associated injuries:
- rib fractures
- tracheobronchial tree rupture
- esophageal injury
- alveolar disruption
- open pneumothorax
- tension pneumothorax

Diagnostic study

- chest radiography—confirms the presence of air in the pleural cavity

Nursing diagnosis

Potential for impaired gas exchange related to lung collapse and compression secondary to air accumulation in the pleural space.

GOAL: Establish and maintain an adequate airway and optimize gas exchange.

Interventions

1. Ensure the availability and proper functioning of equipment for humidified oxygen administration, intubation, and mechanical ventilation. (See "Endotracheal Intubation" in Section VII.)

2. Assist with chest radiography.

Rationale

A pneumothorax results from air entering the pleural space, causing lung collapse. Normally, the chest cavity is filled by the fully expanded lung. Air enters the chest cavity most commonly from a lacerated lung, trachea, or bronchus, or from chest wall disruption. A pneumothorax results from both penetrating and blunt chest trauma. Blood circulating to the collapsed lung is not oxygenated because of impaired lung ventilation. Establishing and maintaining an airway and administering humidified oxygen increase oxygen availability. **Note:** *Any patient with a pneumothorax is at risk for a life-threatening tension pneumothorax. (See "Tension Pneumothorax" in Section II.)*

A radiograph confirms the diagnosis and size of the pneumothorax. Chest radiographs of all trauma patients should be taken as early as possible.

3. Ensure the availability of equipment for a closed-tube thoracostomy. Assist as necessary. (See "Closed-Tube Thoracostomy" in Section VII.)

The treatment for a pneumothorax consists of inserting a chest tube connected to an underwater seal, closed drainage suction device to reexpand the collapsed lung. A chest radiograph should be taken after insertion to check chest tube placement and to evaluate lung reexpansion. A chest tube may not be necessary in a healthy patient with a small pneumothorax who:
- has no other injuries
- is not in respiratory distress
- is not a surgical candidate.

However, this patient will require close observation and monitoring with serial ABG studies and chest radiographs.

4. Monitor the closed drainage suction device for large or continuous air leaks. If they are present, prepare the patient for bronchoscopy. (See "Bronchoscopy" in Section VII.)

Massive or continuous air leaks may indicate tracheobronchial tree rupture. Bronchoscopy confirms the diagnosis.

5. Prepare the patient for possible surgery as indicated. (See "Preparation for Surgery" in Section VII.)

Surgical repair of a lacerated trachea or bronchus may be required. (See "Tracheobronchial Tree Rupture" in Section II.)

Nursing diagnosis

Potential for impaired gas exchange and infection related to lower airway obstruction secondary to retained secretions and atelectasis.

GOAL: Prevent or minimize retained secretions.

Interventions

1. Ensure the availability and anticipate use of supplemental humidified oxygen.

2. Auscultate breath sounds frequently. Provide optimal pulmonary hygiene, including:
- frequent suctioning
- turning the patient every 2 hours
- placement in semi-Fowler's position (unless contraindicated)
- chest physiotherapy
- incentive spirometry.

Rationale

A patient in any degree of respiratory distress requires supplemental oxygen before, during, and after airway establishment to promote optimal gas exchange. Lower airway obstruction from retained secretions or atelectasis decreases alveolar function and impairs gas exchange.

Rales and wheezes on auscultation indicate lower airway obstruction. Pulmonary hygiene must be initiated early during resuscitation to optimize aeration and prevent complications from aspirated and retained secretions. These measures mobilize secretions, prevent pooling, and promote full lung expansion. Prompt and consistent removal of pulmonary secretions reduces the risk of infection, pneumonia, and other pulmonary complications.

Associated care plans

Tension Pneumothorax
Tracheobronchial Tree Rupture
Lower Airway Obstruction

Associated procedures and study

Closed-Tube Thoracostomy
Preparation for Surgery
Bronchoscopy

RESPIRATORY

Medical diagnosis

HEMOTHORAX

Assessment

Note: *A massive hemothorax is a life-threatening emergency because it severely compromises the cardiopulmonary system. Resuscitation, diagnosis, and treatment should be performed simultaneously.*

Mechanism of injury/ etiology:
- penetrating chest trauma
- blunt chest trauma, deceleration injuries
- iatrogenic injury

Physical findings:
Respiratory
- varying degrees of respiratory distress, depending on the extent of the hemothorax
- chest tightness or pain
- dyspnea

- cyanosis
- tachypnea
- decreased or absent breath sounds on the affected side†
- dullness to percussion†
- unequal chest expansion
- tracheal deviation to the unaffected side (massive hemothorax)
- apical pulse displacement to the unaffected side (massive hemothorax)

Cardiovascular
- varying degrees of shock, depending on the extent of the hemothorax
- tachycardia
- hypotension
- pallor
- diaphoresis
- unrelenting shock†
- possible neck vein distention—if the patient suffered significant blood loss, neck vein distention is usually not apparent

Classification of hemothoraces:
- small: < 400 cc of blood
- moderate: 500 to 1,500 cc of blood
- massive: > 1,500 cc of blood

Associated injuries:
- rib fractures
- lung laceration
- systemic or pulmonary vessel disruption
- tension pneumothorax

†The combination of these assessment findings is a classic indicator of a moderate to massive hemothorax.

Diagnostic study

- chest radiograph—upright chest film provides a more accurate assessment of the size of the hemothorax

Nursing diagnoses

1. Potential for impaired gas exchange related to interference in ventilation secondary to progressive hemorrhage into the chest cavity, causing ipsilateral, and eventually contralateral, lung compression.

2. Potential for decreased tissue perfusion related to fluid volume deficit secondary to hemorrhage into the chest cavity from the disruption in the integrity of intrathoracic organ or vasculature.

*3. *Potential for further decrease in cardiac output, tissue perfusion, and hypoxia related to:*
  - *vena cava compression, leading to decreased diastolic filling*
  - *mediastinal shift to the unaffected side, resulting in compression and angulation at the cavoatrial junction and causing further decrease in diastolic filling*
  - *decreased hematocrit, lowering the blood's oxygen carrying capacity, all secondary to the progressive massive hemorrhage into the pleural cavity.*

GOAL #1: Maintain a patent airway and adequate gas exchange.

*Supplemental nursing diagnosis

Interventions

1. Ensure the availability and proper functioning of equipment for humidified oxygen administration, intubation, and mechanical ventilation. (See "Endotracheal Intubation" in Section VII.)

2. Monitor the patient for signs of hemorrhagic shock; monitor vital signs every 5 to 15 minutes, and monitor ECG rhythm and neurologic status.

Rationale

A patient with a small hemothorax may be asymptomatic, showing little or no change in appearance, respiratory effort, or vital signs. A patient with a moderate to massive hemothorax suffers varying degrees of cardiopulmonary distress. A massive hemothorax is life-threatening, requiring immediate recognition and treatment. The cardiovascular and respiratory systems are both severely compromised. The patient's cardiac output falls, leading to peripheral hypoxia and metabolic acidosis. As the chest fills with blood, the mediastinum shifts to the unaffected sides. This causes angulation at the cavoatrial junction, impairing venous return to the heart. Ventilatory function is severely compromised owing to lung compression on both the affected and contralateral sides. The combination of hemorrhagic shock and hypoxia is usually fatal unless promptly corrected.

GOAL #2: Restore and maintain a normovolemic state.

Interventions

1. Ensure adequate I.V. access with at least two large-bore peripheral catheters; administer fluids as ordered.

2. Obtain baseline laboratory studies and monitor trends in hemoglobin, hematocrit, serum electrolytes, ABGs, and coagulation profiles.

3. Ensure the availability of adequate amounts of packed RBCs (PRBCs) and clotting factors for early transfusions. Follow hospital policy for infusion, filtration, and blood warming. **Note:** *The situation's urgency may require the use of uncrossmatched blood.*

4. Ensure the availability and proper functioning of equipment for autotransfusion. (See "Autotransfusion" in Section VII.)

5. Assist with chest radiography as required.

Rationale

Early, aggressive volume replacement with colloid and crystalloid products is necessary to combat hemorrhagic shock. Trend analysis of laboratory data helps assess tissue perfusion, fluid balance, and the overall effectiveness of resuscitation. Prolonged clotting times frequently develop and require early detection and aggressive therapy.

Early, aggressive blood replacement is a major component of effective care. Also, associated injuries can precipitate further blood loss and complicate the shock state. Early initiation of blood component therapy with PRBCs and clotting factors, such as fresh-frozen plasma and platelets, may prevent potentially lethal coagulopathies. If not detected early, or if allowed to persist, they aggravate the hemorrhagic process and may lead to death.

Blunt or penetrating chest trauma with acute blood loss is an indication for autotransfusion. Blood in the chest cavity can be collected, filtered, and reinfused for rapid replacement of intravascular volume loss.

If the patient shows signs and symptoms of a massive hemothorax, a chest radiograph may not be taken before chest tube insertion. If the patient's condition is more stable, an upright radiograph is routine, unless contraindicated. The radiograph confirms the diagnosis and extent of the hemothorax and helps identify associated injuries. A radiograph is always taken after chest tube insertion to visualize tube placement and lung reexpansion and to assess fluid drainage. Serial radiographs should be taken to ensure adequate hemothorax drainage.

GOAL #3: Relieve compression and pressure within the pleural cavity.

Interventions

1. Ensure the availability and proper functioning of equipment for a closed-tube thoracostomy; assist as necessary. (See "Closed-Tube Thoracostomy" in Section VII.)

2. Monitor tube drainage every 5 to 15 minutes. Record and report trends.

3. Initially "milk," or strip, the chest tube in short sections every 5 to 15 minutes, depending on drainage volume.

4. Prepare the patient for possible surgical intervention. (See "Preparation for Surgery" in Section VII.)

Rationale

A patient with a small hemothorax and no accompanying pneumothorax generally needs no mechanical ventilation. If his condition is stable, he should be observed for several days and monitored with serial chest radiographs, laboratory studies (hemoglobin/hematocrit and coagulation profiles), and frequent checking of vital signs. If delayed bleeding occurs, a chest tube is inserted. In a moderate to massive hemothorax, a 36 to 40 French chest tube is inserted and connected to an underwater seal, closed drainage suction device. This evacuates blood from the chest cavity, thus relieving lung compression and promoting reexpansion. A large-bore chest tube minimizes tube occlusion by blood clots. *A chest tube is inserted after I.V. lines are in place.* Resuscitation continues as the chest is decompressed and fluid drained.

Accurate monitoring is vital for a patient with a hemothorax because the extent of chest tube bleeding helps determine if the patient requires surgical intervention to control hemorrhage.

"Milking," or stripping, the chest tube in short sections from the patient to the closed-drainage suction system helps maintain tube patency. This prevents occlusion from blood clots without creating a marked increase in intrapleural pressure, which can damage lung tissue.

The rapid evacuation of 800 to 1,500 cc of chest cavity blood does not always mandate surgical intervention to control bleeding. Most patients with a moderate hemothorax are successfully treated with fluid resuscitation and closed-tube thoracostomy. The patient may require a thoracotomy if chest tube bleeding:
- is > 300 to 500 cc/hour
- is > 200 cc/hour for 3 to 4 hours
- increases over 3 to 5 hours.

Other indications for surgery are an increase in the hemothorax as seen by either follow-up radiography or unrelenting hypotension despite adequate fluid resuscitation.

Nursing diagnosis

Potential for impaired gas exchange and infection related to lower airway obstruction secondary to retained secretions and atelectasis.

GOAL: Prevent or minimize retained secretions.

Interventions

1. Ensure the availability and anticipate the use of supplemental humidified oxygen.

Rationale

A patient in any degree of respiratory distress needs supplemental oxygen before, during, and after airway establishment to promote optimal gas exchange. Lower airway obstruction from retained secretions or atelectasis impairs alveolar function and gas exchange.

2. Auscultate breath sounds frequently. Provide optimal pulmonary hygiene, including:
- frequent suctioning
- turning the patient every 2 hours
- placement in semi-Fowler's position (unless contraindicated)
- chest physiotherapy
- incentive spirometry.

Auscultation of rales and wheezes generally indicates lower airway obstruction. Start pulmonary hygiene early in resuscitation to optimize aeration and prevent complications from aspirates and retained secretions. These measures mobilize secretions, prevent pooling, and promote full lung expansion. Prompt and consistent pulmonary secretion removal lowers the risk of infection, pneumonia, and other pulmonary complications.

Additional considerations

It is not uncommon for a trauma patient to have a combined hemothorax and pneumothorax (hemopneumothorax). The treatment of these patients is the same except for the insertion of an additional chest tube for the drainage of air from the pleural cavity. One is placed anteriorly for the drainage of air and the other is placed posteriorly for the drainage of fluid.

Associated care plans

Lower Airway Obstruction
Tracheobronchial Tree Rupture
Pneumothorax
Tension Pneumothorax
Penetrating Chest Trauma
Traumatic Rupture of the Aorta or Great
    Vessels

Associated procedures and study

Closed-Tube Thoracostomy
Preparation for Surgery
Autotransfusion
Bronchoscopy
Endotracheal Intubation

Medical diagnosis

PULMONARY CONTUSION

Assessment

Mechanism of injury/etiology:
- blunt chest trauma as from rapid deceleration, compression, or blast injury
- penetrating trauma—contused area may surround the high-velocity projectile tract

Physical findings:
Respiratory
- hypoxia-induced restlessness
- dyspnea
- tachypnea
- rales and wheezes
- copious secretions
- hemoptysis
- chest pain—usually from chest wall injury
- ineffective cough

Cardiovascular
- tachycardia

Associated injuries:
- flail chest
- pneumothorax
- tension pneumothorax
- hemothorax
- rib fractures
- cardiac tamponade

Diagnostic studies

- ABG results—may reveal hypoxia, hypercarbia
- chest radiography—may identify contused or atelectatic areas

Nursing diagnosis

Potential for impaired gas exchange and infection related to lower airway obstruction and atelectasis secondary to pulmonary contusion.

> **GOAL #1:** Maintain a high index of suspicion; recognize early signs of pulmonary contusion.

Interventions

1. Suspect a pulmonary contusion in any patient with blunt chest trauma, especially if he has:
- flail chest
- fractured ribs
- pneumothorax
- tension pneumothorax
- hemothorax.

2. Monitor the patient for:
- tachypnea
- tachycardia
- hemoptysis
- rales and wheezes.

Rationale

Pulmonary contusion is the most common potentially lethal chest injury and is frequently seen in the multiple trauma patient. It may not be evident initially and is commonly masked by more immediately life-threatening injuries, such as flail chest, tension pneumothorax, or hemothorax.

With time, progressive pulmonary failure develops and may be fatal. Keeping a high index of suspicion and making a prompt diagnosis improve the prognosis. A pulmonary contusion is bruising to lung parenchyma. Injury causes not only bleeding into the alveoli but also alveolar wall and small blood vessel rupture, prompting interstitial and intraalveolar edema. Blood and fluid accumulations obstruct the lower airway, cause atelectasis, and augment tracheobronchial secretions. Atelectasis worsens, usually because the patient cannot rid himself of pulmonary secretions because of severe chest wall pain. The interruption in ventilation/perfusion ratios results in systemic hypoxia. The lungs' elasticity deteriorates, increasing the work of breathing and oxygen consumption. This exacerbates hypoxia and respiratory acidosis. Attempting to increase oxygenation, the circulatory system increases cardiac output and pulse rate. If the cycle is not corrected, myocardial failure ensues, decreasing tissue perfusion and producing metabolic acidosis. The combination of hypoxia, respiratory acidosis, and metabolic acidosis can be lethal. The prognosis depends on the pulmonary injury's severity and on early, aggressive therapy.

GOAL #2: Maintain a patent airway; optimize gas exchange.

Interventions

1. Ensure the availability and proper functioning of equipment for administration of humidified oxygen, intubation, and mechanical ventilation. (See "Endotracheal Intubation" in Section VII.)

2. Obtain baseline ABG levels. Monitor and report trends.

3. Closely monitor and restrict I.V. intake as ordered.

4. Assist with chest radiography as required.

Rationale

A patient with any degree of respiratory distress requires supplemental humidified oxygen or intubation and mechanical ventilation. Depending on the severity of the contusion, the patient may need only supplemental humidified oxygen for 24 to 36 hours, or he may need immediate intubation and mechanical ventilation with positive end-expiratory pressure to improve his gas exchange.

Early, definitive diagnosis of pulmonary contusion may be difficult in a patient with multiple system injuries, and the contusion may not be clinically evident. Therefore, serial ABG results can determine gas-exchange efficiency. A PaO_2 lower than 60 mm Hg on room air and lower than 300 mm Hg on 100% FiO_2 signals impaired gas exchange. An increase in $PaCO_2$ in the hypoxic patient indicates impaired pulmonary function and the need for intubation and mechanical ventilation. The hypoxic patient would be expected to have a decreased $PaCO_2$ from hyperventilation.

Judicious administration of I.V. fluids helps control interstitial pulmonary edema.

Serial chest radiographs are indicated if pulmonary contusion is suspected as an associated injury. A clinically significant pulmonary contusion can usually be seen on the initial chest radiograph, but its appearance can be delayed 4 to 8 hours. Radiographic assessment of contusion severity is difficult. Pulmonary compliance and ABGs are more sensitive indicators of contusion severity.

GOAL #3: Prevent or minimize secretion retention; minimize the risk of infection.

Interventions

1. Auscultate breath sounds frequently; provide optimal pulmonary hygiene, including:
- frequent suctioning
- tracheal lavage if secretions are thick and difficult to suction
- turning the patient every 2 hours
- positioning in semi-Fowler's (unless contraindicated)
- chest physiotherapy every 2 to 4 hours.

Rationale

Detecting rales and wheezes on auscultation indicates lower airway obstruction. Pulmonary hygiene must be initiated early during resuscitation to optimize aeration and minimize retained secretions and atelectatic complications. These measures help mobilize secretions, prevent pooling, and promote full lung expansion. Also, promptly and consistently removing pulmonary secretions reduces the risk of microbial infection, such as pneumonia, and other pulmonary complications. The key to managing pulmonary contusions effectively is optimal pulmonary hygiene.

2. Administer bronchodilators, as ordered.

Widespread bronchospasms are not unusual in a patient with a pulmonary contusion.

3. Prepare the patient for bronchoscopy, as indicated. (See "Bronchoscopy" in Section VII.)

Bronchoscopy is performed if adequate secretion removal by the interventions just cited is not possible.

Nursing diagnosis

Potential for ineffective breathing patterns and airway clearance related to painful ventilatory effort secondary to associated chest injuries.

GOAL: Minimize pain and discomfort.

Interventions

Rationale

1. Administer analgesics as ordered. Assist with intercostal nerve block if indicated.

Fractures of the bony thorax are common with a pulmonary contusion. They cause severe chest wall pain, prohibiting adequate lung expansion and ventilation. The work of breathing and oxygen consumption are increased, leading to hypoxia. Inadequate expansion and ventilation also contribute to ineffective airway clearance and increased retained secretions. Pain control is key in managing the pulmonary contusion patient.

2. Use a transcutaneous electrical nerve stimulator (TENS) unit as ordered.

The TENS unit lessens or eliminates pain and improves muscle function with minimal use of narcotic agents. The unit's effectiveness is based on the:
- analgesic amount the patient is receiving
- inspiratory capacity of the patient breathing spontaneously
- patient's ability to cough and deep-breathe effectively
- ventilated patient's maximum inspiratory force and vital capacity.

3. Assist with placement of an epidural catheter as needed.

An epidural catheter is placed, usually by the anesthesiologist, at the appropriate spinal level according to the thoracic fracture. Epidural opioids provide an excellent way to control pain. Injecting opioids at the site where they affect the pain's central transmission decreases their common side effects.

Associated care plans

Flail Chest
Pneumothorax
Tension Pneumothorax
Hemothorax
Acute Pericardial Tamponade

Associated procedure and study

Bronchoscopy
Endotracheal Intubation

RESPIRATORY

FLAIL CHEST

Assessment

Note: *Flail chest is defined as the fracture of several ribs on either side of the point of impact, with or without associated sternal fractures or anterior or lateral costochondral separation. The multiple rib fractures disrupt chest wall continuity, and the "flail" segment becomes subject to changes in intrathoracic pressure as it "floats" independently, moving inward on expiration and outward on inspiration.*

Mechanism of injury/ etiology:
- blunt chest trauma—rapid deceleration, crushing injury, assault, sporting accident

Physical findings:
Respiratory
- dyspnea
- tachypnea
- respiratory failure
- cyanosis
- multiple rib fractures

or sternal fracture on palpation
- paradoxical chest wall movement
- splinting of the chest wall on respiration
- subcutaneous emphysema and bony crepitation on palpation
- severe chest wall pain on inspiration or palpation
- abrasions, lacerations, or ecchymoses

- possible tracheal deviation toward the unaffected side

Cardiovascular
- hypotension
- tachycardia

Associated injuries:
- pulmonary contusion
- myocardial contusion
- intraabdominal injury (resulting from lower rib

fractures)
- lung laceration or perforation
- pneumothorax
- hemothorax
- hemopneumothorax

Note: *Associated injuries to intrathoracic structures are common as a result of the great force required to produce this type of crushing chest wall injury.*

Diagnostic studies

- ABG measurements—may reveal hypoxia, hypercarbia and may indicate severity of injury

- chest radiography—shows rib or sternal fractures and aids diagnosis of associated injuries

Potential for ineffective breathing patterns related to mechanical dysfunction of the chest wall and pain secondary to multiple rib or sternal fractures.

GOAL #1: Restore normal breathing patterns.

Interventions

1. Monitor the patient continuously for signs and symptoms of respiratory distress:
- dyspnea
- tachypnea
- cyanosis
- respiratory failure.

2. Obtain baseline ABGs; monitor and report trends in serial ABGs.

Rationale

Suspect possible flail chest in any patient who has sustained a rapid deceleration or crushing chest injury. The patient may not present with signs of respiratory distress or paradoxical chest wall movement on admission because of tissue swelling or a chest wall hematoma. Also, guarding may prevent the patient from breathing deeply enough to create a noticeable pressure gradient.

Baseline ABGs aid evaluation of the severity of the patient's condition on admission and provide a baseline for analysis of further trends.

RESPIRATORY

3. Ensure the availability and proper functioning of equipment for supplemental humidified oxygen administration, endotracheal intubation, and mechanical ventilation. (See "Endotracheal Intubation" in Section VII.)

A patient may initially present in one of two ways: with severe respiratory distress—requiring immediate airway management—or with minimal or no respiratory distress. As his condition progressively deteriorates, compensatory mechanisms fail. A patient with severe paradoxical chest wall movement or with a PaO$_2$ below 60 mm Hg on room air requires endotracheal intubation and mechanical ventilation to ensure a patent airway, decrease the work of breathing (which in turn decreases oxygen demand), and provide internal stabilization of the flail segment.

4. Assist with chest radiography.

A chest radiograph identifies rib or sternal fractures and aids diagnosis of associated injuries.

5. Suspect and assess for associated underlying chest injuries.

Commonly associated intrathoracic, extrathoracic, and intraabdominal injuries occur because of the great amount of force required to produce the flail injury. Associated injuries require rapid diagnosis and treatment to decrease mortality and morbidity.

GOAL #2: Minimize pain and discomfort.

Interventions

Rationale

1. Administer analgesics as ordered. Assist with an intercostal nerve block, if indicated.

Fractures of the bony thorax produce severe chest wall pain, which inhibits adequate lung expansion and ventilation. The work of breathing and oxygen consumption increases, leading to hypoxia. Inadequate lung expansion and impaired ventilation also contribute to ineffective airway clearance and secretion retention. Pain relief is primary in the management of this patient.

2. Utilize a transcutaneous electrical nerve stimulator (TENS) unit, as ordered.

The TENS unit decreases or eliminates pain and improves respiratory muscle function with minimal use of narcotic agents. Evaluation of the unit's effectiveness includes assessment of:
• analgesic dosage
• inspiratory capacity of spontaneous breathing
• maximum inspiratory force and vital capacity in ventilated patients
• ability to cough and deep-breathe.

3. Assist with placement of an epidural catheter, as needed.

An epidural catheter placed to deliver opioids to the spine at the level of the flail segments is an excellent method of pain management without the usual side effects of opioid administration. Catheter placement is usually done by an anesthesiologist.

Nursing diagnosis

Potential for impaired gas exchange and infection related to lower airway obstruction secondary to retained secretions and atelectasis.

GOAL: Prevent or minimize secretion retention.

Interventions

1. Provide supplemental humidified oxygen as ordered.

2. Auscultate breath sounds frequently; provide optimal pulmonary hygiene, including:
- frequent suctioning
- turning every 2 hours
- placement in semi-Fowler's position (unless contraindicated)
- chest physiotherapy
- incentive spirometry.

Rationale

The patient in any degree of respiratory distress requires supplemental oxygen before, during, and after the establishment of an airway to promote optimal gas exchange. Lower airway obstruction from retained secretions or atelectasis decreases alveolar function and impairs gas exchange.

Rales and wheezes indicate probable lower airway obstruction. Pulmonary hygiene must be initiated early in resuscitation to optimize aeration and prevent complications from aspirated and retained secretions. These measures mobilize secretions, prevent pooling, and promote full lung expansion. Prompt and consistent removal of pulmonary secretions reduces the risk of infection, pneumonia, and other pulmonary complications.

Associated care plans

Pulmonary Contusion
Myocardial Contusion
Pneumothorax
Hemothorax
Lower Airway Obstruction
Intraabdominal Trauma: Blunt and
    Penetrating

Associated procedure

Endotracheal Intubation

Medical diagnosis

RUPTURED DIAPHRAGM

Assessment

Mechanism of injury/ etiology:
- penetrating chest or upper abdominal trauma
- blunt trauma—a severe and sudden increase in abdominal pressure may cause diaphragmatic rupture
- rapid deceleration
- compression and crushing trauma

The left side is more often involved because the liver protects the diaphragm on the right side.

Physical findings:
Respiratory
- dyspnea
- decreased breath sounds
- possible tracheal deviation
- apical pulse displacement
- left-sided chest pain or referred shoulder pain
- bowel sounds heard in the chest

Cardiovascular
- shock state

Gastrointestinal
- abdominal or upper left quadrant pain
- displacement of the gastric tube into the chest cavity

Rupture size:
- penetrating trauma— the tear is usually 2 cm or less, depending on the penetrating object
- blunt trauma—the tear may be 2 to 10 cm long, depending on the force exerted; in large tears, the abdominal viscera may herniate into the chest cavity

Associated injuries:
- tension pneumothorax
- pelvic fractures
- lower rib fractures
- pneumothorax
- hemothorax
- pulmonary contusion
- intraabdominal trauma

Note: *Signs and symptoms depend on the size of the tear and the degree of abdominal viscera herniation into the chest cavity. There is a high incidence of associated injuries with diaphragmatic ruptures because of the magnitude of force required to cause the disruption.*

RESPIRATORY

Diagnostic studies

- chest radiography—may reveal gastric tube in chest; massive herniation may appear as a tension pneumothorax

- positive contrast study of the esophagus and stomach—identifies defect

Nursing diagnoses

1. Potential for impaired gas exchange related to interference in ventilation secondary to possible lung compression by herniated abdominal viscera.

2. Potential for decreased cardiac output and decreased tissue perfusion related to compression of the vena cava and mediastinal shift secondary to abdominal viscera herniation into the chest cavity.

> **GOAL:** Recognize the signs of a diaphragmatic rupture; establish and maintain a patent airway.

Interventions

1. Suspect that patients with either penetrating or blunt chest or abdominal trauma have diaphragmatic injuries.

2. Ensure the availability and proper functioning of equipment for humidified oxygen administration, intubation, and mechanical ventilation. (See "Endotracheal Intubation" in Section VII.)

Rationale

Signs and symptoms vary greatly, depending on the degree of diaphragmatic injury and the extent of abdominal viscera herniation. The blunt trauma patient may have sustained severe multiple system injuries. They typically dominate the initial clinical picture and make early diagnosis of a ruptured diaphragm more difficult. In severe cases, namely those involving massive abdominal viscera herniation into the chest cavity, lung compression, decreased ventilation, mediastinal shift, and decreased cardiac output may occur.

RESPIRATORY

3. Assist with chest radiography and positive contrast dye studies as necessary.

The diaphragm should be carefully evaluated in all patients with severe blunt abdominal or chest trauma. Typically, the radiograph shows the gastric tube in the chest cavity. A questionable diagnosis can be confirmed by giving a contrast imaging agent either orally or via the gastric tube and repeating the chest radiograph. If massive herniation is seen, the chest radiograph may appear similar to that of a tension pneumothorax. In penetrating trauma, the tear is usually small and herniation is not evident. Many diaphragmatic ruptures are not seen on a radiograph. Of ruptured diaphragm patients, 50% have normal chest radiographs. For this reason, maintaining a high index of suspicion and knowing the mechanisms of injury are important for early diagnosis and treatment.

4. Prepare the patient for surgery. (See "Preparation for Surgery" in Section VII.)

Surgical repair is the treatment of choice for a confirmed diaphragmatic rupture. It cannot be assumed that this injury will heal without surgical intervention. If the diaphragmatic rupture is not life-threatening, the repair should be done as soon as possible after the patient is hemodynamically stable. If the patient has a severe rupture with massive abdominal viscera herniation into the chest, he must undergo immediate operative intervention to relieve lung compression and mediastinal displacement. Hemodynamic stabilization continues throughout surgery. Close diaphragmatic examination during exploratory laparotomy is essential because many patients with this injury are asymptomatic clinically and radiologically.

Associated care plans

Tension Pneumothorax
Massive Pelvic Injury
Intraabdominal Trauma: Blunt and
    Penetrating
Pulmonary Contusion
Pneumothorax
Hemothorax

Associated procedures and study

Preparation for Surgery
Positive Contrast Study
Endotracheal Intubation

Medical diagnosis

PENETRATING CHEST TRAUMA

Assessment

Note: *Never remove an impaled object in the field or on admission to the emergency department! The object may be embedded in the heart, a lung, or a large blood vessel and—by filling the wound—may actually be preventing hemorrhage. Therefore, the object should be secured and the patient resuscitated and stabilized before transfer to the operating room for removal of the object and hemorrhage control.*

Mechanism of injury/ etiology:
• stab wounds or impalement—as by knives, ice picks, fragments, rib fractures, poles, or stakes—generally causes less cellular damage, lacerating only the tissue contacted by the penetrating object

Assessment tip: *For stab wounds and impaled objects, determine the following, in addition to the* wound site, to help assess severity:
• *weapon type*
• *weapon size*
• *location and angle of entry.*

• gunshot wounds—single missile or shotgun blast—cause marked cellular destruction from the release of kinetic energy and produce laceration, cavitation, and possibly combustion burns (usually in close-range shots when smoke and unburned powder follow the bullet into the wound, where combustion continues)

Assessment tip: *For gunshot wounds, determine the following, in addition to the wound site, to help assess severity:*
• *weapon and missile type*
• *missile velocity*
• *victim's distance from the weapon*
• *location of entrance and exit wounds.*

Physical findings:
• penetrating wound to the chest or upper abdomen (may include entry and exit wounds)
• bleeding
• severe shock state

Associated injuries:
• open pneumothorax
• massive hemothorax
• pericardial tamponade
• pulmonary contusion
• myocardial contusion
• fractures of the bony thorax
• intraabdominal injuries

RESPIRATORY

Diagnostic study

• radiography—helps determine size and location of projectiles, fragments, or impaled objects and may reveal associated injuries

Nursing diagnosis

Potential for decreased tissue perfusion and hypoxia related to fluid volume deficit and impaired gas exchange secondary to injuries resulting from penetrating trauma to the chest.

GOAL #1: Maintain a high index of suspicion.

Interventions

1. Assess all trauma patients for external signs of penetrating trauma to the chest and upper abdomen, including possible entrance and exit wounds. Assess and assist with treatment of associated injuries, such as:
• open pneumothorax
• pneumothorax
• hemothorax

Rationale

This rapid assessment should be performed for all trauma patients; it may reveal a significant injury not even suggested by the initial description of the incident. It is not unusual for a patient involved in a rapid deceleration accident to sustain injuries resulting from blunt *and* penetrating trauma. Also, penetrating injuries may be caused by fractures of the bony thorax or penetration by any object incidental to the accident. In stabbings, details of the weapon's type and size aid estimation of possible underlying dam-

*Supplemental nursing diagnosis

• pericardial tamponade
• pulmonary contusion
• myocardial contusion
• fractures of the bony thorax
• intraabdominal injury.
(See individual care plans for specific information.)

2. Obtain an accurate history of the accident, including the type of weapon used, from prehospital care providers, the police, or family members.

age. Similarly, in gunshot wounds, identifying the firearm type, the missile velocity, and the victim's distance from the weapon suggests the mechanism and possible severity of the injury.

Tissue damage in all types of gunshot wounds occurs not only along the missile tract but also around the tract. As the missile penetrates, the tissues are pushed rapidly away from the bullet, forming a large, temporary cavity. The cavity size is directly proportional to the missile velocity. This rapid expansion can fracture bone and damage muscle, nerves, and blood vessels. Low-velocity missiles usually cause less tissue damage from cavity formation, but they tend to cause more damage from ricochet and laceration. A high-velocity missile usually passes directly through all tissue in its path. The tract of a high-velocity missile can usually be estimated by hypothesizing a straight line between the entrance and exit wounds.

Note: *In any penetrating trauma, the injury's location provides vital clues for determining possible associated injuries. Assess the injury site and assume underlying organ, vessel, and tissue damage until proven otherwise. For example, for any penetrating chest wound*
• *between the midclavicular line on the right and the midaxillary line on the left, assume cardiac involvement.*
• *above the nipple line, assume cervical involvement.*
• *below the nipple line, assume intraabdominal involvement.*

GOAL #2: Establish and maintain a patent airway and optimize gas exchange.

Interventions

1. Ensure the availability and proper functioning of equipment for humidified oxygenation, intubation, and mechanical ventilation. (See "Endotracheal Intubation" in Section VII.)

Rationale

Patients in any degree of cardiopulmonary distress require supplemental oxygen administration and possible intubation and mechanical ventilation to provide a patent airway and improve gas exchange.

GOAL #3: Restore and maintain normovolemia.

Interventions

1. Monitor the patient for signs of hemorrhagic shock. Monitor and document:
• vital signs every 5 to 15 minutes
• ECG rhythm
• neurologic status.
(See "Hemorrhagic Shock" in Section II.)

2. Ensure adequate I.V. access with at least two large-bore peripheral catheters; administer fluids as ordered. **Note:** *This patient may require uncrossmatched blood.*

3. Ensure the availability and proper functioning of equipment for autotransfusion. (See "Autotransfusion" in Section VII.)

Rationale

Penetration of solid organs, lungs, and vasculature causes hemorrhage and may rapidly progress to cardiopulmonary arrest. Trend analysis of cardiovascular, pulmonary, and neurologic system status helps determine the severity of the shock state. Table 2.1 in "Hemorrhagic Shock" lists signs of early and late shock.

Hemorrhagic shock requires rapid, aggressive fluid resuscitation with colloid and crystalloid products. Early institution of component therapy with blood, fresh-frozen plasma, and platelets may effectively prevent coagulation disorders, which commonly occur with massive blood transfusions.

Chest trauma with acute blood loss is an indication for autotransfusion. Blood in the chest cavity can be collected, filtered, and reinfused for rapid replacement of intravascular volume loss resulting from a moderate to massive hemothorax.

4. Prepare for a possible thoracotomy in the emergency department. Assist as necessary. (See "Thoracoabdominal Tray" in Appendix 3.)

If the patient has a penetrating injury to the chest and has had a cardiac arrest or is about to arrest, a thoracotomy may be performed to relieve a possible pericardial tamponade, control intrathoracic hemorrhage, and institute internal cardiac massage. If the heart has been penetrated, hemorrhage is usually controlled initially by direct digital pressure. Fluid resuscitation continues as digital pressure is applied under direct visualization. The wound is closed by suture repair under the occluding finger. Teflon (a fluorocarbon) or Dacron (a polyester fiber) pledgets should be used as buttresses under the suture to prevent further tissue damage.

5. Prepare the patient for surgery and transfer him to the operating room. (See "Preparation for Surgery" in Section VII.)

Once the hemorrhage is under initial control, the patient is transferred to the operating room for further hemorrhage control, repair, and possible reconstruction. The type of surgical repair depends on the extent of injury. If the patient remains stable and does not require an emergency thoracotomy, surgical wound debridement or, possibly, thoracic and abdominal exploration is usually necessary.

Nursing diagnosis

Potential for infection related to penetration of the chest or abdominal cavity by a foreign object, with introduction of pathogens into those cavities.

GOAL: Prevent or minimize further wound contamination and reduce the risk of infection.

Interventions

1. Apply all wound dressings using sterile technique.

2. Obtain the patient's medication, allergy, and tetanus immunization history; administer antibiotics and tetanus, as ordered.

Rationale

Dressings provide a mechanical barrier to environmental contaminants, minimizing the introduction of additional organisms.

Antibiotics, rarely ordered prophylactically, are most commonly initiated after a positive culture has been obtained. However, if the patient has sustained associated abdominal injuries with a suspected bowel perforation, antibiotics are given preoperatively. All patients with open wounds require appropriate immunization against tetanus.

Associated care plans

Open Pneumothorax
Hemothorax
Acute Pericardial Tamponade
Pulmonary Contusion
Myocardial Contusion
Hemorrhagic Shock
Intraabdominal Trauma: Blunt and
    Penetrating

Associated procedures

Preparation for Surgery
Autotransfusion
Endotracheal Intubation

RESPIRATORY

Medical diagnosis

TRAUMATIC RUPTURE OF THE AORTA OR GREAT VESSELS

Assessment

Mechanism of injury/etiology:
- penetrating chest or upper abdominal trauma
- blunt chest trauma—primarily rapid deceleration and chest compression
- horizontal deceleration with or without chest compression, as in motor vehicle (car, truck, motorcycle) accidents:
  - ☐ greater risk for the driver than for the passenger because the driver's chest is compressed against the steering wheel
  - ☐ greater risk for a person ejected from the vehicle than for one not ejected

- chest compression:
  - ☐ pedestrian/vehicle collisions
  - ☐ kicks in the chest by an animal
- vertical deceleration with or without chest compression:
  - ☐ falls from great heights
  - ☐ airplane crashes
- crushing injuries:
  - ☐ burial by landslide

Most common sites of injury
- descending aorta at the aortic isthmus just distal to the origin of the left subclavian artery
- ascending aorta, including the aortic arch
- aortic hiatus

Types of injury
- intimal tear
- partial rupture
- complete vessel transsection causing exsanguination and sudden death

Physical findings:
Respiratory
- restlessness
- dyspnea
- tachypnea
- cyanosis
- hoarseness from hematoma-induced laryngeal compression
- dysphagia from hematoma-induced esophageal compression
- stridor
- retrosternal or interscapular pain

Cardiovascular
- upper extremity hypertension
- pulse or blood pressure differences between arms
- palpable difference in pulse amplitude between upper and lower extremities
- decreased or absent femoral pulses
- tachycardia
- hypotension
- pallor
- unrelenting shock

Associated injuries:
- hemothorax
- pericardial tamponade
- flail chest
- fractured sternum
- pulmonary contusion

Note: *The patient may have no physical signs or symptoms. Knowing the mechanisms of injury and maintaining a high index of suspicion are vital in the assessment of patients injured by blunt or penetrating trauma.*

Diagnostic studies

- 105-degree true erect chest radiography—to visualize superior mediastinal structures
- aortography (definitive study)

Nursing diagnosis

Potential for decreased tissue perfusion related to fluid volume deficit secondary to hemorrhage from aortic or great vessel rupture.

GOAL #1: Maintain a high index of suspicion.

Interventions

1. Suspect aortic or great vessel rupture in all patients injured as the result of:
- horizontal deceleration with or without chest compression
- chest compression
- vertical deceleration with or without chest compression
- crushing chest injuries
- penetrating chest or upper abdominal trauma.

Rationale

Traumatic rupture of the aorta or great vessels is a *life-threatening* emergency. An estimated 80% to 90% of these injuries, if caused by blunt trauma, are fatal at the accident scene, and 10% to 15% of traffic deaths result from aortic rupture. The incidence of traumatic aortic rupture has increased over the last 20 years because of increases in high-speed vehicular collisions. The number of patients surviving transport to a hospital for definitive care has increased because of improved rapid transportation systems. Patients who survive the initial injury frequently can be treated successfully if the diagnosis is made early. Rapid deceleration accidents classically produce multiple injuries to the head, face, abdomen, pelvis, and extremities. The patient may not exhibit external signs of thoracic trauma. Internally, however, upon impact, the relatively mobile ascending aorta continues to move forward as the descending aorta remains in a relatively fixed position. A shearing force is produced, injuring the descending aorta at the aortic isthmus. Tears involving all layers of the aortic wall and overlying parietal pleura cause exsanguination and lead to sudden death. Tears extending into the adventitia without free rupture into the pleural space usually result in an aneurysm and hematoma formation. Knowing the mechanisms of injury and maintaining a high index of suspicion are essential for rapidly diagnosing and treating this life-threatening injury.

CARDIOVASCULAR

GOAL #2: Maintain a patent airway and adequate gas exchange.

Interventions

1. Ensure the availability and proper functioning of equipment for humidified oxygen administration, intubation, and mechanical ventilation. (See "Endotracheal Intubation" in Section VII.)

Rationale

Patients in any degree of cardiopulmonary distress require supplemental oxygen or, if indicated, an artificial airway and mechanical ventilation.

GOAL #3: Restore and maintain normovolemia.

Interventions

1. Monitor the patient for signs of hemorrhagic shock; monitor vital signs every 5 to 15 minutes; monitor ECG rhythm and neurologic status.

2. Obtain baseline laboratory studies and monitor trends in CBC, electrolytes, ABG, and coagulation profiles.

3. Ensure the availability of adequate amounts of packed RBCs (PRBCs) and clotting factors for early transfusions. Follow the hospital's policy for infusion, filtration, and blood warming.

Rationale

Early, aggressive volume replacement with colloid and crystalloid products is necessary to combat hemorrhagic shock. Trend analysis of laboratory data helps evaluate tissue perfusion, fluid balance, and the overall effectiveness of resuscitation. Prolonged clotting times often develop and require early detection and aggressive therapy.

Early, aggressive blood replacement is a major component of effective care. The patient may also have associated injuries that may cause further blood loss and complicate the shock state. Early initiation of component therapy with PRBCs and clotting factors, such as fresh-frozen plasma and platelets, may prevent development of a potentially lethal coagulopathy. If coagulation disorders are not detected early, or if they persist, they aggravate the hemorrhagic process and may lead to death.

4. Ensure the availability and proper functioning of autotransfusion equipment. (See "Autotransfusion" in Section VII.)

Blunt or penetrating chest trauma causing acute blood loss is an indication for autotransfusion. Blood in the chest cavity can be collected, filtered, and reinfused for rapid replacement of intravascular volume loss.

GOAL #4: Confirm the diagnosis of a ruptured aorta or great vessels.

Interventions

Rationale

1. Assist with 105-degree erect chest radiography.

Several team members may be needed to position the patient safely and to maintain the position if the patient is unconscious, sedated, or intubated and mechanically ventilated. An erect chest radiograph is taken to assess superior mediastinal structures and to detect a possible mediastinal hematoma. This diagnosis is suspected if the aortic knob is poorly defined or the mediastinum appears to be widened. If an erect chest radiograph is contraindicated because of cervical, thoracic, or lumbar spine injury, a supine chest radiograph must be taken.

2. Prepare the patient for aortography. (See "Aortography" in Section VII.)

Inability to define superior mediastinal anatomy by chest radiography indicates the need for aortography. An aortogram is the only method that establishes a definitive diagnosis of aortic rupture. Some experts recommend performing an aortogram on all patients with blunt chest trauma or rapid deceleration injuries. Aortography is also performed to locate the site(s) of vessel injury and should be done prior to a thoracotomy, unless the patient requires immediate surgical intervention.

3. Prepare the patient for surgery. (See "Preparation for Surgery" in Section VII.)

Aortic or great vessel injury necessitates immediate surgical repair.

Associated care plans

Hemothorax
Flail Chest
Acute Pericardial Tamponade
Pulmonary Contusion
Hemorrhagic Shock

Associated procedures and study

Closed-Tube Thoracostomy
Aortography
Preparation for Surgery
Endotracheal Intubation
Autotransfusion
Intrahospital Transport of the Shock Trauma Patient

CARDIOVASCULAR

Medical diagnosis

ACUTE PERICARDIAL TAMPONADE

Assessment

Note: *Acute cardiac tamponade presents a life-threatening emergency requiring immediate intervention. Assume that any penetrating chest trauma involves the heart, until proven otherwise. Maintain a high index of suspicion in any patient suffering blunt chest trauma if the degree of circulatory collapse is disproportionate to the injury's apparent severity or if the patient does not respond to resuscitation efforts.*

Mechanism of injury/ etiology:
- primarily penetrating chest trauma
- blunt chest trauma

Physical findings:
Cardiovascular
- hypotension†
- distant or muffled heart sounds†
- distended neck veins† (not usually evident if the patient has had significant blood loss)
- tachycardia
- elevated central venous pressure (above 12 mm Hg)
- pulsus paradoxus (systolic blood pressure decrease of 10 mm Hg or more during inspiration)
- narrowing pulse pressure

Respiratory
- respiratory distress
- air hunger

Associated injuries:
- coronary artery laceration
- myocardial laceration
- myocardial rupture

†These classic signs of pericardial tamponade are referred to as Beck's triad.

Diagnostic study

- pericardiocentesis

Nursing diagnosis

Potential for decreased tissue perfusion related to decreased cardiac output secondary to compression of the myocardium by blood accumulation in the pericardial sac.

GOAL #1: Maintain a patent airway and adequate gas exchange.

Interventions

1. Ensure the availability and proper functioning of equipment for humidified oxygen administration, intubation, and mechanical ventilation. (See "Endotracheal Intubation" in Section VII.)

Rationale

Patients with any degree of cardiopulmonary distress require supplemental oxygen and possibly an artificial airway and mechanical ventilation. Pericardial tamponade increases myocardial oxygen demand, thus increasing the respiratory effort. Supplying additional oxygen helps meet the demand and reduces stress on the myocardium.

GOAL #2: Restore or maintain normovolemia.

Interventions

1. Ensure adequate I.V. access with at least two large-bore peripheral catheters; administer I.V. fluids and blood products, as ordered.

Rationale

Rapid, high-volume resuscitation with colloid and crystalloid restores hemodynamic stability. Early institution of blood component therapy helps improve cardiac output by elevating venous pressure and increasing venous return to the heart.

GOAL #3: Recognize the early signs and symptoms of a cardiac tamponade.

Interventions

1. Monitor all patients with penetrating trauma to the chest or upper abdomen or with blunt chest trauma for the following signs and symptoms:
• persistent hemodynamic instability
• Beck's triad (hypotension, distended neck veins, and muffled or distant heart sounds)
• shock out of proportion to apparent blood loss.

Rationale

In blunt trauma patients, acute pericardial tamponade may be difficult to diagnose because coexisting multiple-system injuries may produce hypotension, tachycardia, and peripheral vasoconstriction. Cardiac tamponade results from a cardiac wound that causes bleeding into the pericardial sac. The pericardial sac, a fibrous, inelastic membrane surrounding the heart, can accommodate only a small amount of blood pooling (150 to 200 cc) before cardiac activity becomes compromised. As the pericardial sac rapidly fills with blood, the expansion compresses the atria and ventricles. This prevents adequate filling, decreasing cardiac output. The mechanical backup of blood produces an increase in central venous pressure and neck vein distention. As the intracardiac pressure continues to increase, coronary blood flow is further decreased, resulting in myocardial hypoxia and failure.

GOAL #4: Relieve cardiac compression and increase cardiac output.

Interventions

1. Ensure the availability of equipment for pericardiocentesis; assist as necessary. Closely monitor the patient's condition and vital signs before, during, and after the procedure.

Rationale

Pericardiocentesis involves needle aspiration of pericardial fluid to diagnose and/or relieve a cardiac tamponade. The physician uses a subxiphoid approach to insert an over-the-catheter needle (16G to 18G, 6″ or longer) attached by a three-way stopcock to a 35-cc syringe. Before, during, and after the procedure, monitor the patient's vital signs closely. The patient requires constant ECG monitoring during the procedure. A precordial lead attached to the needle by an alligator clamp reflects the needle's position. If the needle is advanced too far, contacting or puncturing the myocardium, the ECG will show a widened and enlarged QRS complex or extreme ST-T wave changes.

Aspirating 10 to 20 cc of blood may be enough to dramatically improve the patient's condition. After aspiration relieves the intrapericardial pressure, the catheter, stopcock, and syringe may be taped securely and left in place. This facilitates rapid decompression if cardiac tamponade symptoms recur en route to surgery or during transfer to a definitive care facility. If the pericardiocentesis is negative but a strong suspicion of cardiac tamponade persists, or if the patient develops repeated pericardial effusions, pericardiectomy (creating a pericardial "window") may be performed to promote drainage.

2. Prepare for a possible thoracotomy in the emergency department; assist as necessary.

If the patient becomes bradycardic or hypotensive (systolic pressure below 90 mm Hg) or suffers cardiac arrest, an immediate thoracotomy is usually performed to allow pericardial sac evacuation, hemorrhage control, and internal cardiac massage.

CARDIOVASCULAR

3. Prepare the patient for surgical intervention. (See "Preparation for Surgery" in Section VII.)

Upon confirmation of pericardial tamponade, the patient requires immediate surgery to control the source of bleeding and permit complete drainage of the pericardium.

Associated care plans

Tension Pneumothorax
Traumatic Rupture of the Aorta or Great Vessels
Penetrating Chest Trauma

Associated procedure

Preparation for Surgery

CARDIOVASCULAR

Medical diagnosis

ACUTE MYOCARDIAL INFARCTION (A.M.I.)

Assessment

Note: *Although AMI is not a traumatic injury, it is included in this book because AMI is associated with trauma: it may precipitate or result from a traumatic incident. For example, the patient may have had an AMI while driving and has been admitted because of the resultant automobile accident. Conversely, the patient may experience an AMI resulting from an increase in myocardial oxygen requirements created by his injuries, or he may be unable to maintain myocardial oxygen supply because of blood loss or pulmonary injury.*

Suspect AMI in trauma patients complaining of chest pain inconsistent with injuries, having one or more of the risk factors listed below, or having dysrhythmias not associated with possible cardiac contusion. Use this plan in combination with plans addressing the patient's traumatic injuries, balancing trauma and AMI treatment to provide the best patient outcome.

Mechanism of injury/ etiology:
- acute imbalance in myocardial oxygen demand and supply, caused by either an increase in demand beyond the patient's ability to increase supply or a decrease in oxygen supply caused by injury, blood loss, or blockage of coronary arteries

Precipitating factors
- male patient
- age (risk increases with age)
- family history of atherosclerosis
- hypertension
- diabetes mellitus
- elevated cholesterol levels
- smoking
- sedentary life-style

Physical findings:
Respiratory
- shortness of breath

Cardiovascular
- chest discomfort/pain (ranging from mild discomfort to "crushing" pain but usually described as a pressurelike sensation)

- signs of catecholamine release, including diaphoresis, hypertension followed by hypotension, anxiety/restlessness

Gastrointestinal
- nausea
- vomiting
- indigestion

Diagnostic studies

- serial ECG—characteristic changes help identify site and extent of AMI
- serum enzyme levels—serial measurements over several days show enzyme elevation and return to normal levels. Enzyme elevations have a standard pattern in AMI patients, the presence of which is diagnostic. Enzyme MB bands are more specific to myocardial injury than total enzyme levels, as the total level may rise with large-muscle trauma. It must be remembered, however, that MB bands will also reflect myocardial contusion.
- multiple-gated acquisition scan—helps reveal mechan-

ical alterations in pump efficiency from regional abnormalities of cardiac wall movement; measures ejection fraction, cardiac output, and other parameters. This study is more useful later in the course of AMI, after left ventricular function is impaired.
- technetium pyrophosphate scan—can detect damaged tissue within 1 to 2 days
- thallium scan—can detect ischemic and infarcted areas
- cardiac catheterization—helps evaluate patency of coronary arteries; may disclose underlying cause of AMI

Nursing diagnosis

Alteration in comfort related to activation of bradykinin or mechanical stimulation of cardiac pain receptors secondary to myocardial ischemia or infarction, formation of edema in myocardial tissue, or changes in myocardial contractility in ischemic area.

GOAL: Relieve or minimize chest pain/discomfort; prevent extension of muscle damage.

CARDIOVASCULAR

Interventions

1. Assess the following characteristics of the patient's chest pain:
- location
- radiation
- duration
- intensity
- frequency
- aggravating and relieving factors.

Rationale

The majority of patients with AMI experience chest pain or discomfort. Characteristics of this pain vary greatly. The intensity varies from mild discomfort to pain described as "crushing" or "heavy." Pain may radiate to one or both arms (usually the left), the neck or mandible, the back, or the epigastrium (causing indigestion not relieved by antacids). Pain usually lasts 5 to 10 minutes but may last 30 minutes or longer. The pain is usually not relieved by nitrate administration or rest, which may differentiate this pain from angina (usually relieved by nitrates or rest). Careful assessment of these factors assists differential diagnosis of AMI from other disorders that may present with chest pain.

2. Administer appropriate pain medications, as ordered.

Chest pain may cause anxiety, which increases myocardial oxygen requirements. Low-dose morphine (1 to 5 mg I.V.) reduces chest pain and provides sedation. Morphine is generally contraindicated in patients with bradycardia or heart block because it increases vagal tone and may further decrease heart rate.

3. Anticipate the use of nasal oxygen at 2 to 6 liters/minute. **Note:** *Patients with chronic obstructive pulmonary disease (COPD) require special precautions, generally limiting oxygen rates to 2 to 3 liters/minute.*

Chest pain in AMI may be caused in part by an imbalance between myocardial oxygen supply and demand. Supplemental oxygen increases the oxygen available to the myocardium. In patients with COPD, the normal PCO_2-based respiratory drive is impaired, requiring caution. These patients breathe not because PCO_2 levels are increased, but because PO_2 levels are decreased. Providing these patients with supplemental oxygen, which raises their PO_2 levels, may result in hypoventilation or apnea.

4. Place the patient on bed rest with the head of the bed elevated 30 to 45 degrees or to accommodate the patient's comfort. Increase exercise (for example, dangling, walking to the bathroom) as patient tolerance increases.

An initial period of bed rest decreases cardiac effort while the myocardium begins to recover. Exercise periods are increased as soon as the patient can tolerate more effort, because the cardiovascular and musculoskeletal systems are prone to rapid deterioration with prolonged bed rest. Mild physical activity for short periods can promote an early return of cardiovascular tone. An early resumption of normal activities may also improve the patient's emotional state.

Nursing diagnosis

Potential for decreased cardiac output related to altered myocardial contractility secondary to myocardial infarction or dysrhythmias.

GOAL: Support cardiac output; prevent or minimize dysrhythmias.

Interventions

1. Monitor the patient's cardiac rhythm continuously, from admission.

2. Identify dysrhythmias and treat them according to protocol or as ordered. Notify the physician.

3. Administer prophylactic antidysrhythmics, as ordered.

Rationale

AMI decreases cardiac output by two mechanisms. Infarcted cardiac tissue decreases myocardial contractility, resulting in decreased stroke volume and cardiac output. Irritable tissue in the infarcted area, inadequate cardiac tissue perfusion, and (occasionally) electrolyte imbalances cause dysrhythmias. Ectopic beats and irregular rhythms may cause a decrease in effective stroke volume and result in decreased cardiac output. This effect increases with the number of ectopic beats.

These interventions are designed to decrease dysrhythmia occurrence through prophylactic medication, permit early recognition

CARDIOVASCULAR

4. Monitor vital signs at least every 4 hours or more frequently, as dictated by the patient's condition.

5. Administer vasopressors, as ordered.

6. Monitor laboratory values:
- electrolytes
- hemoglobin/hematocrit
- ABGs.

and treatment of dysrhythmias, and support cardiac output in the seriously compromised patient. Altered electrolytes, hypoxia, acid-base imbalances, and decreased oxygen-carrying ability (from decreased hemoglobin/hematocrit) may cause dysrhythmias and further decrease cardiac output.

Nursing diagnosis

Potential for extension of myocardial infarction related to inadequate myocardial oxygen supply.

> **GOAL:** Prevent or minimize extension of the infarcted area; promote optimal myocardial healing.

Interventions

1. Place the patient on bed rest with the head of the bed elevated or in a comfortable position.

2. Provide supplemental oxygen, as ordered.

3. Reduce environmental stress, such as:
- bright lights
- sudden noises
- excessive staff/visitor conversation (at bedside, in hallways, lounges, nurses' station).

4. Monitor ABG results and notify the physician of deterioration.

Rationale

AMI occurs as a result of coronary artery occlusion or trauma to the heart causing an imbalance between myocardial oxygen supply and demand. AMI creates three areas of progressively worsening tissue damage: the areas of myocardial ischemia, injury, and infarction. Failure to correct the supply/demand imbalance rapidly may cause the infarction to extend into the areas of injury and ischemia or beyond. Placing the patient on bed rest with his head elevated reduces myocardial oxygen requirements by decreasing venous return to the heart, thereby decreasing the amount of blood the heart must pump. Oxygen supply is enhanced by decreasing upward abdominal pressure on the diaphragm, which helps to increase tidal volume by providing more area for lung expansion. Supplemental oxygen improves myocardial oxygen supply. Minimizing environmental stress helps reduce the stress response, which increases myocardial oxygen demand. Evaluating ABG results monitors the adequacy of ventilation and oxygenation and indicates therapeutic effectiveness or the need for further intervention.

Additional considerations

The patient with AMI requires a cardiovascular rehabilitation plan. This program usually begins in the cardiac care unit and continues as the patient progresses to the telemetry or step-down unit, the medical floor, and home. The rehabilitation program should be customized, with each patient assessed for activity and exercise tolerance and response. This program's goals should be to return the patient to, at least, his pre-AMI level of functioning and to prevent future infarctions. To accomplish cardiovascular conditioning, exercises are gradually introduced—and the activity level progressively increased—until the patient can perform the activities of daily living independently. To help reduce the risk of future infarctions, patient education should stress positive life-style changes. Also, during all phases of the rehabilitation process, the positive aspects of the patient's condition and abilities should be stressed in an attempt to offset the patient's probable negative feelings about his future.

In the trauma patient with AMI, these cardiac rehabilitation goals must be coordinated with the trauma-related rehabilitation goals. This may present a serious challenge, as recovery from traumatic disabilities may require a great deal of physical effort, placing the myocardium under considerable stress. If the patient's rehabilitation program is not carefully designed with the AMI in mind, the patient's risk for another infarction could actually be increased.

Associated care plans	Associated procedures
Cardiogenic Shock	Pulmonary Artery Catheterization
Myocardial Contusion	Intraaortic Balloon Pump

*Supplemental nursing diagnosis

Medical diagnosis

MYOCARDIAL CONTUSION

Assessment

Note: *A high index of suspicion is essential for detecting this potentially life-threatening injury. Initially, the patient may be asymptomatic with signs of myocardial contusion appearing 24 to 48 hours after injury.*

Mechanism of injury/ etiology:
● blunt chest trauma:
horizontal deceleration:
  ☐ motor vehicle, including motorcycle, accidents—steering wheel injuries are most common
vertical deceleration:
  ☐ falls from great heights
chest compression:
  ☐ animal kicks
  ☐ severe blows to the chest—from a fist, ball, or club
  ☐ shotgun blast injuries
● penetrating trauma:
  ☐ gunshot wounds to the chest—produce shock-wave effects

Physical findings:
Cardiovascular

● precordial pain—unrelieved by coronary vasodilating agents
● external signs of chest trauma—contusions, lacerations, ecchymoses (especially over the sternum or left side of the chest)
● tachycardia—the most common sign, but it may also be associated with other injuries in the multiple-trauma patient
● dysrhythmias—may include multiple premature ventricular contractions or ventricular tachycardia, atrial fibrillation, conduction blocks

● ECG changes—characteristic of myocardial ischemia or infarction; may be evident shortly after the injury or may not appear for 24 to 48 hours; most common changes are in the ST segment and T wave
● pericardial friction rub
● cardiogenic shock

Associated injuries:
● sternal fractures
● flail chest
● pericardial tamponade

CARDIOVASCULAR

Diagnostic studies

● serial creatine phosphokinase (CPK) isoenzymes— may reveal an elevated CPK-MB level, indicating myocardial damage
● serial 12-lead ECGs—document ECG changes, which help determine the extent of the contusion

● multiple-gated acquisition scan—helps determine mechanical alterations in pump efficiency from regional abnormalities of cardiac wall movement; measures ejection fraction, cardiac output, and other parameters

Nursing diagnosis

Potential for decreased cardiac output related to pump failure and possible electrical instability secondary to myocardial contusion and ischemia.

GOAL: Improve and support cardiac output; prevent or minimize dysrhythmias.

Interventions

1. Suspect all blunt chest trauma patients of having sustained a myocardial contusion.

Rationale

Myocardial contusion is a common injury occurring in nonpenetrating chest trauma. Its most frequent cause is vehicular accidents. The mechanism of injury is rapid deceleration, the driver being thrown forward, hitting his chest against the steering wheel. Internally, the heart is thrown forward against the internal chest wall and may be compressed between the sternum and the vertebral column.

CARDIOVASCULAR

2. Ensure the availability and proper functioning of equipment to administer humidified oxygen, endotracheal intubation, and mechanical ventilation. (See "Endotracheal Intubation" in Section VII.)

3. Ensure the placement of at least two large-bore peripheral I.V. catheters. Administer I.V. fluids as ordered. Monitor and record fluid intake closely.

4. Monitor the patient's cardiac rhythm continuously from the time of admission. Identify dysrhythmias and treat them according to your hospital's protocol or as ordered.

5. Assist with insertion of a pulmonary artery catheter as necessary. Monitor and report trends.

6. Administer inotropic agents as ordered.

7. Monitor the following laboratory values:
- electrolytes
- hemoglobin/hematocrit
- ABGs
- serial cardiac enzymes.

A patient with any degree of cardiopulmonary distress needs supplemental oxygen. A patient with multiple-system injuries is commonly hypotensive and hypoxic because of hypovolemia. Myocardial contusions result in decreased cardiac output, thereby compounding hypovolemia and increasing hypoxia. The combination of hypoxia, hypovolemia, and reduced cardiac output increases myocardial oxygen demand and predisposes the heart to dysrhythmias. Treatment focuses on correcting the hypoxia and hypovolemia and preventing or treating dysrhythmias. Rapid volume restoration and ventilatory support are vital because of the pump failure caused by the myocardial contusion. The patient's I.V. intake must be judiciously monitored to prevent fluid overload.

A pulmonary artery catheter helps monitor and manage the myocardial contusion patient.

Inotropic agents may be instituted to increase cardiac output if it is still inadequate after fluid resuscitation.

Altered electrolyte levels, hypoxia, acid-base imbalances, and decreased oxygen-carrying ability (from decreased hemoglobin/hematocrit) can cause dysrhythmias and further lower cardiac output. Cardiac enzyme levels may be of limited diagnostic value, since the values are already high because of associated musculoskeletal injuries.

Nursing diagnosis

Potential for alteration in comfort related to pain secondary to myocardial contusion and ischemia.

GOAL: Promote patient comfort and reduce pain.

Interventions

1. Administer the appropriate pain medication as ordered.

2. Administer oxygen as ordered, and place the patient on bed rest.

Rationale

Chest pain can cause anxiety, increasing myocardial oxygen requirements.

Supplemental oxygen increases oxygen availability in the myocardium, whereas bed rest decreases cardiac work load, thus decreasing oxygen demand.

Associated care plans

Cardiogenic Shock
Acute Myocardial Infarction
Acute Pericardial Tamponade

Associated procedures

Pulmonary Artery Catheterization
Endotracheal Intubation

INTRAABDOMINAL TRAUMA:
Blunt and Penetrating

Assessment

Note: *Suspect a blunt intraabdominal injury whenever significant injuries exist above and below the abdomen, for example, lower extremity fractures with chest trauma. Suspect a penetrating intraabdominal injury whenever there is penetrating trauma to the chest. Make sure a penetrating object is well secured and left in place until the surgical team is prepared to deal with potential consequences of removal.*

Mechanism of injury/ etiology:
Blunt

- deceleration, compression, crushing, or other blunt forces to the abdomen

Penetrating

- shooting, stabbing, explosive, or other penetrating mechanisms to abdomen, chest, back
- pelvic or rib fractures

Physical findings:
Gastrointestinal

- contusions, abrasions, road burns, penetrating wounds (entrance and possibly exit) on the abdomen, chest, back, flank
- evisceration of abdominal contents from penetrating wounds
- local or generalized abdominal pain/tenderness—onset may be sudden or gradual
- abdominal guarding, rebound tenderness
- radiating or referred pain
- Kehr's sign (pain referred to shoulder)
- low-back pain
- palpable intraabdominal mass; organ enlargement
- abdominal or flank distention and rigidity
- Grey Turner's sign (ecchymosis in flank areas)
- Cullen's sign (ecchymosis around umbilicus)
- nausea and vomiting
- blood in emesis/gastric contents, urine, stool
- decreased or absent bowel sounds

Cardiovascular

- tachycardia
- hypotension
- diaphoresis
- shock state

Respiratory

- shallow, rapid respirations

Associated injuries:
- lower rib fractures
- thoracic injuries
- pelvic fractures
- thoracic/lumbar spine fractures
- genitourinary injuries

Diagnostic studies

- laboratory data—initial data may reflect no significant abnormalities; however:
  - [ ] hemoglobin/hematocrit levels—reveal downward trend
  - [ ] WBC count—rises
  - [ ] platelet count—rises (may fall later)
  - [ ] serum amylase levels—may rise
  - [ ] prothrombin time/partial thromboplastin time—become prolonged
  - [ ] total bilirubin levels—may rise
- manual wound exploration—may confirm peritoneal penetration
- radiography
  - [ ] abdominal films—may help locate a foreign object, such as a bullet, but usually prove inconclusive for either intraabdominal injury type (blunt or penetrating)
  - [ ] chest film—reveals diaphragm integrity
- diagnostic peritoneal lavage (indicated in blunt abdominal trauma; may be indicated in penetrating abdominal injuries if the peritoneum seems intact; usually indicated with penetrating trauma to the thorax, back, pelvis)—determination of positive results varies with mechanism of injury
- abdominal computerized tomography (CT) scan—may help locate bullet or other foreign object; provides quantitative analysis of intraabdominal fluid or air collection; allows visualization of retroperitoneal space. A CT scan may not be appropriate for acutely ill or injured patients who require rapid evaluation.
- ultrasonography, radionuclide scans—may provide valuable data concerning intraabdominal structures, but may not be appropriate or readily available in acute evaluation phase
- contrast studies—excretory urography or intravenous pyelography (IVP) and cystography may be indicated in the presence of hematuria

GASTROINTESTINAL

Nursing diagnosis

Potential for fluid volume deficit related to hypovolemia secondary to evisceration or disruption in intra-abdominal organ and vascular integrity.

GOAL #1: Optimize cellular perfusion; restore and maintain a normovolemic state.

Interventions

1. Monitor the patient for signs of hemorrhagic shock; monitor and document vital signs every 5 to 15 minutes; monitor ECG rhythm and neurologic status.

2. Ensure adequate intravenous access with at least two large-bore peripheral catheters; administer fluids as ordered.

3. Obtain baseline laboratory studies and monitor trends in CBC, electrolyte levels, ABGs, and coagulation profiles.

4. Monitor and document respiratory status and trends; anticipate the need for supplemental oxygen.

5. Apply a sterile, occlusive dressing to open abdominal wounds.

6. In the presence of evisceration:
- minimize unnecessary patient movement and stimulation
- apply a wet saline dressing to exposed abdominal contents
- notify the appropriate physician immediately
- notify operating room staff.

7. Insert an indwelling urinary catheter using aseptic technique; monitor and document ongoing intake/output balance; test urine for occult blood and specific gravity.

Rationale

Disruption and penetration of solid intraabdominal organs and vasculature cause hemorrhage and decreased tissue perfusion, potentially producing rapid deterioration leading to cardiopulmonary arrest. Trend analysis of cardiovascular and neurologic status helps determine the severity of the shock state. Table 2.1 in "Hemorrhagic Shock" in Section II lists signs of early and late shock.

Hemorrhagic shock requires rapid, aggressive fluid resuscitation with colloid and crystalloid products. Early institution of component therapy with packed red blood cells, fresh-frozen plasma, and platelets may effectively prevent coagulation disorders (which often occur with massive blood transfusions).

Trend analysis of laboratory data helps evaluate tissue perfusion, fluid balance, and the overall effectiveness of resuscitative efforts. Prolonged clotting times may develop when severe hemorrhage necessitates massive blood transfusions. Early and appropriate therapy can prevent clotting disorders from aggravating the hemorrhagic process.

Tachypnea (>20 breaths/minute) develops with Class II shock, and rates increase as the shock progresses. Supplemental oxygen enhances tissue perfusion by increasing oxygen availability at the alveolar/capillary membrane. When administered early, oxygen therapy may minimize secondary pulmonary complications.

An occlusive dressing may help control bleeding and may prevent evisceration of abdominal contents.

Evisceration causes further volume depletion and may worsen the shock state. Any movements or procedures that increase intraabdominal pressure must be avoided to prevent additional evisceration. Covering exposed viscera with moist dressings eliminates drying and further injury. Evisceration requires emergency surgical intervention. Early notification of the operative team facilitates the patient's transfer to the operating suite.

Urine output helps evaluate the resuscitative effect because it reflects the degree of tissue perfusion; urine output falls as the shock state progresses. A finding of microscopic hematuria indicates the need for further diagnostic studies, such as IVP and cystography.

GASTROINTESTINAL

8. Prepare the patient for diagnostic peritoneal lavage (DPL):
• explain the procedure to the patient
• assemble necessary equipment
• ensure insertion and proper placement of a gastric decompression tube and urinary catheter prior to DPL
• make certain that the team follows the procedure for sterile technique, including wearing a mask, hat, and gloves. (See "Diagnostic Peritoneal Lavage" in Section VII.)

DPL aids rapid diagnosis of intraabdominal bleeding and determines the need for exploratory laparotomy. Gastric and bladder decompression lessens the risk of complications during the procedure. Sterile technique minimizes the risk of contamination and subsequent infection.

9. Prepare the patient for surgical interventions. (See "Preparation for Surgery" in Section VII.)

Positive DPL results, the presence of a penetrating intraperitoneal wound, evisceration, and a persistent shock state of undetermined etiology indicate the need for an exploratory laparotomy for accurate diagnosis and repair.

GOAL #2: Recognize early signs of persistent or occult bleeding.

Interventions

1. Monitor the patient continuously for signs of occult bleeding, including:
• increasing abdominal girth
• Grey Turner's or Cullen's sign
• complaints of low-back or abdominal pain, discomfort, tightness
• classic signs of shock. (See "Hemorrhagic Shock" in Section II.)

Rationale

Initial DPL or other diagnostic studies may reveal inconclusive or borderline results. Patients who do not require emergency surgery on admission need close observation and trend analysis to detect subtle or sudden deteriorating changes.

Nursing diagnosis

Potential for infection related to penetration of the abdominal cavity by foreign object and/or peritoneal inflammation by the presence of free blood, urine, gastric contents, bile, feces.

GOAL: Prevent or minimize further wound contamination and reduce the risk of infection.

Interventions

1. Apply a sterile dressing to the abdominal wound.

Rationale

Dressings provide a mechanical barrier to environmental contaminants, thereby reducing the introduction of additional organisms.

2. Obtain the patient's history of medication allergies and tetanus immunizations; administer antibiotics and tetanus toxoid, as ordered. (See Appendix 6, "Tetanus Prophylaxis.")

Preoperative antibiotics are usually ordered for penetrating abdominal injuries. All patients with open wounds require tetanus immunization.

3. Monitor and document vital signs (including temperature); note trends or changes from baseline physical examination, especially in pain level, abdominal girth, and bowel sounds; send lavage return sample for WBC count; note trends in laboratory data, especially WBC counts.

Trauma to the stomach, bladder, bowel, or ductal system may cause rupture and visceral content spillage, which provides an ideal medium for bacterial growth.

GASTROINTESTINAL

Nursing diagnosis

Alteration in bowel elimination related to paralytic ileus secondary to disruption in visceral integrity, peritoneal inflammation, and shock state.

GOAL: Prevent or minimize paralytic ileus.

Interventions

1. Ensure cautious and proper placement of a gastric decompression tube; auscultate over the left lower rib border while instilling 30 cc of air into the suction port to check position; maintain the patient NPO.

2. Maintain decompression with 80 to 120 mm Hg (intermittent) or 30 to 40 mm Hg (continuous) suction.

3. Irrigate the air vent with 30 cc of air and the suction port with 30 cc of normal saline solution (NSS) every 2 hours (more frequently if using continuous suction). Manually aspirate the suction port gently to ensure return of air and NSS.

4. Assess and document the amount and characteristics of gastric secretions; document initial pH and monitor every 2 to 4 hours; test drainage for occult blood; include gastric drainage in output totals.

5. Monitor and document trends in quality and quantity of bowel sounds.

6. Measure and document abdominal girth; monitor trends.

Rationale

Most gastric injuries resulting from blunt or penetrating trauma are associated with a distended stomach. (The empty stomach is less prone to injury because of its protected location and natural mobility.) Therefore, anticipate gastric decompression. The gastric tube must be inserted gently and with great caution to avoid further injury. This may become a physician responsibility if a gastric or esophageal injury is suspected. Decompression and maintaining NPO status lessen the risk of aspiration of acidic or bloody gastric contents should vomiting occur. They also prevent ileus aggravation by relieving gastric pressure on the bowel. Proper tube positioning is essential to proper functioning.

Controlled and carefully monitored suction levels lessen the risk of gastric mucosa injury. Continuous suction, although not the optimal method, can be used initially (until the stomach is emptied) if recommended suction levels are adhered to and the lumen is irrigated frequently. For ongoing gastric decompression, only those tubes with built-in air vent systems are recommended.

Frequent irrigation ensures patency and proper functioning of both ports. Air vent obstruction increases the risk of mucosal damage.

This baseline and diagnostic information helps detect gastric injury and evaluate the ileus. Gastric pH levels less than 5 to 7 usually require future therapy with an antacid or other alkalinizing agent. Include gastric drainage when balancing intake/output levels and estimating blood loss.

This provides a baseline assessment and aids ongoing evaluation of GI function. Hypoactive bowel sounds usually accompany paralytic ileus.

Abdominal distention indicates intraabdominal accumulation of blood, gas, or other fluids. Baseline measurements aid continuing ileus evaluation.

Associated care plans

Hemorrhagic Shock
Vasogenic Shock
Paralytic Ileus
Peritonitis
Renal System Injury
Malnutrition in the Trauma Patient

Associated procedures and study

Diagnostic Peritoneal Lavage
Preparation for Surgery
Intrahospital Transport of the Shock Trauma Patient
Positive Contrast Study
The Pneumatic Antishock Garment

GASTROINTESTINAL

Medical diagnosis

ABDOMINAL TRAUMA DURING PREGNANCY: Blunt and Penetrating

Assessment

Mechanism of injury/ etiology:
- blunt—as from deceleration or crushing forces, assault, fall
- penetrating—as from missile, blast, or impaling injury

Physical findings:
Note: *When assessing the pregnant trauma patient,* *keep in mind the many changes normal to pregnancy (such as increased heart and respiratory rates and laboratory value changes). Evaluate her for shock or injuries in light of these expected changes. To review these changes, see Table 2.6 and Table 2.7 in Section II.*

Associated injuries:
This patient risks the same injuries as a non-pregnant patient with abdominal trauma (see "Intraabdominal Trauma: Blunt and Penetrating" in Section II), plus the following:
- bladder rupture—upward displacement from normally protected position within the pelvis increases injury risk
- diaphragm tear—uterine enlargement increases injury risk

Diagnostic studies

- laboratory data—to evaluate, compare with normal values during pregnancy; see Table 2.8 in Section II.
- diagnostic peritoneal lavage (DPL)—confirms intraabdominal hemorrhage (DPL preceded by urinary bladder and stomach decompression and uterine size estimation, to help prevent complications)
- radiography—helps determine associated injuries (not usually indicated or conclusive for intraabdominal injuries)

Nursing diagnosis

Potential for ineffective airway clearance related to nasal and oropharyngeal mucosa engorgement.

GOAL: Establish and maintain an adequate airway.

Interventions

1. Monitor respiratory status carefully. Promote safe airway maintenance by gently inserting a small, well-lubricated oropharyngeal or endotracheal airway.

Rationale

During pregnancy, vascularization normally increases, causing nasal and upper airway engorgement. Thus, trauma to the pregnant patient may precipitate serious respiratory complications. A small, well-lubricated airway reduces the risk of further respiratory compromise and of upper airway trauma and hemorrhage during intubation.

Nursing diagnosis

Potential for decreased gas exchange related to decreased functional residual capacity secondary to diaphragmatic elevation, and vomiting and aspiration secondary to decreased gastric motility.

GOAL #1: Optimize gas exchange and oxygenation.

GASTROINTESTINAL

Interventions

1. Administer supplemental oxygen or assist ventilation as ordered.

Rationale

The pregnant patient has an elevated diaphragm, which decreases her functional residual capacity and makes her less tolerant of hypoxic episodes. Fetal distress rapidly results from maternal hypoxia; so prompt supplemental oxygen therapy or ventilatory assistance optimizes maternal and fetal outcomes.

GOAL #2: Minimize the risk of aspiration.

Interventions

1. Insert a gastric decompression tube. Maintain the proper position, patency, and appropriate suction levels. Keep the patient NPO.

Rationale

Presume the pregnant trauma patient has a full stomach because of delayed gastric emptying time. Prompt gastric decompression can decrease the risk of vomiting and possible aspiration.

Nursing diagnosis

Potential for decreased fetal and maternal tissue perfusion related to fluid volume deficit secondary to hemorrhage from abruptio placentae or uterine damage.

GOAL #1: Optimize cellular perfusion; restore and maintain a normovolemic state.

Interventions

1. Monitor maternal vital signs and fetal heart rate every 5 to 15 minutes, or as the patient's condition warrants. Evaluate trends for signs of shock (see "Hemorrhagic Shock" in Section II).

Rationale

Maternal hypervolemia may mask early signs of shock; maternal tachycardia and supine hypotension may further confuse the clinical picture. Uterine perfusion decreases as an initial vasoconstrictive response to shock, so *the fetus may be the first to evidence decreased perfusion.* Continuous monitoring and trend analysis of maternal vital signs and fetal heart rate help detect subtle changes.

2. Use a continuous fetal monitor, whenever available (normal fetal heart rate: 120 to 160 beats/minute).

Fetal tachycardia and (more gravely) bradycardia require early recognition and prompt treatment.

3. Ensure placement of two large-bore, peripheral I.V. catheters and administer fluids, as ordered.

By the time fetal or maternal vital signs reflect shock, significant blood loss has already occurred. Survival of both the mother and the fetus requires rapid volume replacement.

4. Obtain baseline laboratory results and compare them with normal pregnancy values and, when possible, the patient's preinjury values.

Laboratory values alter significantly during pregnancy. Therefore, accurate evaluation requires comparison of postinjury laboratory data with values normal during pregnancy (see Table 2.8). Further comparison with the patient's most recent preinjury results (obtainable from her obstetrician) enhances an accurate assessment.

5. Monitor coagulation profile trends.

Coagulation normally changes during pregnancy, predisposing the pregnant trauma patient to disseminated intravascular coagulation, particularly with placental disruption. **Note:** *A placental separation of more than 50% greatly endangers fetal viability and significantly increases maternal risk of coagulopathy.*

GASTROINTESTINAL

6. Position the patient in the left lateral position or direct a team member to displace the uterus manually.

When the patient is supine, the enlarged uterus compresses the vena cava and the aorta. This impedes venous return to the heart and decreases cardiac output. Positioning the patient on her left side (or manually displacing the uterus) minimizes uterine pressure, improves venous return, and increases cardiac output. Use manual displacement with a suspected cervical spine injury.

7. Apply a pneumatic antishock garment, but do not inflate the abdominal section. (See "The Pneumatic Antishock Garment" in Section VII.)

This garment may benefit the shock patient and, when used cautiously, can be safe for the pregnant patient. However, inflating the abdominal section may impede uterine blood flow.

8. Either avoid inotropic agents or administer them only in low doses, as ordered, when necessary for maternal survival.

These drugs cause severe vasoconstriction, minimizing uterine blood flow and causing fetal hypoxia and distress.

GOAL #2: Recognize early signs and symptoms of abruptio placentae and uterine damage.

Interventions

Rationale

1. Monitor the patient for signs and symptoms of abruptio placentae, including:
• vaginal bleeding
• abdominal pain
• uterine tenderness
• uterine tetany or rigidity
• rising fundal height
• maternal hemorrhage and shock
• fetal distress.

Abruptio placentae—*the most common obstetric cause of fetal death following automobile accidents*—can develop as late as 48 hours after trauma. Therefore, the pregnant trauma patient requires continuous assessment for early detection of this injury. A mild abruption may exhibit only vague signs, making detection difficult.

2. Measure and record fundal height every 30 minutes (measure from the symphysis pubis to the top of the fundus).

A rising fundal height may indicate abruptio placentae.

3. Monitor the patient's pad count.

An accurate pad count helps estimate blood loss and helps detect a sudden change in vaginal drainage.

4. Monitor the patient for signs of uterine damage, including:
• abdominal pain or rigidity
• vaginal bleeding
• uterine tenderness
• loss of fetal movement or heart tones
• maternal hemorrhage and shock.

Detecting and repairing minor uterine damage early can prevent maternal hemorrhage and fetal compromise. More severe uterine damage requires rapid identification and treatment to prevent both maternal and fetal death.

5. Prepare the patient for DPL:
• explain that this test will not hurt her baby but rather helps diagnose injuries, thus maximizing both maternal and fetal survival
• assemble equipment at the patient's bedside
• insert a urinary catheter, using aseptic technique
• insert a gastric tube.
(See "Diagnostic Peritoneal Lavage" in Section VII.)

A DPL can be safely performed during pregnancy after defining uterine size and decompressing the stomach and bladder. If evidence indicates abdominal perforation and a shock state, DPL may be omitted and the mother taken directly to the operating suite.

GASTROINTESTINAL

6. Prepare the patient for surgical intervention and possible emergency cesarean section:
• notify operating room personnel
• notify the pediatrician of possible delivery.
(See "Preparation for Surgery" in Section VII.)

Exploratory laparotomy helps identify the extent of uterine damage and other intraabdominal injuries. Surgical repair of uterine lacerations, tears, or other organ or vessel injuries can be accomplished without uterine disruption. Emergency cesarean section may be necessary in:
• uterine rupture
• fetal distress related to abruptio placentae
• severe cases, for better visualization of other intraabdominal injuries.
Fetal viability, according to gestational age (should be at least 26 weeks), and current fetal status help determine the need for a cesarean section. An infant who is premature or in distress needs resuscitation immediately after delivery. Early notification of operating room personnel facilitates availability of specialized equipment and appropriate consultants, such as the pediatrician or neonatologist. **Note:** *The last menstrual period, when known, provides the best estimate of gestational age. Other general indicators include auscultation of fetal heart tones, quickening, and fundal height. An ultrasound examination, when available and if immediate surgery is not required, also supplies valuable data on gestational age.*

Nursing diagnosis

*Potential for premature labor and delivery related to altered uterine perfusion or uterine disruption.

GOAL #1: Identify signs of premature labor.

Interventions

1. Monitor the patient for early signs of premature labor, including:
• back pain
• altered vaginal discharge.

2. Monitor her for late signs of premature labor, including:
• contractions every 10 minutes or less, of 30-second duration and causing cervical dilation.

Rationale

Early identification of premature labor is essential to successful labor intervention. Premature labor may suggest uterine or fetal injuries.

GOAL #2: Inhibit premature labor.

Interventions

1. Administer medications to inhibit premature labor, as ordered.

2. Administer I.V. fluids, as ordered.

Rationale

Medication may successfully inhibit labor if the cervix is dilated less than 3 cm and if concomitant injuries have been ruled out as the precipitating cause of labor.

Dehydration may cause uterine irritability and trigger premature labor.

GOAL #3: Promote safe delivery of a premature infant.

*Supplemental nursing diagnosis

GASTROINTESTINAL

Interventions

1. Monitor the labor process and use a continuous fetal heart rate monitor. Have obstetric personnel interpret the labor process.

2. Notify pediatric and neonatal staff of impending delivery. Obtain necessary resuscitation equipment.

Rationale

Obstetric personnel can help identify potential neonatal problems. Their observations are most important if labor has progressed too far to inhibit or has been medically inhibited, or if delivery is imminent.

A premature infant's survival may depend on aggressive resuscitation at birth.

Nursing diagnoses

Potential for infection related to premature rupture of membranes secondary to blunt trauma.
Potential for infection related to disruption in skin integrity and peritoneal contamination by free blood, feces, urine, or bile secondary to penetrating trauma.

GOAL #1: Identify ruptured membranes.

Interventions

1. Prepare the patient for a sterile speculum examination.

2. Assess for signs of ruptured membranes, including:
• sudden fluid gush
• vaginal pH between 7 and 7.5
• positive fern test.

Rationale

This examination enables determination of vaginal pH and sampling of vaginal fluid for use in the fern test (both of which confirm the presence of amniotic fluid). Ruptured membranes increase the risk of infection by allowing bacteria direct entrance to the uterus. Sterile technique during the examination minimizes further bacterial contamination of the birth canal.

GOAL #2: Recognize early signs of infection.

Interventions

1. Monitor the patient for signs of infection. Record temperatures with vital signs at least every 2 hours. Monitor trends in leukocyte counts.

Rationale

Promptly detecting signs of infection in the pregnant trauma patient is essential. A fever $> 101°$ F. and a WBC count $> 22,000$, in the presence of ruptured membranes, suggest amnionitis.

GOAL #3: Prevent or minimize further risk of infection.

Interventions

1. Obtain the patient's history of medication allergies and tetanus immunization.

2. Administer antibiotics and tetanus prophylaxis, as ordered.

Rationale

Most medications are contraindicated and require caution during pregnancy. Fetal risks, however, must be weighed against maternal benefits. Tetanus toxoid can be given safely during pregnancy.

GASTROINTESTINAL

Nursing diagnosis

Potential for fetal distress related to direct fetal injury secondary to blunt or penetrating trauma.

GOAL: Detect early signs of fetal distress.

Interventions

1. Assess fetal status with each maternal assessment, including fetal heart rate and activity.

2. Prepare the patient for diagnostic ultrasonography.

Rationale

Early signs of fetal injury may include changes in fetal movement and fetal tachycardia or bradycardia.

Ultrasound serves several purposes for the pregnant trauma patient; it may:
- identify fetal injuries, such as skull and clavicle fractures
- locate foreign objects, such as a bullet
- aid estimation of gestational age to help determine fetal viability.

An emergency cesarean section is deemed inappropriate for an immature infant (as identified in the Table 2.5) with direct injuries because of the decreased chance for fetal survival; the fetus should remain in utero.

Table 2.5

Classification	Weight	Approximate weeks of gestation
Premature infant	1,500 to 2,500 grams	> 28 weeks
Immature infant	500 to 1,500 grams	20 to 28 weeks
Abortion	< 500 grams	< 20 weeks

Nursing diagnosis

Potential for anxiety related to potential fetal injury or death.

GOAL: Reduce the patient's anxiety and support her coping mechanisms.

Interventions

1. Provide explanations in terms the patient can understand. Ask her for feedback. Reinforce information as necessary. Include the father, when possible, in information-sharing sessions.

2. Reassure the mother that the best chance for fetal survival lies in prompt, aggressive maternal care.

Rationale

Clear communication, positive feedback, and reinforcement aid understanding and help reduce anxiety. Providing the father with current, accurate information may relieve some of his anxiety concerning the mother and baby.

The mother's anxiety may lessen and her cooperation improve if she understands the reasons for, and benefits of, aggressive care directed at her needs and injuries.

*Supplemental nursing diagnosis

3. Let the mother hear fetal heart tones with a Doppler device, when appropriate.

This measure may alleviate her anxiety concerning the baby's well-being.

4. Encourage the mother to verbalize her feelings.

Allowing the mother to react and ventilate shows her that you acknowledge, understand, and accept her feelings.

5. Permit visits or telephone calls from the father, family, and friends, when possible.

This promotes the patient's use of her established support systems.

6. Ensure the opportunity for religious rites, such as baptism, in cases of fetal death, as requested. Arrange for the parents and family to see the baby in privacy.

Acknowledgment and acceptance of the patient's religious beliefs and facilitating requests for or performing specific rites, such as baptism, offer the parents spiritual support. Allowing the parents and other family members to see and hold the baby may facilitate the grieving process and their acceptance of the baby's death. Ensuring privacy promotes family interaction and natural expression of feelings.

Additional considerations

Comprehensive anticipation of this patient's needs must include a system that ensures quick access to specialty consultants, such as obstetricians, pediatric surgeons, pediatricians, neonatologists, and specialized nursing resources. For example, a list of telephone numbers, affixed to the pediatric crash cart, promotes immediate access to appropriate consultants. The pregnant trauma patient usually requires rapid transfer to a regional referral center with neonatology capabilities. Established, written transfer guidelines facilitate this process. Guidelines should include the mechanism for notifying the transport vehicle and trained personnel to accompany the patient.

Associated care plans

Intraabdominal Trauma: Blunt and
    Penetrating
Hemorrhagic Shock
Peritonitis
Paralytic Ileus
Psychosocial Support of the Trauma Patient
Vasogenic Shock
Disseminated Intravascular Coagulation

Associated procedures

Preparation for Surgery
Diagnostic Peritoneal Lavage
The Pneumatic Antishock Garment

GASTROINTESTINAL

Table 2.6
Signs and Symptoms of Pregnancy

- Palpable uterus (at 12 to 14 weeks)
- Auscultation of fetal heart tones (at 9 to 12 weeks)
- Quickening—fetal movement

- Last menstrual period > 4½ weeks prior to admission
- Breast changes, such as engorgement
- Morning sickness

Table 2.7
Normal Assessment Changes During Pregnancy

Neurologic:
- Gait and balance changes (particularly in the third trimester)

Cardiovascular:
- Syncope and fatigue (first trimester)
- Hypervolemia: 35% to 50% increase in circulating volume can mask a 10% to 15% acute or 30% gradual blood loss
- Heart rate increase of 15 to 20 beats above pre-pregnancy rate
- Supine hypotension (vena cava syndrome)

Respiratory:
- Upper respiratory passage engorgement
- Respiratory rate increase of about 15%

Gastrointestinal:
- Hypoactive bowel sounds and delayed gastric emptying

Genitourinary:
- Increased urinary frequency
- Glycosuria

Table 2.8
Comparing Normal Laboratory Values

Study	Nonpregnancy	Pregnancy
Hematocrit	37% to 48%	32% to 42%
Hemoglobin	12 to 16 g/dl	10 to 14 g/dl
Leukocytes	4,300 to 10,000/mm³	5,000 to 15,000 mm³
Fibrinogen	250 to 400 mg %	600 mg %
Platelets	150,000 to 350,000/mm³	Same or slightly ↓
Arterial pH	7.38 to 7.44	7.40 to 7.45
PCO₂	35 to 50 mm Hg	25 to 30 mm Hg
PO₂	98 to 100 mm Hg	101 to 104 mm Hg
Base excess	0.7 mEq/liter	3 to 4 mEq/liter
Bicarbonate	24 to 30 mEq/liter	17 to 22 mEq/liter

GASTROINTESTINAL

ACUTE UPPER GASTROINTESTINAL BLEEDING (Esophageal Varices, Peptic Ulcer)

Assessment

Mechanism of injury/ etiology:

Esophageal varices

- responsible for about 17% of GI bleeding episodes
- directly related to liver disease and portal hypertension
- associated with recent or chronic history of hepatitis, alcoholism, cirrhosis of the liver

Peptic ulcers

- responsible for 50% to 80% of GI bleeding episodes
- linked to precipitating factors or conditions including excessive alcohol intake, gastric-irritating drugs, excessive caffeine intake, gastritis, stressful environment

- associated with such injuries or conditions as head injuries, central nervous system trauma, multisystem trauma, severe shock, sepsis, respiratory insufficiency, hypoxia, severe peritonitis, burns, multisystem organ failure, coagulopathies
- associated with such genetic factors or chronic

diseases as tuberculosis, chronic obstructive pulmonary disease, cirrhosis of the liver, rheumatoid arthritis

Physical findings:
Table 2.9 summarizes symptoms and manifestations of peptic ulcers and esophageal varices.

Diagnostic studies

The patient's history and physical findings often provide adequate data for diagnosis.

Esophageal varices

- esophagogastroscopy—identifies bleeding site(s)

Peptic ulcers

- esophagogastroscopy/duodenoscopy—directly visualize bleeding site and help in biopsy procedure

- contrast studies—upper GI series may identify duodenal defect or active ulcer
- arteriography—identifies bleeding site(s)
- laboratory studies—identify elevated serum amylase level, low hemoglobin/hematocrit level, stool sample positive for occult blood
- chest radiography—although not a diagnostic tool for ulcers, may reveal subdiaphragmatic free air, which is consistent with ulcer perforation

Potential for impaired tissue perfusion related to fluid volume deficit secondary to excessive upper GI bleeding.

GOAL #1: Restore and maintain normovolemia; optimize tissue perfusion.

Interventions

1. Monitor the patient closely for signs of hemorrhagic shock, including:
- hypotension
- tachycardia
- pallor
- sluggish capillary refill time
- diaphoresis
- tachypnea
- decreased urine output
- altered level of consciousness.

Monitor and document vital signs every 5 to 15 minutes as long as the patient is unstable and every hour thereafter or as his condition warrants.

2. Ensure the placement of at least two large-bore peripheral I.V. catheters. Administer fluid replacement as ordered. Assemble equipment for and assist with arterial pressure line and pulmonary artery (PA) catheter placement. (See "Pulmonary Artery Catheterization" in Section VII.) Ensure chest radiograph after insertion of PA catheter.

3. Obtain baseline and serial laboratory studies for CBC, electrolytes, coagulation profile, serum amylase levels, liver function tests, and ABGs. Monitor trends.

4. Administer vitamin and electrolyte replacements as ordered.

5. Ensure that a blood sample is sent promptly for typing and cross matching. Administer blood component replacement, including packed RBCs, fresh-frozen plasma, and platelets, as ordered. Notify blood bank personnel of the probable need for large volumes of blood and clotting factors.

6. Monitor the patient's respiratory status closely and administer supplemental oxygen as ordered. Ensure the availability of equipment necessary for intubation and mechanical ventilation. (See "Endotracheal Intubation" in Section VII.)

Rationale

Esophageal varices and gastric or duodenal ulcers can cause massive blood loss. Increased portal system resistance and pressure causes development of collateral circulation. The fragile, dilated, valveless veins, usually arising in the esophagus, are easily injured when pressure increases, as from vomiting. Peptic ulcers are mucosal erosions that can disrupt the integrity of large arteries, commonly the gastroduodenal or pancreaticoduodenal. Arterial invasion precipitates significant blood loss. Early recognition of hemorrhagic signs should trigger prompt intervention to prevent hemorrhagic shock.

Rapid fluid resuscitation is essential to prevent deterioration in the shock state. An arterial pressure line provides consistent blood pressure monitoring and easy access for blood sampling. PA catheter data helps direct further volume resuscitation. Proper placement of the catheter is confirmed by chest radiograph.

Baseline and ongoing serial laboratory data help analyze resuscitation effectiveness, tissue perfusion, and oxygenation; identify preexisting liver or clotting disorders; and direct further therapy.

Multivitamin supplements, usually indicated in patients with preexisting deficiencies, are commonly given soon after hemodynamic stability is achieved. Potassium and sodium are lost through excessive vomiting and gastric suction.

Early blood transfusion and component therapy may prevent or minimize shock-related complications. Anticipating the need for large volumes of blood and clotting factors and notifying the blood bank early during patient admission facilitate blood availability.

Supplemental oxygen can minimize hypoxia-related complications associated with excessive blood loss and shock states.

GOAL #2: Estimate blood loss.

Interventions

1. Determine the patient's blood loss by:
• obtaining information on the blood he lost before admission from the patient, his family, and prehospital care providers
• estimating the volume of blood on clothing, linen, stretcher.

2. Document the volume and source of ongoing bleeding.

Rationale

Estimating blood loss helps determine the degree of hypovolemia and blood replacement needs.

GOAL #3: Identify the bleeding site.

Note: *Although promptly determining the specific bleeding site is essential, resuscitation aimed at correcting existing or impending hemorrhagic shock must always take precedence over diagnostic procedures.*

Interventions

1. Ensure gastric decompression tube placement. Document gastric secretion volume, pH, and characteristics.

2. Prepare the patient for and help with such diagnostic studies as gastroscopy, esophagogastroscopy, and arteriography. (See "Endoscopy" in Section VII.)

Rationale

Gastric decompression provides diagnostic and therapeutic information. Gastric secretion analysis, including pH, color, and consistency, helps determine the GI bleeding site. For example, fresh blood usually reflects ulcer-related bleeding, whereas darker blood or coffee-ground secretions may reflect bleeding from a source proximal to the stomach. Gastric decompression helps prevent aspiration of irritating gastric secretions should the patient vomit. The tube also helps slow bleeding since clot and gastric secretions evacuation stimulates gastric contraction, constricting the flow through gastric vessels. Accurate gastric drainage monitoring ensures accuracy of blood loss and output records. This information is valuable to confirm the need for surgery.

Identifying the bleeding site promptly is essential for initiating the most appropriate, effective therapy. Arteriography can be both diagnostic and therapeutic for bleeding ulcers.

GOAL #4: Prevent or minimize further bleeding.

Interventions

1. Perform a gastric lavage with cool saline solution or water, as ordered, for a patient with suspected or confirmed bleeding ulcers. Administer norepinephrine via gastric tube as ordered. Closely monitor the irrigating solution return and include amounts greater than the instillation in output totals.

Rationale

Gastric lavage helps control gastric bleeding because the cool solution promotes local vasoconstriction and clot formation. Lavage also dilutes and evacuates acidic secretions and reduces autodigestive enzyme activity. Iced or cold saline solution is no longer popular because the temperature extreme is thought to stimulate hydrochloric acid production. Norepinephrine instillation augments gastric vasoconstriction. Maintaining an accurate record of the blood lost through the gastric tube is essential for overall patient progress evaluation.

GASTROINTESTINAL

2. Assist with placement of a Sengstaken-Blakemore tube in a patient with suspected or confirmed bleeding esophageal varices. Follow your hospital's protocol and the manufacturer's instructions for safe use. Be sure to:
• monitor the patient's respiratory status
• keep scissors at the patient's bedside and on the emergency crash cart when transporting the patient out of the unit
• suction his nose and mouth frequently
• insert a gastric tube above the esophageal balloon
• pad the tube where it touches the patient's nostril
• monitor the nostril closely
• ensure balloon deflation at recommended intervals.

This tube can help differentiate gastric from esophageal bleeding. It obstructs the esophagus and serves as a tamponade for bleeding esophageal varices. Several hazards and complications associated with its use mandate constant tube monitoring. Airway obstruction occurs if the gastric balloon ruptures. External traction on the tube can pull the esophageal balloon up into the airway, causing a sudden obstruction. Rapid detection, cutting all balloon ports, and immediate tube removal restore the patient's airway. He will be unable to swallow oral secretions and therefore will require frequent oral and nasal suctioning. The gastric tube helps remove secretions above the level of the esophageal balloon. Nasal mucosa irritation can develop from the pressure caused by tube traction. Tube padding, where it touches the nostril, minimizes irritation. Both esophageal and gastric balloons can cause mucosal irritation or erosion if they remain inflated beyond the recommended time of 24 to 48 hours.

3. Administer anticholinergics, antacids, agents that promote ulcer healing and reduce pain, vasopressin, and vitamin K as ordered. See the hospital formulary or other reference work for information on drug effects, dosages, and contraindications.

Anticholinergics block vagal nerve stimulation, decrease gastric motility, reduce gastroduodenal spasms, and shunt blood away from the gastric mucosa. Antacids administered via the gastric tube help neutralize gastric secretions and may alleviate pain. Drugs such as cimetidine, ranitidine, and sucralfate augment ulcer therapy since they decrease gastric acid secretion and promote healing and may reduce discomfort. Vasopressin may be used after arteriography identifies the bleeding site. Direct intraarterial or I.V. infusion through a pump into the superior mesenteric or gastric artery causes splanchnic vasoconstriction and may lower portal pressure. Vasopressin may reduce the bleeding from both ulcers and esophageal varices. Vitamin K administration enhances production of prothrombin and Factors VII, IX, and X and augments coagulation.

4. Prepare the patient for surgical intervention. (See "Preparation for Surgery" in Section VII.)

Unrelenting bleeding from ulcer disease or esophageal varices that is intractable to medical therapy may require surgical intervention. Procedures such as vagotomy, ulcerative-area resection, ulcer oversewing, or gastrectomy may be necessary. Surgical intervention for esophageal varices—for example, direct ligation of uncontrollable bleeding varices—generally has a high mortality. Medical management remains the treatment of choice during acute bleeding episodes. Later operative procedures are aimed at reducing and controlling portal pressure.

Nursing diagnosis

Potential for infection related to spillage of gastric or duodenal contents into the peritoneum or erosion of surrounding viscera secondary to ulcer penetration.

GOAL: Recognize peritonitis early and initiate therapy promptly.

GASTROINTESTINAL

Interventions

1. Monitor the ulcer patient closely for signs of peritoneal inflammation, including:
- sudden pain onset that rapidly reaches maximal intensity
- pain in the right upper quadrant or epigastrium that rapidly becomes generalized and may radiate to the shoulder
- rebound tenderness
- abdominal distention or rigidity
- patient lying motionless
- hypoactive or absent bowel sounds
- hypotension, tachycardia
- diaphoresis, pallor
- elevated WBC count and serum amylase level
- fever.

Rationale

Ulcers can erode through the gastric or duodenal mucosa to the peritoneal cavity or continue their erosion into a nearby organ or vessel. The liver, pancreas, greater omentum, and biliary tract are most commonly affected. Sudden development of clinical findings in the ulcer patient heralds peritoneal penetration. This complication may swiftly deteriorate to hypovolemic shock. Vasogenic-septic shock may develop if signs and symptoms go unrecognized.

Additional considerations

This care plan addresses only the acute interventions of upper GI bleeding. Other aspects of both peptic ulcer disease and esophageal varices, however, must be considered. Patient education focusing on knowledge of the specific disease, complications, the need for dietary and behavioral restrictions, and drug therapy is essential for effective, successful care. Patient comfort, although not discussed previously, often directly impinges on dietary, behavioral, and medication compliance. Anxiety about current or future exacerbations may require that the patient receive professional counseling. During an acute bleeding episode, with hemorrhagic shock a possibility, these considerations are not immediate priorities. Special focus on comfort, anxiety, and education becomes more appropriate only after the patient is hemodynamically stable and the acute bleeding is controlled.

Associated care plans	Associated procedures and studies
Hemorrhagic Shock	Intrahospital Transport of the Shock Trauma Patient
Vasogenic Shock	Positive Contrast Studies
Malnutrition in the Trauma Patient	Endoscopy
Psychosocial Support of the Trauma Patient	Pulmonary Artery Catheterization
Peritonitis	Preparation for Surgery
	Endotracheal Intubation
	Aortography

GASTROINTESTINAL

GASTROINTESTINAL

Table 2.9
Gastrointestinal Bleeding

Generalized symptoms

Cardiovascular:
- syncope
- fatigue
- hypotension
- tachycardia
- pallor
- diaphoresis
- shock state
- low-grade fever

Genitourinary:
- decreased urinary output

Gastrointestinal:
- hematemesis
- coffee-ground emesis
- melena

Neurologic:
- anxiety
- altered level of consciousness
- unresponsiveness

Peptic ulcers: Additional symptoms or manifestations

Gastrointestinal:
- pain—pattern as important as location and intensity:
  - ☐ midepigastric—heartburn
  - ☐ right or left upper quadrant
  - ☐ radiating to back
- pain-free intervals that alternate with recurrences:
  - ☐ increased pain when stomach is empty
  - ☐ increased pain at night
  - ☐ pain relieved by food, antacids
  - ☐ anorexia
- nausea/vomiting
- abdominal fullness or distention

- melena
- frank or occult blood in gastric contents
- shock state
> indicate hemorrhage

- sudden onset of acute abdominal pain
- referred pain
- pain increases with movement
- vomiting
- abdominal distention with rigidity
- shock state
- sepsis
> indicate perforation

Esophageal varices: Additional symptoms or manifestations

Gastrointestinal:
- hematemesis
- melena or maroon stools with clots
- jaundice
- signs of liver disease and portal hypertension, including:
  - ☐ ascites
  - ☐ enlarged spleen or liver
  - ☐ spider nevi
  - ☐ anemia
  - ☐ palmar muscle atrophy
  - ☐ hemorrhoids

Cardiovascular:
- generalized weakness
- delirium tremens
- shock state

Neurologic:
- hepatic encephalopathy

Medical diagnosis

RUPTURED ECTOPIC PREGNANCY

Assessment

Mechanism of injury/ etiology:
• 90% of ectopic pregnancies occur within a fallopian tube—usually the right tube
• predisposing factors include tubal abnormalities, adhesions, or obstructions

• diagnosis is usually within the first trimester

Physical findings:
Gastrointestinal
• abdominal or pelvic pain—sudden and acute†
• Cullen's sign—periumbilical ecchymosis
• pain referred to a shoulder

Genitourinary
• vaginal bleeding—scant, dark red†
• palpable mass on the tube or in the cul-de-sac on pelvic examination†
• pelvic distention or feeling of fullness
• pain on pelvic examination

Cardiovascular
• decreased hemoglobin/ hematocrit values
• elevated WBC count
• fever
• postural hypotension
• vertigo, syncope
• shock state

†Comprises one of the three elements of the triad of ectopic pregnancy

Diagnostic studies

• accurate menstrual history and physical examination—often furnish adequate data for a definitive diagnosis
• urine immunologic pregnancy test and serum sample for human chorionic gonadotropin test (beta-subunit assay)—valuable if results are positive but inconclusive if results are negative
• ultrasonography—may reveal a mass or fluid in or around the cul-de-sac, fallopian tube, or adnexa; may visualize an extrauterine gestational sac
• laparoscopy or exploratory laparotomy—may be required to confirm the diagnosis

Nursing diagnosis

Potential for fluid volume deficit related to hemorrhage secondary to rupture of the pregnant extrauterine structure.

GOAL #1: Early recognition of the classic triad of symptoms.

Interventions

1. Assess the patient for classic symptoms of ruptured ectopic pregnancy:
• abdominal or pelvic pain
• scant, dark red vaginal blood
• palpable mass on the tube or in the cul-de-sac.

Rationale

An early differential diagnosis is essential because the patient can abruptly deteriorate to a profound shock state.

GOAL #2: Restore and maintain normovolemia.

Interventions

1. Monitor the patient for signs of hemorrhagic shock; monitor and document vital signs every 5 to 15 minutes or as her condition warrants; monitor ECG rhythm and neurologic and respiratory status.

Rationale

Hemorrhage associated with rupture of a pregnant extrauterine structure can cause the patient to rapidly develop profound shock. Close evaluation of the cardiopulmonary and neurologic systems helps determine the severity of shock. (See Table 2.1 in "Hemorrhagic Shock" in Section II for signs of early and late shock.)

GENITOURINARY

2. Ensure adequate venous access with two large-bore (14- to 16-gauge) catheters; administer fluids as ordered.

Hemorrhagic shock requires rapid, aggressive fluid replacement with colloid and crystalloid products.

3. Obtain baseline laboratory studies and monitor trends in CBC, electrolyte, and ABG levels, and coagulation profile.

Trend analysis of laboratory data helps evaluate tissue perfusion, fluid balance, and overall resuscitative effectiveness. Prolonged clotting times may develop when severe hemorrhage mandates massive blood transfusions.

4. Ensure blood typing and cross matching with Rh determination.

Component therapy can effectively prevent clotting disorders. The Rh factor helps confirm or negate the mother's need for RhoGAM, an $Rh_o(D)$ immune globulin.

5. Prepare the patient for surgery:
- assist with obtaining consent
- assist with physical preparation as needed
- ensure the availability of packed RBCs.
(See "Preparation for Surgery" in Section VII.)

Accurate diagnosis of a ruptured ectopic pregnancy may require a laparoscopy or exploratory laparotomy. Surgical intervention may be necessary to obtain hemostasis. Procedures may include salpingectomy, removal of the pregnancy, and, rarely, hysterectomy.

Nursing diagnosis

Potential for infection related to peritoneal inflammation from extrauterine bleeding.

GOAL: Recognize early signs of infection.

Interventions

1. Monitor and document the patient's temperature and vital signs; monitor pain changes or trends; also note trends in laboratory data, especially the WBC count.

Rationale

Extrauterine rupture causes blood to extravasate into the peritoneal or retroperitoneal spaces. The pooled blood provides an ideal medium for bacterial growth.

Nursing diagnosis

Potential for anxiety related to loss of pregnancy and sudden hospitalization.

GOAL: Reduce anxiety level; maintain established support systems.

Interventions

1. Provide the patient with clear, honest explanations. Accept her emotional responses without judgment.

2. Maintain established support systems:
- encourage a preoperative telephone call or brief visit from the patient's husband, significant other, or friend.

Rationale

Anxiety can impair the patient's ability to comprehend this situation. She may suffer an emotional crisis from the sudden, unexpected hospitalization and abortion.

Personal support systems facilitate the grieving process and help the patient reestablish self-esteem.

GENITOURINARY

Additional considerations

The Rh-negative mother needs an anti-D immune globulin (RhoGAM) injection within 72 hours of the abortion if the products of conception were Rh-positive. RhoGAM prevents isoimmunization, the mother's formation of Rh-positive antibodies, which will develop in reaction to the agglutinogens produced in a subsequent Rh-positive fetus. These antibodies can cross the placenta and destroy fetal cells, potentiating erythroblastosis fetalis in a subsequent pregnancy.

Associated care plans	**Associated procedure**
Hemorrhagic Shock	Preparation for Surgery
Psychosocial Support of the Trauma Patient	
Peritonitis	

GENITOURINARY

SPONTANEOUS ABORTION

Assessment

Mechanism of injury/ etiology
- in first trimester, usually placental or fetal abnormalities, such as congenital or genetic defects
- in second trimester, usually maternal problems, such as uterine dysfunction, endocrine problems, viral infections, cervical incompetence, trauma
- instrumentation, with intent to terminate pregnancy
- complication following amniocentesis

Physical findings:
Note: *Spontaneous abortions are categorized as threatened, inevitable, incomplete, complete, or septic.*

Genitourinary

- threatened
  - [ ] dark, thick vaginal bleeding or spotting
  - [ ] mild cramps (suprapubic, low back)
  - [ ] closed cervix
- inevitable
  - [ ] vaginal bleeding with clot passage
  - [ ] ruptured membranes
  - [ ] uterine contractions, pain

- [ ] dilated cervix
- [ ] no tissue apparent in vagina
- incomplete
  - [ ] bright red vaginal bleeding
  - [ ] increasing uterine contractions
  - [ ] cervical dilation
  - [ ] placental tissue partially separated and present at the os or in the vagina; some fragments remain in utero
- complete
  - [ ] cervical dilation
  - [ ] passage of fetus, membranes, placenta
- septic

- [ ] possible lacerations or puncture marks around or on cervix
- [ ] constant pain; uterine tenderness
- [ ] foul, purulent vaginal discharge
- [ ] cervical pain on palpation (cervical motion tenderness)
- [ ] distention

Cardiovascular

- shock (hemorrhagic, vasogenic-septic)
- fever (100° F./37.8° C.); elevated WBC count (most common with incomplete and septic abortions)

Diagnostic studies

- pregnancy test—may be positive even after complete abortion
- patient history and physical examination (including pelvic examination)—usually confirms diagnosis

- sonography—helps determine stage of abortion and need for dilatation and curettage as evidenced by uterine or placental abnormality; confirms presence or absence of fetal heartbeat

Nursing diagnosis

*Potential for spontaneous abortion related to maternal or fetal abnormality.

GOAL #1: Recognize signs of threatened abortion.

Interventions

1. Evaluate for, and immediately report, signs of threatened abortion, including:
- dark vaginal spotting or bleeding
- pain similar to that of menstrual cramps, following onset of vaginal bleeding
- disappearance of signs of pregnancy (nausea, breast tenderness, urinary frequency) approximately 2 days before bleeding began.

Rationale

Occasional painless vaginal spotting may occur during early pregnancy without further untoward effects. Pain associated with spotting, however, usually signals distress. Significant vaginal bleeding during the first trimester is usually associated with high fetal mortality. These signs of threatened abortion should trigger interventions aimed at averting further deterioration.

GENITOURINARY

*Supplemental nursing diagnosis

2. Prepare the patient for diagnostic ultrasonography, as ordered or according to hospital protocol.

Ultrasonography helps determine the stage of the abortion and placental integrity. Preparation may include I.V. infusion, oral ingestion, or direct bladder insufflation (via a urinary catheter) with 1 liter of fluid, and ensuring that the patient refrains from urinating. This promotes bladder distention, which is necessary for optimal visualization.

GOAL #2: Prevent or minimize the risk of progression to inevitable abortion.

Interventions

1. Provide the patient with clear, concise instructions regarding the need for complete bed rest and abstinence from sexual intercourse.

2. Ensure patient compliance with activity restrictions if hospitalization is required.

3. Administer sedatives, as ordered.

Rationale

For optimal cooperation, the patient must fully understand the rationale behind these restrictions. Complete rest is imperative and often the only therapy effective in preventing progression to abortion. However, there is no guarantee this therapy will be effective.

Mild sedation may be necessary for relief of uterine discomfort and to promote restfulness.

Nursing diagnosis

Potential for fluid volume deficit related to hemorrhage secondary to inevitable, incomplete, or complete abortion.

GOAL #1: Prompt recognition of increasing blood loss.

Interventions

1. Instruct the at-home patient with a threatened abortion to record a pad count and report immediately any increase in vaginal bleeding (particularly if it is as much or more than during regular menstruation) to appropriate personnel.

2. Monitor hospitalized patients for signs of hemorrhage, including:
● sudden increase in pad count and in degree of saturation
● passage of large or numerous clots
● bright red vaginal bleeding
● tachycardia
● hypotension
● diaphoresis
● pallor.

Rationale

The abortive process places the patient at risk for excessive bleeding and deterioration to hemorrhagic shock. Close monitoring of these patients is essential for prompt detection of increased blood loss. The patient with inevitable abortion begins to bleed more heavily as the abortion progresses. An incomplete abortion, when only partial placental separation occurs, interferes with sufficient uterine contraction, which is necessary for adequate hemostasis. Bleeding will continue until complete evacuation is accomplished.

GOAL #2: Restore and maintain a normovolemic state.

GENITOURINARY

Interventions

1. Ensure adequate peripheral I.V. access with large-bore catheters. Administer fluid replacement as ordered.

2. Obtain blood samples for baseline data including hemoglobin/hematocrit levels, WBC and platelet counts, type and cross matching, and Rh determination. Monitor trends.

3. Administer packed RBCs and replace clotting factors, as ordered.

4. Monitor vital signs as frequently as the patient's condition warrants, for example, every 5 to 15 minutes while the patient remains unstable.

5. Insert an indwelling urinary catheter using sterile technique. Monitor urine output hourly during the unstable phase.

Rationale

Anticipating impending blood loss and instituting measures to prevent hypovolemia can avoid the development of hemorrhagic shock. Large-bore I.V. catheters facilitate rapid crystalloid administration and blood replacement necessary to restore normovolemia. Trend analysis of laboratory data, vital signs, and urine output helps evaluate resuscitative efforts and direct further therapy.

GOAL #3: Minimize further blood loss.

Interventions

1. Administer an oxytocin infusion, as ordered. Monitor vital signs and uterine contractions closely during infusion. Administer analgesia, as ordered.

2. Prepare the patient for operative intervention and notify operating room personnel. (See "Preparation for Surgery" in Section VII.)

Rationale

Oxytocin and other oxytocic drugs facilitate the delivery process and the completion of the abortion. They produce contractions with the intensity, frequency, and duration of those seen in spontaneous labor. The uterine contractions aid expulsion of the fetus or the retained placental fragments and thus reduce bleeding. Analgesia is usually required as oxytocin intensifies the pain associated with contractions.

Dilatation and curettage may be necessary if complete abortion does not occur spontaneously. This procedure ensures complete removal of any retained products of conception.

Nursing diagnosis

Potential for infection related to incomplete or instrumentation-induced abortion.

GOAL: Recognize early signs of infection.

Interventions

1. Monitor the patient closely for signs of infection:
- fever
- foul, purulent vaginal discharge
- constant lower abdominal or back pain
- elevated WBC count
- chills, night sweats (48 hours after instrumentation).

Rationale

A patient may seek emergency care for a preexisting infection resulting from an instrumentation-induced abortion. The patient with an incomplete abortion may develop profound sepsis related to intrauterine bacterial infections, caused by retained products.

GENITOURINARY

2. Obtain the patient's medication allergy history; administer antibiotics, as ordered.

Broad-spectrum antibiotics may be instituted either prophylactically or after identification of positive cultures. At least two doses may be ordered prior to dilatation and curettage.

Nursing diagnosis

Potential for anxiety related to sudden hospitalization, termination of pregnancy, and uncertainty of future pregnancies.

GOAL: Reduce the patient's anxiety level and support her coping mechanisms.

Interventions

1. Provide explanations in terms the patient can understand. Ask for patient feedback. Reinforce information as necessary. Include her partner in information-sharing sessions, when possible. Reinforce that a spontaneous abortion at less than 14 weeks is never her "fault."

2. Encourage visitation and phone calls from her family and friends when possible.

3. Facilitate baptism of the fetus if requested by the mother or family. Contact family or hospital clergy as requested.

4. Provide information on available counseling services for both parents, as appropriate. Encourage and discuss the grieving process. Offer information on the possibility or probability of recurrence in a future pregnancy.

Rationale

Clear communication and feedback promote understanding and reduce event-related anxiety.

This promotes use of her established support systems.

Acknowledging religious beliefs and granting requests for or facilitating specific rites, such as baptism, offer spiritual support and comfort.

Patients may experience a variety of psychological effects after an abortion. Guilt, fear for viability of future pregnancies, and severe depression may all require professional counseling.

Additional considerations

The Rh-negative mother requires an anti-D immune globulin (RhoGAM) injection within 72 hours of the termination of the pregnancy if the products of conception were determined to be Rh positive. (Abortion clinics may routinely provide RhoGAM because in early spontaneous abortion there may not be enough products to test.) RhoGAM prevents isoimmunization, the mother's formation of Rh antibodies, which will occur in reaction to the agglutinogens produced in a future Rh-positive fetus. These antibodies can cross the placenta and destroy fetal cells, causing erythroblastosis fetalis in future pregnancies.

Associated care plans	Associated procedure
Abdominal Trauma During Pregnancy: Blunt and Penetrating	Preparation for Surgery
Psychosocial Support of the Trauma Patient	
Hemorrhagic Shock	
Vasogenic Shock	
Disseminated Intravascular Coagulation	

GENITOURINARY

RENAL SYSTEM INJURY
(Kidney, Bladder, Ureter, Urethra)

Assessment

**Mechanism of injury/
etiology:**
• blunt trauma: pedestrian, motor vehicle, motorcycle, bicycle accidents; crushing or straddle injuries (from falls); assaults; industrial accidents
• penetrating trauma to the chest, back, abdomen, flank, or genital or perineal areas

Physical findings:
Genitourinary
• obvious wounds; abrasions; contusions; edema around genitals, perineum, abdomen, flank, pelvis
• pain/tenderness in abdomen, back, flank
• abdominal or bladder distention
• ecchymosis over flanks or around umbilicus
• blood at the urinary meatus
• inability to urinate spontaneously
• no urine output after catheterization
• difficult or unsuccessful catheterization
• hematuria (obvious or microscopic)
• displaced prostate gland

Cardiovascular
• shock state

Associated injuries:
• pelvic fractures
• intraabdominal injury

Diagnostic studies

• contrast studies—evaluate structural integrity and function of urethra, bladder, kidneys, ureters
  ☐ urethrography
  ☐ excretory urography, or intravenous pyelography (IVP)
  ☐ retrograde cystography
• diagnostic peritoneal lavage—may help diagnose intraperitoneal bladder rupture, but usually inconclusive if rupture is extraperitoneal
• abdominal radiograph—may reveal mass, loss of psoas-muscle shadow
• CT scan—evaluates structural integrity and function of the renal system when performed using contrast material, identifies fluid accumulation, hematomas

Potential for fluid volume deficit related to hemorrhage secondary to kidney injury.

GOAL: Restore and maintain a normovolemic state.

Interventions

1. Monitor the patient for signs of hemorrhagic shock; monitor and document vital signs every 5 to 15 minutes; monitor ECG rhythm and neurologic status.

2. Ensure adequate I.V. access with two large-bore peripheral catheters; administer fluids, as ordered.

3. Apply a pneumatic antishock garment (PASG) as indicated. (See "The Pneumatic Antishock Garment" in Section VII.)

Rationale

Disruption or penetration of a solid organ, such as the kidney, can cause significant blood loss and decreased tissue perfusion and may lead rapidly to profound shock. Trend analysis of cardiovascular and neurologic status helps determine the shock state. Table 2.1 in "Hemorrhagic Shock" in Section II lists physical findings in early and late shock stages.

Hemorrhagic shock requires rapid, aggressive fluid replacement with colloid and crystalloid products.

The PASG can act as a tamponade or pressure dressing for penetrating and blunt injuries and may redistribute some portion of the blood from the lower extremities to the vital organs.

GENITOURINARY

4. Obtain baseline laboratory data and monitor trends in CBC, blood urea nitrogen levels, creatinine, electrolyte, and ABG levels, and coagulation profile.

Trend analysis of laboratory data helps evaluate tissue perfusion, renal function, fluid balance, and the overall effectiveness of resuscitative efforts.

5. Monitor the patient's respiratory status and note trends; anticipate the need for supplemental oxygen.

Supplemental oxygen enhances tissue perfusion by increasing oxygen availability at the alveolar/capillary membrane. Early oxygen therapy may prevent or minimize secondary pulmonary complications.

6. Insert an indwelling urinary catheter using aseptic technique; monitor ongoing intake/output balance; test urine for occult blood.

Urine output is a valuable parameter, reflecting tissue perfusion. Microscopic hematuria suggests renal system injury and requires additional diagnostic studies.

Nursing diagnosis

Potential for altered urinary elimination related to disruption in urethral, ureteral, kidney, or bladder integrity.

GOAL: Recognize urinary tract injury and prevent further injury.

Interventions

Rationale

1. Assess the patient for signs of urinary tract injury, including:
- urge, but inability, to void spontaneously
- blood at the urinary meatus
- difficult or unsuccessful catheterization
- no urine output after catheterization
- obvious or microscopic hematuria.

Signs and symptoms of urinary tract injury are usually subtle if not completely occult. A high index of suspicion based on mechanism of injury and signs and symptoms aids early injury detection. All initial urine samples should undergo hematesting.

2. Encourage the patient to urinate spontaneously.

Premature or overzealous attempts to insert a urinary catheter may cause further injury to a partially torn or lacerated urethra.

3. Insert an indwelling urinary catheter if the patient cannot urinate spontaneously but lacks obvious signs of blood at the urinary meatus. Abandon the catheterization attempt if you meet any resistance or obstruction.

Inability to urinate despite urgency and adequate volume replacement may indicate a urinary tract injury. Urinary catheterization should not be tried when there is blood at the urinary meatus because of the high probability of injury. Discontinuing catheterization when you meet resistance minimizes the risk of extending an injury. Instead, consult the urologist for evaluation and diagnosis.

4. Prepare the patient for retrograde urethrography:
- assemble necessary equipment, including contrast material
- notify appropriate radiology personnel
- assist as needed.

Blood at the urinary meatus suggests urinary tract injury, which should be investigated using retrograde urethrography before attempting catheterization. Notifying the radiographer early expedites the diagnostic procedure. This and other studies for urinary tract injury are easily performed at the bedside with portable radiographic equipment.

5. Prepare the patient for an IVP:
- assemble the necessary equipment, including contrast material
- question the patient or family about allergies to iodine-based products, dye, and shellfish
- notify appropriate radiology personnel
- assist as needed.

An IVP is indicated for those patients with signs of kidney or ureteral injury. The study should be performed before retrograde cystography to ensure proper visualization of upper urinary tract structures. If the patient has a history of iodine-product allergy, anticipate untoward effects.

GENITOURINARY

6. Prepare the patient for retrograde cystography:
- assemble necessary equipment, including contrast material
- notify appropriate radiology personnel
- assist as needed.

Retrograde cystography is indicated for those patients with hematuria and other signs of bladder trauma. Early diagnosis of bladder injuries is essential because an undetected accumulation of urine in the intraperitoneal cavity can cause serious complications. The procedure should follow an IVP to ensure adequate ureteral visualization. Extravasated contrast material from a bladder rupture can obscure ureteral injuries. You may need to coordinate this study with the orthopedist because results of additional radiographs for pelvic injuries may also be inconclusive if extravasation from the bladder occurs.

Nursing diagnosis

Potential for infection related to peritoneal inflammation by the presence of free urine and blood secondary to disrupted integrity of the bladder, ureters, or urethra.

> **GOAL:** Recognize early signs of infection.

Interventions

1. Monitor and document temperature with vital signs; note trends in laboratory data, especially the WBC count.

Rationale

Signs of infection may not become evident for several hours after the injury. Trend analysis aids early detection of an infectious process. Trauma to the bladder, ureters, and urethra may cause urine extravasation, furnishing a perfect medium for bacterial growth.

Additional considerations

Except for injury to the kidney, injury to the urinary tract is seldom life-threatening; however, the long-term ramifications of such injuries mandate early recognition and appropriate therapy. Undiagnosed ureteral injuries permit ongoing urinary extravasation and predispose the patient to chronic infections. They are also associated with ureteral strictures, which cause outflow disorders and obstructions and allow urine accumulation in the kidney region. All these complications may require further operative intervention. Urethral injuries, regardless of severity and initial management, may cause strictures and chronic impotence; chronic, long-term infections may plague this patient.

Associated care plans	**Associated procedures and study**
Hemorrhagic Shock	Positive Contrast Study
External Genitalia Injury	Preparation for Surgery
	The Pneumatic Antishock Garment

GENITOURINARY

Medical diagnosis

EXTERNAL GENITALIA INJURY

Assessment

Mechanism of injury/ etiology:
- "power-takeoff" injuries—clothing or skin caught in moving parts of a motor vehicle or of an industrial or farm machine
- bullet or stab wound
- self-inflicted trauma
- straddle injury
- abuse-related assault

Physical findings:
- lacerations
- contusions
- avulsions
- edema
- in women, external genitalia injuries are rare:
  - ☐ abrasions
  - ☐ hematomas
  - ☐ minor lacerations
- in men, testicular injuries involve:
  - ☐ severe pain radiating to groin or flank
  - ☐ nausea or vomiting

Associated injuries:
- pelvic fractures
- renal system injuries

Nursing diagnosis

Impaired skin and tissue integrity related to local trauma.

GOAL: Promote healing and minimize tissue loss.

Interventions

1. Prepare sterile suturing equipment, and assist as needed.

2. Apply cool packs to external genitalia and elevate or support the scrotum, if needed.

3. Prepare the patient for surgery (see "Preparation for Surgery" in Section VII).

Rationale

Suturing lacerations approximates tissue and shortens healing time.

If hematomas, contusions, or edema are present, cool packs minimize bleeding into the tissue. These measures also help ease pain.

Proper debridement and repair require an operative procedure. Rupture must be ruled out or repaired if the testis is to be salvaged. In scrotal tissue avulsion, a thigh pouch may temporarily be used to cover the testes until scrotal skin regenerates. Penile lacerations or loss of skin may require surgical exploration and repair. Some partial avulsion injuries to the penile shaft may require skin grafting. Partial avulsion injuries, if incorrectly managed, can obstruct lymphatic drainage, producing a distal-segment lymphedema.

Nursing diagnosis

Disturbance in self-concept related to altered body and sexual image or sexual function secondary to external genitalia injury.

GOAL: Assist the patient in reconstructing his altered body image.

GENITOURINARY

Interventions

1. Establish trust with the patient:
- encourage his expressions about the injury and himself
- encourage him to ask questions
- provide an environment conducive to ventilation of feelings
- avoid negative criticism
- involve the patient in self-care.

2. Initiate health teaching and referrals, as indicated.

Rationale

All human beings have sexual feelings, and physical manifestations are an integral part of these complex feelings of one's perceived sexuality. Developing a therapeutic relationship with the patient assists him in coping with and resolving the traumatic changes.

Nursing diagnosis

Potential for altered patterns of urinary elimination related to mechanical obstruction or pain secondary to edema or hematoma.

GOAL: Provide a method for urinary elimination; relieve pain related to urinary obstruction or retention.

Interventions

1. Measure the patient's spontaneous urinary output. Report inadequate output, bladder distention, or inability to void (despite urgency) to the physician.

2. Assemble equipment and insert an indwelling urinary catheter, if ordered. Use sterile technique for catheter insertion.

Rationale

Edema or hematoma can make urination difficult, painful, or impossible. Assessments of the patient's ability to void indicate whether or not catheterization is necessary.

Catheterization bypasses obstructions and alleviates urinary retention. The use of sterile technique prevents contamination and possible subsequent urinary tract infection.

Nursing diagnosis

Alteration in comfort related to pain secondary to external genitalia injury.

GOAL: Minimize or alleviate pain.

Interventions

1. Assess the patient's pain level:
- observe changes in his vital signs
- observe his facial expressions
- observe him for guarding of the painful site
- obtain subjective data from the patient.

2. Administer pain medication, as ordered. Observe the patient for side effects.

Rationale

Pain is subjective. However, by careful observation and evaluation, you can assess it in a patient and take measures to alleviate it.

Associated care plans	**Associated procedure**
Psychosocial Support of the Trauma Patient Renal System Injury	Preparation for Surgery

GENITOURINARY

TRAUMATIC AMPUTATION

Assessment

Mechanism of injury/etiology:
• sudden loss of limb or body part caused by cut, crush, or avulsive injury; may be complete or partial

Physical findings:
Musculoskeletal
• cut amputation—wound with well-defined edges, damage is local
• crush amputation—damage to the tissue and arterial intima, either localized or extended some distance
• avulsive amputation—tissue torn and stretched away by force; separation of vascular and neural structures may occur at varying degrees of proximity to the bone/cartilage defect

Cardiovascular
• tachycardia
• hypotension
• pale mucous membranes
• possibly profound hemorrhagic shock

Respiratory
• tachypnea

Psychosocial
• anxiety
• fear

Diagnostic studies

• radiograph of injured area—determines severity of bone injury

• angiogram—determines vascular status of partial amputations

Nursing diagnosis

Potential fluid volume deficit related to hemorrhage.

GOAL #1: Establish hemostasis at the injury site.

Interventions

1. Apply a sterile pressure dressing to the injury site. Do not use a tourniquet unless all other measures to control bleeding prove ineffective.

2. Monitor the patient for signs of hemorrhagic shock. (See Table 2.1 in "Hemorrhagic Shock.")

Rationale

Pressure dressings minimize damage to vascular and neural structures while effecting hemostasis. Tourniquet application can increase neural and vascular damage because of its narrow constricting band. Hemostats can further damage vascular structures by crushing them. "Blind" grabs for bleeders may inadvertently damage nerves, which lie in close proximity to vascular structures.

Hypovolemic shock may indicate ineffective hemostasis. Massive blood loss during the prehospital phase and from associated injuries may account for a persistent shock state.

GOAL #2: Restore and maintain a normovolemic state.

Interventions

1. Ensure adequate venous access with a minimum of two large-bore catheters.

Rationale

Large-bore catheters permit rapid infusion of large fluid volumes, which may be required to restore a normovolemic state.

MUSCULOSKELETAL

2. Establish baseline data and monitor trends in hemoglobin/hematocrit and coagulation studies.

These studies help determine the need for blood and blood component replacement.

3. Monitor the patient for signs of hypovolemic shock.

Persistence of hypovolemic shock indicates inadequate volume replacement, inadequate hemostasis, and possibly additional injury.

Nursing diagnosis

Potential for infection related to wound contamination and devitalized soft tissue secondary to traumatic amputation.

GOAL #1: Prevent or minimize the risk of wound infection.

Interventions

1. Obtain the patient's history regarding allergic reaction to medications.

2. Ensure the availability of supplies for wound culture.

3. Use sterile technique for all wound care.

4. Avoid the use of iodine-based solutions in the open wound.

5. Prepare supplies for wound irrigation under pressure of 7 to 10 psi (35-cc syringe with 18G to 20G needle).

6. Administer antibiotics, as ordered.

7. Pad cool packs used to reduce soft tissue edema.

Rationale

Allergies to specific medications will influence the choice of antibiotic therapy.

Detection of specific organisms in the wound may affect the choice of antibiotic therapy.

Sterile technique minimizes the introduction of pathogens into the wound.

Free iodine can be absorbed by the tissue and may elevate serum iodine levels. Also, iodine is toxic to the cells responsible for tissue repair and local defense.

Mechanical wound cleansing with irrigation at this pressure effectively removes debris and bacteria without forcing microorganisms further into the soft tissue.

Antibiotics must be started as early as possible during the resuscitative period to decrease the risk of postinjury sepsis.

Cool packs are recommended for the treatment of soft tissue edema. Ice packs placed directly against the skin or inadequately padded cause burns and severe vasoconstriction with decreased perfusion. Decreased tissue perfusion increases the risk of infection.

GOAL #2: Prevent the risk of traumatic tetanus.

Interventions

1. Obtain a history of environmental factors involved with the mechanism of injury.

2. Obtain the patient's tetanus immunization history.

Rationale

The organism *Clostridium tetani* is a spore-forming, gram-positive bacillus commonly found in the intestinal contents of humans and animals. Thus, any injury involving farm equipment or occurring in a farm-type environment increases the patient's risk for tetanus.

Immunization must be active to prevent traumatic tetanus. (See Appendix 6, "Tetanus Prophylaxis.")

Nursing diagnosis

Decreased tissue perfusion to limb or appendage related to vascular injury secondary to partial amputation.

GOAL: Optimize tissue perfusion to partially amputated limb or appendage.

Interventions

1. Splint the partially amputated limb or appendage in normal anatomical alignment without twisting or applying tension to the soft tissue flap.

2. Elevate the affected part, but not higher than the level of the heart. Apply a cool pack over the wound dressing and the partially amputated limb or appendage. Place loosely wrapped gauze, or a substitute, between the cool pack and the skin.

Rationale

The remaining soft tissue flap may contain intact vascular structures, allowing for some perfusion to the partially amputated part.

Elevation increases venous return, thereby decreasing swelling. Cooling slows the ischemic process, thus increasing tissue viability. Cooling also aids preservation of skin and muscle tissue, which can be used for wound coverage if replantation is not possible. Separating the cool pack from the skin of the amputated part reduces the risk of a cold burn to the tissue.

Nursing diagnosis

*Potential for muscle tissue death of amputated part related to ischemia secondary to partial or complete amputation.

Note: *Two important factors in successful limb replantation are correct care of the limb from the time of injury and the timely transfer of the patient to a replantation center. Preestablished procedures and guidelines for transfer to a replantation center facilitate an effective and efficient transfer process and increase the chances for successful replantation.*

GOAL: Minimize the risk of muscle tissue ischemia.

Interventions

1. Apply sterile saline dressings to exposed soft tissue on the amputated part and stump. Avoid the use of iodine-based solutions.

2. Wrap the partially or completely amputated part in loose, bulky gauze and apply cool packs to the entire area.

3. Ascertain from the patient, his family, or prehospital care providers the time of injury and when cooling of the amputated part began.

4. Communicate with operating room personnel regarding preparation of the patient for surgery.

5. Prepare the patient for transfer to a replantation center, if required. Send copies of the patient care records with the patient.

Rationale

Moistened dressings help prevent dessication of the exposed tissue. Free iodine can be absorbed and can elevate serum iodine levels. Iodine is toxic to those cells responsible for tissue repair and local host defense.

Cooling increases tissue viability by slowing the ischemic process responsible for muscle tissue death. Bulky gauze placed between the tissue and the cool pack eliminates the risk of freezing, which would prevent revascularization.

The replantation team will need to know the estimated warm ischemic time to determine the part's viability.

Coordination with operating room personnel can facilitate a timely transfer to the operating room.

Replantation of an amputated part requires a center capable of microvascular surgery. The replantation team will need documentation of medications and fluids administered, warm/cool ischemic time of the limb or body part, and the patient's history.

*Supplemental nursing diagnosis

MUSCULOSKELETAL

Nursing diagnosis

Potential for fear and anxiety related to change in body image secondary to sudden, unexpected amputation.

GOAL: Decrease the patient's anxiety level. Support the patient's coping mechanisms.

Interventions

1. Maintain family contact via telephone or by allowing visiting prior to surgery.

2. Explain all procedures to the patient using comprehensible terms; repeat explanations as needed.

3. Monitor the bedside conversation of health care personnel; restrict conversation concerning sensitive topics, such as the wound, stump, and blood loss.

Rationale

This allows the patient access to his established support systems.

Anxiety may alter the patient's ability to comprehend events. The patient's short-term memory may also be affected, requiring repeated explanations.

The patient may misinterpret conversations, resulting in an increase in anxiety.

Associated care plans

Hemorrhagic Shock
Soft Tissue Injuries
Fractures: Open/Closed
Psychosocial Support of the Trauma Patient
Hand Injuries

Associated procedure

Preparation for Surgery

Medical diagnosis

MASSIVE PELVIC INJURY

Assessment

Mechanism of injury/ etiology:
- blunt trauma as from a fall, crushing mechanism, deceleration injury, pedestrian/vehicle collision, ejection from motorcycle
- penetrating mechanisms as from a gunshot, explosion

Physical findings:
Cardiovascular
- hypotension
- tachycardia
- obvious hemorrhage from pelvic wounds
- shock state

Musculoskeletal
- pain, the most common sign of injury; continuous and aggravated by palpation, pelvic compression, or movement; complaints of low-back pain
- crepitus, pelvic instability or unusual movement on palpation
- obvious rotation, shortening, or malalignment of lower extremities
- open wounds, abrasions, contusions
- impaired movement and sensation in the lower extremities
The patient may be asymptomatic initially.

Abdominal
- abdominal pain and tenderness

Genitourinary
- edema and ecchymosis of the perineum, genitals, rectum, and upper thighs
- perineal or genital pain from bleeding into the surrounding tissue
- hematuria, frank or occult
- blood at the urinary meatus
- inability to urinate

Associated injuries:
- intraabdominal injuries
- bladder injuries
- urethral injuries
- genital injuries
- sciatic nerve injuries
- injury to major pelvic blood vessels
- retroperitoneal hematoma

Diagnostic studies

- anteroposterior radiography of the pelvis, including both hips—should be a standard admission radiograph on all blunt trauma patients
- inlet, outlet, and judet (oblique) views—help determine the amount of pelvic-ring displacement and bony fragment location
- computed tomography of the pelvis—aids evaluation of pelvic-ring and retroperitoneal hematoma
- pelvic arteriogram—is diagnostic for locating bleeding vessels and therapeutic for embolizing bleeding vessels
- diagnostic peritoneal lavage, cystography, intravenous pyelography (IVP), and urethrography—may be performed to diagnose intraabdominal, bladder, and urinary tract injuries

Nursing diagnosis

Potential for decreased tissue perfusion related to fluid volume deficit secondary to massive pelvic hemorrhage.

> **GOAL:** Optimize cellular perfusion; restore a normovolemic state.

Interventions

1. Monitor the patient for signs of hemorrhagic shock; monitor vital signs every 5 to 15 minutes; monitor ECG rhythm and neurologic status.

Rationale

The primary cause of early death after massive pelvic injury is exsanguination. The rich arterial and venous networks lie close to the bony pelvis. The venous plexus consists of fragile, thin-walled vessels, which are easily disrupted by trauma and pelvic fractures. Also, the pelvic basin and retroperitoneal space can accommodate as much as 4 liters of blood before the formation of a tamponade, making it difficult to accurately estimate blood loss. Close monitoring is essential because the patient may appear stable initially but can deteriorate rapidly. Table 2.1 in "Hemorrhagic Shock" in Section II summarizes the signs of early and late shock.

MUSCULOSKELETAL

2. Ensure adequate I.V. access with at least two large-bore peripheral catheters; administer fluids as ordered.

Early, aggressive volume replacement with colloid or crystalloid products is necessary to combat hemorrhagic shock. Trend analysis of laboratory data aids accurate evaluation of tissue perfusion, fluid balance, and overall effectiveness of the resuscitative efforts. Prolonged clotting times often develop and require early detection and aggressive therapy.

3. Obtain baseline laboratory studies and monitor trends in CBC, electrolyte, and ABG levels, and coagulation profiles.

4. Ensure the availability of adequate amounts of packed red blood cells (PRBCs) and clotting factors for early transfusions; follow hospital policy for filtering, warming, and infusing blood.

Early, aggressive blood replacement is a major component of effective care. A patient with a massive pelvic injury may also have associated intraabdominal injuries, causing additional blood loss and complicating the shock state. Early initiation of component therapy with PRBCs and clotting factors, such as fresh-frozen plasma and platelets, may prevent a potentially lethal coagulopathy. If coagulation disorders are not detected early, or if they persist, they aggravate the hemorrhagic process and may lead to the patient's death.

5. Monitor and document the patient's respiratory status and trends; anticipate the need for supplemental oxygen.

Tachypnea (> 20 breaths/minute) develops in Class II shock, and rates increase as the shock deepens. Supplemental oxygen administration improves tissue perfusion and, when started early, may minimize later pulmonary complications.

Nursing diagnosis

Potential for persistent fluid volume deficit related to hemorrhage secondary to coagulopathy and fracture site disruption.

> **GOAL #1:** Recognize early signs of persistent bleeding.

Interventions

1. Monitor the patient continuously for signs of hemorrhagic shock.

Rationale

Coagulopathies may develop early if the patient requires aggressive and numerous blood transfusions; they create a vicious and potentially lethal cycle. The patient with a massive pelvic injury may lose a significant yet undetected volume of blood. Continuous monitoring of all hemodynamic and laboratory parameters is essential for accurate evaluation of resuscitative efforts.

> **GOAL #2:** Minimize or halt further bleeding; immobilize fractures.

Interventions

1. Use caution when moving, lifting, or transporting the patient.

Rationale

Early rehabilitation measures include preventing further injury and maintaining existing function. To reduce the risk of greater neurovascular injury from mobile bone ends, the patient should be gently and safely moved by a sufficient number of personnel. Sudden, exaggerated movement can release a retroperitoneal hematoma, causing rapid deterioration in the patient's condition. A long wooden backboard and the logroll and total body lift techniques can lower the risks of all exaggerated movement.

2. Apply a pneumatic antishock garment (PASG) as indicated; follow protocols for proper application, maintenance, and removal. (See "The Pneumatic Antishock Garment" in Section VII.)

Despite the controversy surrounding the actual effects of a PASG on blood redistribution, its ability to provide a tamponade or pressure dressing effect remains undisputed. Bleeding may be controlled or minimized since the PASG provides compression and immobilization of the fractured bone ends. It also serves as an excellent pressure dressing for patients with extensive, open wounds associated with pelvic disruption. In essence, a PASG buys time for transporting the patient to the hospital and carrying out initial resuscitative attempts.

3. Anticipate application of an external pelvic fixator; follow protocols for emergency surgery preparation. (See "Preparation for Surgery" in Section VII.) Notify operating room personnel.

The external pelvic fixator can control or stanch bleeding. Application of this metallic device requires surgical insertion of pins into both iliac wings. The pins are then connected to a trapezoid metal frame that aligns and compresses the bones of the pelvic ring. Decreased movement of bone ends reduces blood loss, release of particulate matter, the risk of further vascular injury, and the development of compartment syndrome. This compression frame facilitates early patient mobilization in the postoperative and recovery phase as well. Application of the fixator is usually performed in the operating suite and requires operative preparation, including informed consent from the patient or family.

4. Anticipate the need for pelvic embolization; ensure the availability of an adequate number of personnel and adequate equipment to provide safe transport of the patient to the angiography suite. (See "Therapeutic Embolization" in Section VII.)

Identifying and successfully embolizing bleeding vessels are lifesaving procedures for the patient with a massive pelvic injury. Pelvic embolization is a major and often lengthy procedure, requiring careful planning and coordination with all team members. Adequate supplies and equipment and sufficient personnel must be on hand for continuous patient monitoring and possible emergency interventions.

5. Anticipate the need for an emergency operative procedure. (See "Preparation for Surgery" in Section VII.)

In addition to the external pelvic fixator, the patient may need more extensive surgical intervention. Packing of the pelvis, direct embolization, or repair or ligation of bleeding vessels may increase morbidity and mortality risks but may be attempted in grave situations. Associated intraabdominal or genitourinary injuries may also necessitate surgical management.

Nursing diagnosis

Potential for decreased tissue perfusion and sensorimotor deficit related to compression of neurovascular bundles secondary to compartment syndrome in the pelvic and/or gluteal muscle groups.

GOAL: Recognize the early signs of compartment syndrome; initiate prompt therapy.

*Supplemental nursing diagnosis

MUSCULOSKELETAL

Interventions

1. Monitor the patient for signs of compartment syndrome:
- pelvic:
  - ☐ pain in the inguinal ligament and on passive hip extension after flexion
  - ☐ paresthesia around the medial aspect of the lower leg
  - ☐ paresis
  - ☐ firm fascial compartment on palpation
- gluteal:
  - ☐ pain after hip flexion or adduction
  - ☐ paresthesia of sciatic nerve–innervated muscles
  - ☐ paresis
  - ☐ firm fascial compartment on palpation.

Report positive findings immediately.

2. Ensure availability of equipment and assist with intracompartment pressure measurements. (See "Intracompartment Pressure Measurement" in Section VII.)

Rationale

Both the iliacus compartment in the pelvis and the gluteal compartment in the buttocks can develop increased pressures leading to compartment syndrome. Delayed therapy or persistent bleeding from injured pelvic vessels can precipitate this serious complication. Increased muscle tissue fluid pressures can occlude intracompartment microcirculation, leading to muscle ischemia and muscle and nerve necrosis. Early recognition facilitates prompt surgical intervention to reduce the compartment pressure, thus minimizing damage.

Intracompartment pressure measurements supplement the clinical examination and confirm the diagnosis.

Nursing diagnosis

Potential for altered urinary elimination related to disruption of urinary tract secondary to pelvic injury.

GOAL #1: Recognize the high-risk patient early.

Interventions

1. Assess the patient for signs of urinary tract injury, including urine hematest.

Rationale

Renal injuries, urethral lacerations or transections, and bladder perforations or ruptures, commonly associated with massive pelvic injuries, require rapid detection and prompt therapy to reduce later morbidity.

GOAL #2: Prevent further injury to, and promote early diagnosis of disruption of, the urinary tract.

Interventions

1. Use caution when inserting an indwelling urinary catheter; do not insert a catheter if blood is detected at the urinary meatus; stop at once if you meet resistance.

2. Ensure the availability of appropriate contrast materials and catheters for:
- urethrography
- IVP
- cystography.

Rationale

Urethral injuries represent significant, potentially long-term problems because they often cause strictures and may cause impotence in the male patient. Inserting a urinary catheter into a covertly injured urethra may extend a laceration.

A patient with symptoms of renal, bladder, or urethral injuries requires further diagnostic studies.

Nursing diagnosis

Potential for decreased sensory perception and motor function related to nerve disruption secondary to pelvic fracture.

GOAL #1: Recognize sciatic nerve involvement early.

Interventions

1. Assess the patient for signs of sciatic nerve damage, including:
- altered or impaired sensation in the affected leg
- footdrop
- inability to plantar- or dorsiflex foot.

Rationale

Detecting a sciatic nerve injury can be difficult during resuscitation. Altered level of consciousness or decreased sensation from concomitant injuries, shock, and chemical intoxication can obscure clinical findings.

GOAL #2: Prevent further sciatic nerve injury.

Interventions

1. Maintain proper pelvic and limb alignment and immobilization as much as possible. Ensure sufficient staff to move the patient safely and gently.

Rationale

Further disruption of fractured pelvic bones, as from excessive movement, can increase injury severity. Although detection and therapy for sciatic nerve damage are not high priorities during resuscitation, prevention of further injury is essential since it may prolong and complicate rehabilitation.

Additional considerations

The patient with a massive pelvic injury and trauma to other major systems often poses a tremendous challenge to the trauma team. Accurately determining treatment priorities, even in the most prepared and best-staffed facility, may be difficult. The patient can quickly deplete a blood bank's supply with his urgent need for massive volumes of blood and clotting factors. Angiographic facilities may be unavailable at night or on weekends. For these and other reasons, the patient often requires rapid transfer to a more sophisticated health care facility. Established protocols for patient transfer and rapid transportation help make the process smooth and efficient.

The patient with an injury to the posterior, or weight-bearing, portion of the pelvis, including bony and ligamentous structures, usually requires extensive rehabilitation. Associated sciatic nerve injury or other extremity fractures may also complicate the patient's return to mobility and self-care. All efforts should be made both to preserve existing function and to prevent further injury or complications. They should be initiated immediately after injury and maintained throughout the patient's hospital stay.

Associated care plans

Hemorrhagic Shock
Intraabdominal Trauma: Blunt and
   Penetrating
Renal System Injury
Compartment Syndrome
Disseminated Intravascular Coagulation

Associated procedures and study

Therapeutic Embolization
Diagnostic Peritoneal Lavage
Intrahospital Transport of the Shock Trauma Patient
The Pneumatic Antishock Garment
Preparation for Surgery
Intracompartment Pressure Measurement
Positive Contrast Study

MUSCULOSKELETAL

FRACTURES: Open/Closed

Assessment

Mechanism of injury/ etiology:
Closed fracture

- blunt trauma: pedestrian/vehicular accident, fall, sporting accident

Open fracture

- those mechanisms listed for closed fracture
- penetrating trauma, as from a gunshot wound

Physical findings:
Musculoskeletal

Open and closed fracture:
- pain
- muscle spasm
- crepitus
- ecchymosis
- edema
- angulation/rotation
- shortening of affected

extremity
- altered skin color
  □ pale indicates arterial compromise
  □ bluish indicates venous congestion
- decreased capillary refill time (CRT)
- decreased motor strength
- decreased range of motion
- altered sensation

Open fracture:
- exposed bone
- open wound within zone of injury (open wound not always directly over fracture site)
- fat globules in the wound

Classification of fractures:
- type of fracture line—transverse, spiral,

oblique, greenstick
- number of fracture lines—comminuted, multiple fracture lines with bone fragment(s); simple, one-fracture line
- location of fracture line along bone structure—diaphyseal, metaphyseal, epiphyseal, intraarticular
- displacement of fracture—impacted, distracted, angulated, degree of translation
- presence or absence of direct communication between fracture and external environment

Grades of open fractures:
- I—low-energy wound, < 1 cm long, minimal soft tissue damage

- II—wound > 1 cm long, higher energy than in Grade I, moderate soft tissue damage
- III—high-energy wound, > 10 cm long, with significant avulsion, soft tissue damage, muscle devitalization, or wound flap; includes high-velocity gunshot or shotgun wounds, bumper mechanism wounds, open-segment fractures, wounds with neurovascular involvement, and those occurring on a farm or in a barnyard

Associated injuries:
- neurovascular disruption
- soft tissue injury
- compartment syndrome
- fat embolism syndrome

Diagnostic studies

Open fracture:
- clinical findings—may alone determine diagnosis
- wound exploration—may be required to determine if direct communication exists between fracture and external environment

Closed and open fracture:
- radiography (anterior-posterior, lateral, oblique views)—helps classify the fracture
- computed tomography scan—provides additional information in diagnosing fractures, especially fractures involving articulating surfaces
- tomograms

Nursing diagnosis

Potential for further impairment of tissue integrity related to mobility of fractured bone ends and fragments.

GOAL: Prevent further soft tissue disruption.

Interventions

1. Immobilize the fracture site, including joints above and below it. Assist the physician and other personnel in establishing fractured bone alignment by using traction apparatus as necessary.

2. Apply a cool pack over the suspected zone of injury and elevate the fracture site when possible.

3. Maintain fracture immobilization during any procedure in which movement of the fracture site is necessary.

Rationale

The sharp ends of fractured bones can cause considerable damage to surrounding soft tissue. Immobilization, the first treatment step for any fracture, minimizes bone movement. Traction prevents overriding of bone ends caused by muscle spasm.

Edema from the soft tissue injury and the fracture can increase pressure on neurovascular structures, causing more damage. Cooling and elevation help reduce the edema. Think of any fracture in terms of the zone of injury: that is, as an injury to both bone and soft tissue. Fractured bone ends can override each other and then transect through a considerable amount of soft tissue, creating a large area of soft tissue injury.

Movement of the affected site is sometimes necessary to complete diagnostic procedures and treatments. Assigning specific personnel to maintain immobilization and traction minimizes further soft tissue injury.

Nursing diagnosis

Potential for fluid volume deficit related to disruption of vascular supply in bone and surrounding soft tissue secondary to fracture.

Note: *Significant blood can be lost in open and closed fractures. In a closed fracture, the volume of blood lost before tamponade depends on the potential space available. More blood can be lost from an open than from a closed fracture. Potential estimated blood loss from fractures follows:*

Table 2.10

Fracture site	Closed fracture	Open fracture
Humerus	1 to 2 units	
Ulna/radius	½ to 1 unit	Estimate an additional 1 to 3 units for all fracture sites.
Pelvis	2 to 12 units	
Tibia/fibula	½ to 4 units	
Ankle	½ to 2 units	

GOAL: Restore and maintain normovolemia.

Interventions

1. Ensure venous access with large-bore catheters; administer fluids as ordered.

2. Apply a sterile dressing to the open wound. Continue to estimate blood loss.

3. Obtain baseline and serial hemoglobin/hematocrit levels and monitor heart rate and blood pressure. Anticipate the need for RBC replacement.

4. Maintain immobilization and traction of the fracture.

Rationale

Large-bore catheters permit rapid replacement of fluid volume necessitated by significant blood loss.

A secure, nonconstricting dressing helps control bleeding. Continued bleeding indicates ineffective hemostasis.

Bleeding associated with fractures can cause hemorrhagic shock. RBCs may be required as part of the total fluid volume replacement. (See "Hemorrhagic Shock" in Section II.)

Moving fractured bone ends can aggravate soft tissue injury, increase bleeding, and disrupt a tamponade.

MUSCULOSKELETAL

Nursing diagnosis

Potential for infection related to wound contamination and devitalized soft tissue secondary to open fracture.

> **GOAL #1:** Prevent or minimize the risk of wound infection.

Interventions	Rationale
1. Obtain the patient's history of allergic reactions to medications.	Allergies to specific medications can alter antibiotic therapy.
2. Ensure availability of necessary supplies for wound culture.	Specific organisms in the wound can also alter antibiotic therapy.
3. Use sterile technique in all wound care.	This decreases the introduction of pathogens into the wound.
4. Avoid iodine-based solutions in the open wound.	The tissue can absorb free iodine and elevate serum iodine levels. Iodine is also toxic to the cells responsible for tissue repair and local antimicrobial defense.
5. Prepare supplies for wound irrigation under a pressure of 7 to 10 psi (35-cc syringe with an 18G to 20G needle).	Wound irrigation at this pressure effectively removes debris and bacteria without forcing microorganisms deeper into the soft tissue.
6. Administer antibiotics as ordered.	Antibiotics must be administered as early as possible during resuscitation to reduce the risk of postinjury sepsis.
7. Prepare the patient for possible transfer to the operating room.	Extensive soft tissue wounds require irrigation and surgical debridement.

> **GOAL #2:** Minimize the risk of traumatic tetanus.

Interventions	Rationale
1. Obtain the history of the environmental factors involved in the mechanism of injury.	The microorganism *Clostridium tetani* is a spore-forming, gram-positive bacillus often found in the intestinal contents of humans and animals. Any injury either involving farm or barnyard equipment or occurring on a farm or in a barnyard increases the patient's risk of tetanus.
2. Obtain the patient's tetanus immunization history; administer appropriate immunization as ordered.	Immunization must be active to prevent traumatic tetanus. (See Appendix 6, "Tetanus Prophylaxis.")

Nursing diagnosis

Potential for decreased tissue perfusion in affected extremity related to progressive arterial occlusion secondary to tearing and stretching of the arterial intima at the time of injury.

> **GOAL:** Recognize early signs of vascular compromise; prevent further vascular injury.

Interventions

1. Assess and document the quality of pulses above and below the fracture, CRT, and skin temperature every 30 minutes. Compare findings with those for the opposite extremity. Immediately report abnormal findings to the physician.

2. Maintain immobilization and traction of the fracture.

3. Prepare the patient for arteriography if arterial damage is suspected.

Rationale

At the time of fracture, arterial stretching and tearing can occur. This damage often causes the intimal lining to tear without occluding the lumen. Initially, pulse quality may be normal. Constant arterial pressure against the intimal flap, however, can lead to intimal lining dissection, causing gradual occlusion. Occlusion, in turn, decreases tissue perfusion, slows CRT, and lowers skin temperature. The zone of injury extends above and below the fracture site. The zone's extent depends on the amount of energy applied and absorbed to cause the injury. Vascular injuries can occur proximal as well as distal to the fracture site.

Immobilization and traction further constrain movement, including overriding caused by muscle spasm.

Arteriography can confirm vascular damage.

Nursing diagnosis

Potential for motor and sensory deficit related to nerve damage secondary to fracture.

> **GOAL:** Recognize a patient with nerve damage; minimize further damage.

Interventions

1. Assess and document the patient's ability to differentiate among a sharp, dull, and light touch above and below the level of the fracture.

2. Assess and document the patient's motor ability by testing muscle groups above and below the level of the fracture.

3. Ensure immobilization and traction of the fracture.

Rationale

Inability to discriminate between contrasting stimuli reflects injury to the peripheral nerve's sensory component.

Decreased motor strength against active and passive resistance reflects injury to the peripheral nerve's motor component.

Further neural compression, tearing, and stretching can occur if movement and overriding of bone ends continue.

Nursing diagnosis

Potential for altered tissue perfusion and sensorimotor deficit related to compression of neurovascular bundles secondary to compartment syndrome.

> **GOAL #1:** Recognize early signs of compartment syndrome; minimize the risk of associated complications.

*Supplemental nursing diagnosis

MUSCULOSKELETAL

Interventions	Rationale
1. Assess patients with fractures for signs of increased compartment pressure: • pain—out of proportion to injury or occurring on passive stretching of muscle groups • firmness of fascial compartments on palpation • paresthesia • paralysis. Immediately report earliest physical findings of compartment syndrome to the physician.	Patients with open or closed fractures are at risk for compartment syndrome. Even minor injuries can subject muscle groups within fascial compartments to increased pressure from bleeding or edema. External sources, such as a cast, air splints, a pneumatic antishock garment, and dressings can also cause increased compartment pressures. Pain is the earliest symptom. Treatment must be initiated early to prevent irreversible muscle damage. (See "Compartment Syndrome" in Section IV.) **Note:** *Intracompartment pressures of 30 to 60 mm Hg can cause muscle ischemia. Because the diastolic pressure of the main artery traveling through the compartment is greater than 30 to 60 mm Hg, the quality of pulses and CRTs distal to the compartment are usually not affected. Therefore pulse quality and CRTs are not useful as assessment criteria. The exception to this is in compartment syndrome of the hands and feet, where the normal distal end arterial pressures are lower. In these situations the compartment pressures above can easily impair arterial flow and diminish CRTs.*
2. Ensure the availability and proper functioning of equipment needed to remove external causes of compartment syndrome. Prepare the patient for transfer to the operating room if surgical intervention is required. (See "Preparation for Surgery" in Section VII.)	Treatment is aimed at reducing intracompartment pressure by accommodating tissue swelling. Early decompression restores adequate tissue perfusion and prevents muscle necrosis. Often, treatment may be as simple as removing a cast, splint, or dressings that have prevented the fascial compartment from expanding to its maximum size. Surgical intervention involves opening the fascial sheath, releasing the pressure on the neurovascular bundles caused by tissue swelling.

GOAL #2: Minimize the risk of compartment syndrome.

Interventions	Rationale
1. Apply a cool pack to the zone of injury; elevate the extremity, when possible; and maintain immobilization of the fracture.	Cooling and elevation reduce swelling. Immobilization minimizes further soft tissue injury and bleeding into fascial compartments.

Nursing diagnosis

Potential for decreased tissue perfusion related to occlusion of pulmonary vasculature secondary to mobilization of fat globules and altered fat metabolism.

GOAL: Minimize the risk of fat embolism syndrome.

Interventions	Rationale
1. Monitor the patient closely for early signs of fat embolism syndrome: rapid onset of respiratory distress, altered mentation, and fever.	Recognizing fat embolism syndrome early and initiating proven therapeutic measures promptly help reduce patient morbidity. (See "Fat Embolism Syndrome" in Section IV.)
2. Maintain immobilization of the fracture. Handle the fracture gently when movement is necessary.	Immobilization reduces movement of bone ends or fragments, which release fat globules from the marrow into the circulation after injury.

Nursing diagnosis

Alteration in comfort secondary to fracture.

GOAL: Promote patient comfort.

Interventions

1. Apply a cool pack to the zone of injury. Elevate the extremity when possible. Maintain immobilization and traction.

2. Administer analgesics as ordered. Assess and document their effectiveness.

Rationale

Immobilization, traction, cooling, and elevation all reduce the pain associated with edema, soft tissue injury, and muscle spasm.

Besides the measures already cited, analgesia may be required. If pain continues or is out of proportion to what would be expected, suspect neurovascular compromise.

Nursing diagnosis

Impaired physical mobility related to mechanical or medical restrictions secondary to fracture.

GOAL: Mobilize the patient as early as possible.

Interventions

1. Educate the patient concerning methods to prevent immobility-related complications. Elicit his cooperation in maintaining as much mobility as conditions permit.

2. Assist in preparations needed for fracture treatment, for example:
• ensure availability of supplies and equipment for casting, splinting, and traction
• communicate with operating room personnel about preparing the patient for surgical repair (internal/external fixation).

Rationale

The most common risks of immobility can be prevented by simple interventions, such as turning, coughing, deep breathing, and range-of-motion exercises.

The method of fracture stabilization is determined by considering the patient's other injuries, potential complications, and physiologic status. Treatment must be aimed not just at the fracture but at the whole patient. Methods promoting early patient mobility reduce the risk of immobility-related complications.

Associated care plans

Compartment Syndrome
Fat Embolism Syndrome
Soft Tissue Injuries

Associated procedures

Intracompartment Pressure Measurement
Preparation for Surgery

MUSCULOSKELETAL

Medical diagnosis

DISLOCATIONS

Assessment

Mechanism of injury/ etiology:
- blunt trauma as from a fall or a vehicular or sports-related accident
- twisting injury

Physical findings:
Musculoskeletal
- deformity
- soft-tissue edema
- pain (localized)
- decreased range of motion

- decreased motor strength
- decreased sensation
- rotation of extremity
- shortening of extremity
- prolonged capillary refill time (CRT)

- pallor
- alteration in distal pulse quality

Associated injuries:
- neurovascular injuries
- fractures

Diagnostic studies

- radiography—several views needed to determine type of dislocation
- computerized tomography—to provide more information on joint condition
- arteriogram—to identify and evaluate vascular injury

Nursing diagnosis

Potential for further impairment of tissue integrity related to stretching, tearing, contusion, and compression of soft tissue structures secondary to movement of dislocated joint.

GOAL: Minimize further soft tissue disruption.

Interventions

1. Immobilize and splint the dislocated joint in the position of deformity. Apply a cool pack to the area. Monitor the underlying skin for a cold burn.

Rationale

Immobilizing the joint minimizes further soft tissue, including neurovascular disruption. Applying a cool pack reduces soft tissue edema. Ice is not recommended because it severely vasoconstricts and impairs local tissue perfusion.

Nursing diagnosis

Potential for impaired physical mobility related to inadequate return of joint function secondary to delayed reduction of dislocation.

GOAL: Maximize physical mobility.

Interventions

1. Assist the orthopedist and radiographic technician as needed to obtain radiographs.

2. Administer analgesics and muscle relaxants as ordered.

Rationale

Radiographs are necessary to complete the diagnosis and help determine treatment.

Severe muscle spasms cause intense pain, hindering joint reduction. Analgesics and muscle relaxants may be required to reduce spasms, facilitating reduction.

MUSCULOSKELETAL

3. Assist with reduction and postreduction immobilization as needed.

Early reduction provides the most effective treatment and the best chance of regaining joint function. Complete or partial joint immobilization postreduction prevents redislocation and promotes soft tissue healing.

4. Anticipate transferring the patient to the operating room. (See "Preparation for Surgery" in Section VII.)

General anesthesia may be required to achieve full muscular relaxation to permit closed reduction. Open joint reduction is required if interposing soft tissue or bone fragments prevent reduction.

Nursing diagnosis

Potential for decreased tissue perfusion and impaired sensorimotor function related to disruption of neurovascular structures secondary to joint dislocation.

GOAL: Recognize signs and symptoms of neurovascular compromise. Prevent or minimize the risk of permanent injury.

Interventions

Rationale

1. Assess and document the neurovascular status of the affected extremity hourly, including:
- skin color and temperature
- pulse quality
- CRT
- ability to differentiate among a sharp, dull, and light touch
- two-point discrimination
- motor strength.

Potential or actual neurovascular compromise renders some joint dislocations true orthopedic emergencies. Elbow dislocations can disrupt the brachial artery and the median and ulnar nerve. Shoulder dislocations can cause brachial plexus and axillary arteriovenous injuries. Hip dislocations can disrupt the integrity of the sciatic and femoral nerves and the femoral artery and vein. Hip dislocations can also cause aseptic necrosis of the femoral head; the incidence is higher in posterior than in anterior dislocations. Knee dislocations greatly increase the risk of injury to the common peroneal nerve and the popliteal artery.

Intervention must be immediate to prevent or minimize permanent damage, including sensorimotor deficit, loss of joint function, and loss of the limb.

2. Prepare the patient for an arteriogram, if required.

An arteriogram is necessary to confirm or rule out vascular injury. A popliteal artery arteriogram is commonly performed based on the mechanism of injury alone, because the incidence of vascular injury with knee dislocations is so high. Signs and symptoms of vascular compromise are not always evident in vascular disruption. A one-shot arteriogram can determine the popliteal artery's structural integrity.

3. Prepare the patient for surgery. (See "Preparation for Surgery" in Section VII.)

Damage to neurovascular structures requires surgical repair.

Associated care plan	Associated procedure and study
Fractures: Open/Closed	Preparation for Surgery Positive Contrast Study

MUSCULOSKELETAL

*Supplemental nursing diagnosis

SOFT TISSUE INJURIES

Assessment

Note: *Soft tissue injuries—including those to blood and lymphatic vessels, nerves, muscles, and tendons—are classified by causes, associated injuries, extent of contamination, and whether primary wound healing will occur. In a tidy wound, the wound is clean, risk of infection low, soft tissue loss minimal or absent, and damage to the wound edge limited. In an untidy wound, the mechanism of injury includes crushing or avulsive forces with extensive soft tissue damage and loss, devitalized tissue, a high infection risk, and necrosis.*

Mechanism of injury/ etiology:
- blunt trauma—from shearing, crushing, or avulsive forces as caused by a vehicular or sports-related accident, bumper injury, fall
- penetrating trauma—from shotgun blasts, gunshot wounds, impaling injuries, stabbings
- burns

Physical findings:
Musculoskeletal
- wound (from avulsion, degloving, laceration, crushing injury)
- ecchymosis
- fracture (open or closed)
- burn (thermal, chemical, electrical)

Cardiovascular
- tachycardia
- hypotension

- pallor
- change in pulse quality
- prolonged capillary refill time (CRT)
- paresthesia
- paresis

Respiratory
- tachypnea

Genitourinary
- hemoglobinuria
- myoglobinuria
- oliguria
- anuria

Associated injuries:
- fractures

Diagnostic studies

- clinical examination—determines neurovascular status
- radiograph—to identify foreign objects and associated injuries
- angiogram—to assess potential vascular injuries

- laboratory data—hemoglobin/hematocrit, coagulation studies, urine hemoglobin and myoglobin—help identify complications associated with soft tissue injuries (for example, shock, coagulopathy, myoglobinuria)

Potential for fluid volume deficit related to hemorrhage and fluid loss into third space secondary to soft tissue injury.

GOAL: Restore and maintain normovolemia.

Interventions

1. Monitor vital signs, including heart rate, blood pressure, and urine output. Estimate blood loss. Ensure venous access with at least two large-bore catheters. Administer fluid replacement as ordered.

2. Apply or maintain a sterile pressure dressing to the wound. Continue estimating blood loss.

Rationale

Significant blood loss leads to hypovolemia, requiring fluid-volume replacement. Large-bore catheters permit rapid infusion of fluid.

A pressure dressing helps control bleeding without aggravating damage to neurovascular structures. Continued bleeding reflects ineffective hemostasis.

MUSCULOSKELETAL

3. Obtain baseline and serial hemoglobin/hematocrit and coagulation studies and analyze trends. Anticipate the need for RBC and blood product replacement. (See "Hemorrhagic Shock" in Section II.)

Soft tissue injury bleeding can cause hypovolemic shock and coagulation defects. RBCs and blood products may be needed as part of the total fluid volume replacement. With massive crushing injuries, redistribution of plasma into the third space can induce hypovolemia and hemoconcentration.

Nursing diagnosis

Potential for soft tissue necrosis related to decreased tissue perfusion secondary to excessive manipulation of soft tissue segment.

> **GOAL:** Prevent or minimize soft tissue necrosis.

Interventions

1. Assess vascular status of the soft-tissue flap, including CRT and skin temperature.

2. Maintain the soft-tissue flap in near-anatomic alignment. Minimize handling of the flap.

Rationale

Alteration in the vascular supply to the flap lowers skin temperature and prolongs CRT.

Twisting and excessively handling the flap further compromise vascular supply and increase the risk of necrosis.

Nursing diagnosis

Potential for impaired urinary elimination related to tubular necrosis secondary to crush syndrome.

> **GOAL:** Minimize the risk of tubular necrosis.

Interventions

1. Test urine for myoglobin and hemoglobin. Monitor urine output and pH. Administer I.V. fluids, bicarbonate, and an osmotic diuretic as ordered.

Rationale

Muscle ischemia and contusion can result in the release of myoglobin and hemoglobin into the plasma. If untreated, myoglobin and hemoglobin precipitation in the renal tubules can lead to tubular necrosis. Treatment consists of maintaining alkaline urine and promoting an output of at least 100 cc/hour.

Nursing diagnosis

Potential for infection related to wound contamination and devitalized tissue.

> **GOAL #1:** Prevent or minimize wound infection.

Interventions

1. Use sterile technique with all wound care.

2. Immobilize soft tissue with a moist sterile saline dressing. Avoid iodine-based solutions in the wound.

Rationale

This step decreases the introduction of pathogens into the wound.

Immobilizing the soft tissue reduces the spread of microflora by slowing lymphatic flow. Moist sterile saline dressings can prevent tissue desiccation, which compromises antibiotic efficacy. The tissue can absorb free iodine, which is toxic to cells responsible for tissue repair and local antimicrobial defense.

MUSCULOSKELETAL

*Supplemental nursing diagnosis

3. Avoid applying ice directly over the wound.

Ice causes severe vasoconstriction and decreases tissue perfusion, increasing the risk of infection. Cool packs are recommended to help reduce edema. If ice packs are used, ensure adequate padding between the skin and the ice pack.

4. Ensure the necessary supplies for wound culture. Obtain the patient's medication-allergy history.

Wound cultures reflect the bacteria present and signal their antibiotic sensitivities. Antibiotics are most often used in crush injuries or avulsive wounds because of extensive tissue ischemia. Allergies to specific medications limit antibiotic selection.

5. Prepare supplies for irrigation of the wound under pressure of 7 to 10 psi (35-cc syringe with an 18G to 20G needle).

Mechanical wound cleansing at this pressure effectively removes debris and bacteria without forcing microorganisms deeper into the soft tissue.

6. Provide a local anesthetic without epinephrine for contaminated wounds.

Epinephrine's vasoconstrictive effect can promote ischemia and increase the risk of infection.

GOAL #2: Prevent the risk of traumatic tetanus.

Interventions

1. Obtain a history of environmental factors related to the mechanism of injury. Obtain the patient's tetanus immunization history. Administer tetanus toxoid as ordered.

Rationale

The organism *Clostridium tetani* is a spore-forming, gram-positive bacillus often found in the intestinal flora of humans and animals. Any injury involving farm equipment or occurring in a farmyard setting increases the patient's risk for tetanus. The patient's immunization must be active if it is to prevent traumatic tetanus. (See Appendix 6, "Tetanus Prophylaxis.")

GOAL #3: Prevent or minimize delay in wound healing.

Interventions

1. Apply the dressing to the wound after repair in layers—first the porous, nonadherent, then the absorbent—and secure the bandage.

Rationale

The porous, nonadherent layer facilitates blood and fluid drainage from the wound and its absorption by the second layer. This minimizes fluid accumulation within the wound. Otherwise, the site becomes ideal for bacterial growth, which can delay healing.

2. Secure any drains inserted into the wound to prevent accidental dislodging. Monitor drainage type and volume. Notify the physician if the drain becomes dislodged.

Drains are inserted into the wound to prevent blood and fluid accumulation. If blood and fluid accumulate, healing takes longer because the body needs time to reabsorb the fluid. The fluid also provides an excellent medium for bacterial growth. Foul-smelling or purulent drainage indicates infection.

Associated care plans

Hemorrhagic Shock
Fractures: Open/Closed

MUSCULOSKELETAL

HAND INJURIES

Assessment

Mechanism of injury/ etiology:
- crushing forces caused by industrial or farm machinery
- lacerations from sharp instruments or other cutting devices
- infection caused by high-pressure injection

devices, extravasation of I.V. medications, human or animal bite
- electrical, chemical, or thermal burns

Physical findings:
Musculoskeletal
- lacerations

- puncture, crush, or avulsive wound
- soft tissue swelling
- deformity
- discoloration
- foreign body in hand
- absent pulse
- pallor
- prolonged capillary refill time (CRT)

- poikilothermy
- edema
- cyanosis

Neurologic
- paresthesia
- paralysis
- pain

Diagnostic studies

- radiography—identifies fractures, dislocations, and location of radiopaque foreign bodies
- xeroradiography—helpful in identifying nonradiopaque

substances embedded in soft tissue
- angiography—assesses integrity of hand circulation

Potential for sensory and motor deficit related to nerve/tendon damage.

GOAL: Establish presence and extent of sensory/motor impairment.

Interventions

1. Observe the hand at rest. The wrist should be in slight extension, the fingers forming a normal cascade of progressive finger flexion, the small finger being most flexed.

2. Ask the patient or others about the mechanism of injury and the position of the hand and digits when the injury happened.

3. Ask the patient to extend his wrist and digits simultaneously.

4. Assess the patient's ability to abduct his index finger against resistance. Simultaneously palpate his first interosseous muscle, located in the dorsal web space, to confirm its contraction.

Rationale

Normal digital stance may be altered by a tendon injury. This may be the only clue to an injury in a small, uncooperative child or a comatose adult.

A crushing injury usually produces more extensive damage, whereas a sharp laceration produces more localized damage. A tendon lacerated while in flexion travels distally from the skin site when placed in extension. This normal retractive process makes repair complex, requiring a hand surgeon.

Inability to perform strong, full extension indicates potential radial nerve injury and requires further evaluation. Wrist extension is critical for grasping, which is integral to normal hand functioning.

Inability to contract the first dorsal interosseous muscle required to perform this function indicates ulnar nerve impairment. The ulnar nerve is the "nerve of power" and is critical for strong pinching, which is integral to normal hand functioning.

MUSCULOSKELETAL

*Supplemental nursing diagnosis

5. Assess the patient's ability to abduct his thumb toward the ceiling, away from the palm while the palm is turned upward. Simultaneously palpate the thenar muscle, located below the volar surface of the thumb metacarpophalangeal (MP) joint, to confirm its contraction.

Inability to contract the thenar muscle needed to perform this function indicates median nerve impairment. The median nerve is the "nerve of precision" and is critical for accurate sensibility.

6. Test for sensation at the thumb's dorsal web space.

Radial nerve integrity can be discriminately assessed by testing sensation in the hand segment innervated solely by this one nerve.

7. Test for sensation on the tip of the little finger's volar surface.

Ulnar nerve integrity can be discriminately assessed by testing sensation in the hand segment innervated solely by this one nerve.

8. Test for sensation at the tip of the index finger's volar surface.

Median nerve integrity can be discriminately assessed by testing sensation in the area of the hand innervated solely by this one nerve.

9. Assess the patient's ability to flex each digit's distal interphalangeal (DIP) joint while holding the MP and proximal interphalangeal (PIP) joints in extension.

Inability to flex any DIP joint reflects an injury to the flexor digitorum profundus tendon.

10. Assess the patient's ability to flex each digit's PIP joint while all other digits are held in extension.

Inability to flex a digit's PIP joint reflects an injury to the flexor digitorum superficialis tendon. However, this test is unreliable for the index finger, which has an independent profundus tendon. Also, the flexor digitorum superficialis tendon may be weak, absent, or connected to the tendon of the ring finger. So, for an accurate assessment, let the patient flex *both* the ring finger and the little finger simultaneously.

11. Assess the patient's ability to actively extend all fingers.

Asymmetrical extension, usually at the DIP joint, indicates partial or complete disruption of the extensor tendons.

12. Assess the patient's ability to raise his thumb when his hand is placed palm down.

Inability to perform this movement indicates impairment of the extensor pollicis longus tendon, the most important of the thumb's extensor tendons.

13. Assess the patient's ability to discriminate between two points.

The normal digital two-point discrimination is 3 to 5 mm. The points should be initially set 10 mm apart and then brought closer until the patient can no longer discriminate between one or two points. Abnormal two-point discrimination suggests nerve integrity disruption. However, this test is inaccurate when done on the hand's dorsal surface owing to the poor tactile response there. Light touch would be a more reliable method in assessing this aspect.

14. Assess the patient for partial lacerations of the flexor tendons by testing for "PSST":
• **p**ain on active contraction

• **s**light alteration in stance

Normal muscle tone integrity is disrupted, causing pain, especially when the tendon is contracted.
To ease pain, the muscle relaxes slightly, altering the digit's stance.

MUSCULOSKELETAL

- **s**trength diminished

- **t**endon sheath involved.

When flexed against resistance, pain causes an involuntary response, inhibiting the muscle tendon unit and causing weakness. Assessing tendon sheath integrity is the physician's responsibility. A sheath laceration almost certainly points to tendon injury as well. **Note:** *In assessing the flexor tendon only in extension, the examiner may miss a partial laceration of the actual tendon. A partially lacerated flexor tendon is at risk of rupturing several days after injury, when it begins to soften during healing. Rupture usually causes severe disability.*

15. Perform the wrinkle test by immersing the fingers in warm water for 15 minutes. Examine the fingers' volar surface for wrinkling.

Loss of finger pad wrinkling ability reflects a disruption in sympathetic response. This test helps assess neural integrity in a small child or a comatose patient.

Nursing diagnosis

Potential for decreased tissue perfusion related to alteration in the hand's vascular flow.

GOAL #1: Establish hemostasis at the injury site.

Interventions	Rationale
1. Apply direct pressure to the actively bleeding site using a sterile dressing.	Direct pressure effectively maintains hemostasis without risking damage to neurovascular structures.
2. Avoid blind grabs with a hemostat to control active bleeding.	Because of the proximity of arteries to nerves in the hand, most blind grabs at an arterial bleeder result in crushed nerves.
3. Avoid the use of tourniquets during examination to control bleeding.	Histologic evidence shows that trying to control bleeding by pneumatic tourniquet can damage capillaries and striated muscle cells and lead to acidosis-related blood hypocoagulability.
4. Provide a local anesthetic (*without* epinephrine) if needed.	Epinephrine's vasoconstrictive effect further decreases tissue perfusion.

GOAL #2: Determine the presence and extent of vascular impairment.

Interventions	Rationale
1. Assess the hand for edema, color, CRT, and temperature.	A cool, pale hand and finger with poor CRT indicate major arterial insufficiency, whereas an edematous, cyanotic hand indicates venous insufficiency.
2. Assess both radial and ulnar arterial pulses. Perform the Allen's test by compressing both arteries simultaneously, then releasing one artery at a time.	The radial and ulnar arteries form a rich anastomotic network to the entire hand. But in some hands, due to individual variability, necrosis of one or more digits can develop if one of these arteries is compromised. The Allen's test helps identify the presence or absence of collateral arterial filling to the hand.
3. Assess the arteries at the tips of the digits' volar surfaces either by palpation or with a Doppler ultrasound blood flow detector.	Individual digital artery assessment can reveal specific circulatory compromise.

MUSCULOSKELETAL

4. Ascertain from the patient or others the time of injury to determine the ischemic time frames.

Reversing digital ischemia can be successful up to 12 hours after injury. This time is approximately double what is considered optimal for palms and limbs because of the lower digital muscle mass.

GOAL #3: Optimize tissue perfusion.

Interventions

1. Splint the hand in the position of function. The wrist should be in 30° extension, the MP joints in 60° to 80° flexion, the DIP/PIP joints in 5° to 10° flexion, and the thumb abducted 30° to 40° palmward.

2. Leave fingertips exposed.

3. Elevate the injured hand to heart level.

Rationale

Splinting the wrist in extension prevents occlusion of venous outflow across the dorsum of the hand and wrist. Keeping the wrist flexed can cause occlusion and lead to edema. Splinting the digits in the position of function maximizes collateral ligament stretch and minimizes the risk of contractures. Although this position is preferred for most hand injuries, it may have to be altered for isolated tendon injuries requiring other healing considerations.

Fingertip exposure provides easy access for continuing circulation assessment and sensory and motor function monitoring.

Elevation facilitates venous and lymphatic drainage, thereby minimizing venous congestion and the associated pain. Elevation also minimizes adhesion and fibrous tissue formation, which may subsequently restrict movement.

Nursing diagnosis

Potential for infection related to wound contamination and devitalized soft tissue secondary to specific mechanism of injury.

GOAL #1: Minimize the risk of traumatic tetanus.

Interventions

1. Ask the patient or others what environmental factors were associated with the injury.

2. Obtain the patient's tetanus immunization history. Administer tetanus toxoid and tetanus immune globulin if ordered. (See Appendix 6, "Tetanus Prophylaxis.")

Rationale

The risk of traumatic tetanus increases if the injury site was in contact with soil and animal or human waste.

Immunization must be active to prevent traumatic tetanus.

GOAL #2: Minimize the risk of rabies.

Interventions

1. Obtain information about the events surrounding an animal bite.

Rationale

The likelihood that the attacking animal was rabid increases if it was carnivorous, was feral (wild), and attacked without provocation. Details about the event facilitate the decision about initiating rabies prophylaxis. To be most effective, treatment must be initiated within several hours of the attack.

2. Obtain a blood sample for antibody titer if rabies prevention is necessary. Administer human diploid cell rabies vaccine or duck embryo vaccine for active immunization and human rabies immune globulin for passive immunization, as ordered.

Both active and passive immunization should be administered (except to a previously immunized patient) to prevent rabies. The Centers for Disease Control publishes a guide on such treatment.

3. Wash the wound and surrounding skin with soap and water.

Washing removes residual saliva around the wound.

4. Scrub or flush the wound with a 20% soap solution.

Soap solution provides a viricidal environment.

GOAL #3: Minimize the risk of wound infection.

Interventions

Rationale

1. Prepare supplies for scrubbing intact skin and irrigating the wound with copious amounts of sterile saline solution under 7 to 10 psi (35-cc syringe with an 18G to 20G needle).

Mechanical irrigation of the wound at this pressure effectively removes debris and bacteria without forcing microorganisms deeper into the soft tissue.

2. Assist with wound debridement and foreign body removal.

Organic foreign matter, as from wood and plants, has a greater potential for causing tissue reaction than do inorganic materials, such as glass or metal. Early debridement minimizes the risk of infection. Foreign substances injected into the hand by high-pressure injection devices can cause swelling and arterial thrombosis, leading to massive tissue necrosis. These devices are capable of ejection pressures of 1,500 to 12,000 psi, but create only a small, innocuous-looking puncture wound. Early and extensive surgical debridement by a hand surgeon is the treatment of choice.

3. Assist with radiography and xeroradiography as necessary.

Radiography helps identify radiopaque substances, such as paint deposits and metal objects. Xeroradiography helps visualize nonradiopaque substances, such as grease, multiple small glass fragments, and wood.

4. Prepare wound culture supplies before initiating antibiotic therapy.

Gram stains and cultures or specimens obtained from wounds and incised infections help guide antibiotic therapy.

5. Obtain the patient's history of medication allergies. Administer antibiotics as ordered.

Medication allergies influence the antibiotic choice. Administer antibiotics as soon as possible, while the bacterial count is still low.

GOAL #4: Promote wound healing.

Interventions

Rationale

1. Apply sterile saline-moistened gauze or nonadherent gauze directly to the open wound.

This type of dressing is easier and less painful to remove. Moistened or nonadherent gauze promotes blood migration from the wound via a "wicking effect," thereby minimizing the risk of hematoma.

MUSCULOSKELETAL

Nursing diagnosis

Potential for impaired hand mobility related to contracture formation.

GOAL: Preserve function and prevent potential disability.

Interventions

1. Apply a bulky hand dressing consisting of:
- interdigital gauze padding
- large quantities of fluffed gauze in the palm/thumb area
- large quantities of fluffed gauze on the dorsum of the hand.

Rationale

Interdigital gauze padding prevents web maceration. Adequate padding maintains thumb abduction and also supplies an absorbent, protective environment. Dorsal padding provides a mechanism for gentle compression, which is useful in reducing edema. The dorsum is particularly prone to edema because the skin is so loosely attached.

Nursing diagnosis

*Potential for muscle ischemia related to increased capillary permeability secondary to compartment syndrome.

GOAL: Recognize early signs of compartment syndrome to minimize the risk of permanent disability.

Interventions

1. Assess the patient closely for signs and symptoms of compartment syndrome:
- proximal forearm pain on passive finger extension
- palpable compartment firmness
- paresthesia of the hand
- progressive digital flexion contraction.

2. Prepare the patient for surgical decompression of the involved fascial compartments, if necessary. (For further details, see "Compartment Syndrome" in Section IV.)

*Supplemental nursing diagnosis

Rationale

The fascial compartments of the forearm and hand are at risk for compartment syndrome. Early recognition and treatment are necessary to prevent irreversible muscle damage.

Release of the constricted muscle through a fasciotomy may be the only way to reverse the ischemic process. This surgical decompression must be performed early for optimal recovery.

Additional considerations

Help reduce the number and extent of hand injuries by disseminating safety procedure information. Teach patients who operate machinery with moving parts to:
• remove jewelry and avoid wearing loose clothing—moving machine parts can snag on these surfaces and drag the extremity (even the whole body) into the machinery.
• form the habit of cutting off all power before checking machine malfunctions.
• minimize the extent of damage, should an accident occur, by turning off all power immediately and manually reversing gears to disengage the trapped body parts. (If this does not work, disassemble the machine for transport with the patient.)

The list of hazardous industrial equipment is virtually endless, but more familiar equipment presents unexpected dangers. Equipment used around the home that commonly causes injuries includes lawn mowers, hedge trimmers, snowblowers, ice makers, and blenders. Hazardous farm machinery includes tractors, hay balers, corn pickers, auger devices, and power takeoff equipment.

Associated care plans	**Associated procedures**
Fractures: Open/Closed	Preparation for Surgery
Traumatic Amputation	Intracompartmental Pressure Measurement
Soft Tissue Injuries	
Thermal Burns	
Electrical Burns	
Chemical Burns	
Compartment Syndrome	

MUSCULOSKELETAL

REFERENCES

INJURIES—ACUTE ILLNESSES— SHOCK STATES

Shock

American College of Surgeons. *Committee on Trauma Advanced Life Support Student Manual*, 1984.

Ballinger, W.F., II. *The Management of Trauma*, 2nd ed. Philadelphia: W.B. Saunders Co., 1973.

Bordicks, K.J. *Patterns of Shock, Implications for Nursing Care*, 2nd ed. New York: Macmillan Publishing Co., 1980.

Carpenito, L.J. *Nursing Diagnosis, Application to Clinical Practice*. Philadelphia: J.B. Lippincott Co., 1983.

Cowley, R A., and Dunham, C.M. *Shock Trauma/Critical Care Manual*. Baltimore: University Park Press, 1982.

Emergencies. Nurse's Reference Library. Springhouse, Pa.: Springhouse Corp., 1985.

Guthrie, M.M. *Shock*. New York: Churchill Livingstone, 1982.

Hincker, E.A., and Malasanos, L. *The Little-Brown Manual of Medical-Surgical Nursing*. Boston: Little, Brown & Co., 1983.

Lanros, N.E. "Assessment and Intervention in Emergency Nursing," in *Neurological Injuries*. Bowie, Md.: Robert J. Brady Co., 1978.

Perry, A.G., and Potter, P.A., eds. *Shock—Comprehensive Nursing Management*. St. Louis: C.V. Mosby Co., 1983.

Rice, V. "Shock, A Clinical Syndrome," *Critical Care Nurse*, Parts 1, 2, 3, 4, March/April, May/June, July/August, September/October 1982.

Roberts, S.L. *Physiological Concepts and the Critically Ill Patient*. Englewood Cliffs, N.J.: Prentice-Hall, 1985.

Thompson, M. *Shock Syndrome*. Reading, Mass.: Addison-Wesley Publishing Co., 1978.

Thompson, W.L., et al. *The Cell in Shock*. Kalamazoo, Mich.: Scope Publications, 1974.

Thompson, W.L., et al. *The Organ in Shock*. Kalamazoo, Mich.: Scope Publications, 1974.

Weil, M.H. "Current Concepts on Mechanism and Treatment of Cardiogenic Shock," *American Heart Journal* 92:103-13, 1976.

Neurologic

American Association of Critical Care Nurses. *Critical Care Nursing of the Multi-Injured Patient*. Edited by Mann, J.K., and Oakes, A.R. Philadelphia: W.B. Saunders Co., 1980.

Ballinger, W.F., II. *The Management of Trauma*, 2nd ed. Philadelphia: W.B. Saunders Co., 1973.

Carpenito, L.J. *Nursing Diagnosis, Application to Clinical Practice*. Philadelphia: J.B. Lippincott Co., 1983.

Cooper, P.R. *Head Injury*. Baltimore: Williams & Wilkins Co., 1982.

Davis, J.E., and Mason, C.B. "Spinal Cord Injury," in *Neurologic Critical Care*. New York: Van Nostrand Reinhold Co., 1979.

Henry, G.L., and Little, N. *Neurologic Emergencies, A Symptom Oriented Approach*. New York: McGraw-Hill Book Co., 1985.

Hickey, J.B. *The Clinical Practice of Neurological and Neurosurgical Nursing*. Philadelphia: J.B. Lippincott Co., 1981.

Nikas, D.L. "Acute Spinal Cord Injuries: Care and Complications," in *The Critically Ill Neurosurgical Patient*. New York: Churchill Livingstone, 1982.

Ricci, M.M., ed. *Core Curriculum for Neuroscience Nursing*, vols. 1 and 2, 2nd ed. Park Ridge, Ill.: American Association of Neuroscience Nurses, 1984.

Shires, G.T. *Care of the Trauma Patient*, 2nd ed. New York: McGraw-Hill Book Co., 1979.

Zedjik, C.P. *Management of Spinal Cord Injury*. Belmont, Calif.: Wadsworth Inc., 1983.

Respiratory

American College of Surgeons Committee on Trauma. *Advanced Trauma Life Support Student Manual*, 1984.

Asfaw, I., and Arbula, A. "Penetrating Wounds of the Pericardium on a Heart," *Surgical Clinics of North America* 37-48, February 1977.

Attar, S., et al. "The Widened Mediastinum in Trauma," *Annuals of Thoracic Surgery* 435-49, May 1972.

Ayella, R.A., et al. "Ruptured Thoracic Aorta Due to Blunt Trauma," *Journal of Trauma* 199-205, March 1977.

Ayella, R.J. *Radiologic Management of the Massively Traumatized Patient*. Baltimore: Williams & Wilkins Co., 1978.

Bigelow, D.B. "The Choices in Flail Chest," *Emergency Medicine*, May 1983.

Chung, E.K. *Cardiac Emergency Care*. Philadelphia: Lea & Febiger, 1980.

Cowley, R A., and Dunham, C.M. *Shock Trauma/Critical Care Manual*. Baltimore: University Park Press, 1982.

Duncan, C., and Erickson, R. "Pressures Associated with Chest Tube Stripping," *Heart & Lung* 166-71, November 1982.

Giesecke, A.H. "Anesthesia for Trauma Surgery," in *Anesthesia*, vol 2. Edited by Miller, R.D. New York: Churchill Livingstone, 1981.

Hoyt, K.S. "Chest Trauma—When the Patient Looks Bad, Act Fast. When the Patient Looks Good, Act Fast...," *Nursing83* 34-41, May 1983.

Kirsh, M., and Sloan, H. *Blunt Chest Trauma: General Principles of Management*. Boston: Little, Brown & Co., 1977.

Kohn, M.S. "Management of Chest Injuries," *Topics in Emergency Medicine* 79-94, May 1979.

Mann, J., and Oakes, A. *Critical Care Nursing of the Multi-Injured Patient*. Philadelphia: W.B. Saunders Co., 1980.

Maull, K.I. "Complications of Multisystem Trauma Management," in *Complications in Surgery and Trauma*. Edited by Greenfield, L.J. Philadelphia: J.B. Lippincott Co., 1984.

McSwain, N. "To Manage Multiple Injury," *Emergency Medicine* 207-43, November 1982.

Meller, S.M. "Functional Anatomy of the Larynx," *Otolaryngologic Clinics of North America* 17(1): 3-12, 1984.

Mills, J., et al. *Current Emergency Diagnosis and Treatment*, 2nd ed. Los Altos, Calif.: Lange Medical Pubns., 1983.

Nacelerio, E.A. "Axions of Emergency Management of Chest Injuries," *Hospital Medicine* 6-22, March 1969.

Naclerio, E.A. *Chest Injuries: Physiologic Principles and Emergency Management*. New York: Grune & Stratton, 1971.

O'Boyle, C., et al. *Emergency Care—The First 24 Hours.* East Norwalk, Conn.: Appleton-Century-Crofts, 1985.

Perdue, P. "Life-Threatening Respiratory Injuries," *RN* 27-33, April 1981.

Perdue, P. "Stab and Crush Wounds to the Heart," *RN* 63-65, 124, 126, May 1981.

Rich, N., and Spencer, F. *Vascular Trauma.* Philadelphia: W.B. Saunders Co., 1978.

Snow, J.B. "Diagnosis and Therapy for Acute Laryngeal and Tracheal Trauma," *Otolaryngologic Clinics of North America* 17(1): 101-06, 1984.

Stoelting, R.K. "Endotracheal Intubation," in *Anesthesia,* vol 1. Edited by Miller, R.D. New York: Churchill Livingstone, 1981.

Symbas, P.N. *Traumatic Injuries to the Heart and Great Vessels.* Springfield, Ill.: Charles C. Thomas, 1972.

Veise-Berry, S. "Nursing Consideration During Radiologic Examination of the Massively Injured Trauma Patient," *Critical Care Quarterly* 6(1): 55-63, 1983.

White, K.M. "Evaluating the Trauma of Gunshot Wounds," *American Journal of Nursing* 1589-93, October 1977.

Wilson, R.F., et al. "Non-Penetrating Thoracic Injuries," *Surgical Clinics of North America* 17-36, February 1977.

Cardiovascular

Asfaw, I., and Arbula, A. "Penetrating Wounds of the Pericardium on a Heart," *Surgical Clinics of North America* 37-48, February 1977.

Ayella, R.A., et al. "Ruptured Thoracic Aorta Due to Blunt Trauma," *Journal of Trauma* 199-205, March 1977.

Cheitlin, M.D., and Abbott, J.A. "Cardiac Emergencies," in *Current Emergency Diagnosis and Treatment,* 2nd ed. Edited by Mills, J., et al. Los Altos, Calif.: Lange Medical Pubns., 1985.

Chung, E.K. *Cardiac Emergency Care.* Philadelphia: Lea & Febiger, 1980.

Collicott, P. *Advanced Trauma Life Support Course for Physicians—Instructor Manual.* American College of Surgeons, 1984.

Cowley, R.A., and Dunham, C.M. *Shock Trauma/Critical Care Manual.* Baltimore: University Park Press, 1982.

Diseases. Nurse's Reference Library. Springhouse, Pa.: Springhouse Corp., 1981.

Himes, V.J. "Traumatic Cardiac Tamponade," *Journal of Emergency Nursing* 28-32, March/April 1980.

Hoyt, K.S. "Chest Trauma—When the Patient Looks Bad, Act Fast. When the Patient Looks Good, Act Fast...," *Nursing83* 34-41, May 1983.

Janeira, L.F. "Cardiac Tamponade—Relieving Fluid Pressure on the Heart," *Emergency* 44-48, February 1980.

Kirsh, M., and Sloan, H. *Blunt Chest Trauma: General Principles of Management.* Boston: Little, Brown & Co., 1977.

Perdue, P. "Stab and Crush Wounds to the Heart," *RN* 63-65, 124, 126, May 1981.

Rich, N., and Spencer, F. *Vascular Trauma.* Philadelphia: W.B. Saunders Co., 1978.

Sympas, P.N. *Traumatic Injuries to the Heart and Great Vessels.* Springfield, Ill.: Charles C. Thomas, 1972.

Woods, S.L. "Diagnosis and Treatment of the Patient with an Uncomplicated Myocardial Infarction," in *Cardiac Nursing.* Edited by Underhill, S.L., et al. Philadelphia: J.B. Lippincott Co., 1982.

Gastrointestinal

Auerback, P. "Trauma in the Pregnant Patient," in *Priorities in Multiple Trauma.* Edited by Meislin, H. Rockville, Md.: Aspen Systems Corp., 1980.

Baker, P. "Trauma in the Pregnant Patient," *Surgical Clinics of North America* 62(2):275-89, April 1982.

Cowley, R.A., and Dunham, C.M., eds. *Shock Trauma/Critical Care Manual.* Baltimore: University Park Press, 1982.

Cox, E.F. "Blunt Abdominal Trauma," *Annals of Surgery* 199(4): 467-74, April 1985.

Crosby, W. "Traumatic Injury During Pregnancy," *Clinical Obstetrics and Gynecology* 26(4), December 1983.

Elrad, H., and Gleicher, N. "Physiologic Changes in Normal Pregnancy," in *Principles of Medical Therapy in Pregnancy.* Edited by Gleicher, N. New York: Plenum Medical Book Co., 1985.

Foster, C. "The Pregnant Trauma Patient," *Nursing84* 58-63, November 1984.

Frey, C. *Initial Management of the Trauma Patient.* Philadelphia: Lea & Febiger, 1976.

Gunning, J. "For Controlling Intractable Hemorrhage: The Gravity Suit," *Contemporary OB/GYN* 22, 23-32, July 1983.

Higgins, S., and Garite, T. "Late Abrupteo Placentae in Trauma Patients: Implications for Monitoring," *Obstetrics and Gyncology* 63(3): Supp. 105-90, March 1984.

Hillard, P. "Physical Abuse in Pregnancy," *Obstetrics and Gynecology* 66(2):185-90, August 1985.

Marx, J.A., et al. "Limitations of Computed Tomography in the Evaluation of Acute Abdominal Trauma: A Prospective Comparison with Diagnostic Peritoneal Lavage," *Journal of Trauma* 25(10):933-37, October 1985.

Merlotti, G.J., et al. "Use of Peritoneal Lavage to Evaluate Abdominal Penetration," *Journal of Trauma* 25(3):228-31, March 1985.

Moncure, A.C., and Ottinger, L.W. "Abdominal Emergencies," in *MGH Textbook of Emergency Medicine,* 2nd ed. Edited by Wilkins, E.W. Baltimore: Williams & Wilkins Co., 1983.

Myers, R.A.M., et al. "A Safe, Semi-Open Procedure for Diagnostic Peritoneal Lavage," *Surgery, Gynecology and Obstetrics* 153:738-40, November 1981.

Newkick, E., and Fry, M. "Trauma During Pregnancy," *Focus on Critical Care* 12(6):30-39, December 1985.

Santos, O. "The Obstetrical Patient for Non-Obstetric Surgery," *Current Reviews for Nurse Anesthetists,* Lesson 9, vol. 7, 1984.

Shahinpour, N. "Disorders of the Hepatic System and Pancreas," in *Little-Brown Manual of Medical-Surgical Nursing.* Edited by Hincker, E.A., and Malasanos, L. Boston: Little, Brown & Co., 1983.

Sleisenger, M.H., and Fordtran, J.S., eds. *Gastrointestinal Disease: Pathophysiology, Diagnosis, Management.* Philadelphia: W.B. Saunders Co., 1973.

Stafford, P. "Protection of the Pregnant Woman in the Emergency Department," *Journal of Emergency Nursing* 7(3), May/June 1981.

Strange, J.M. "Abdominal Trauma," in *Trauma Nursing.* Edited by Cardona, V.D. Oradell, N.J.: Medical Economics Books, 1985.

Vander Veer, J.B. "Trauma During Pregnancy," *Topics in Emergency Medicine* 6(1):72-77, April 1984.

Waitkoff, B. "Disorders of the GI System," in *Little-Brown Manual of Medical-Surgical Nursing.* Edited by Hincker, E.A., and Malasanos, L. Boston: Little, Brown & Co., 1983.

Young, B., et al. "Pregnancy after Spinal Cord Injury: Altered Maternal and Fetal Response to Labor," *Obstetrics and Gynecology* 62(1):59-63, July 1983.

Genitourinary

Ballinger, W.F., II. *The Management of Trauma*, 2nd ed. Philadelphia: W.B. Saunders Co., 1973.

Chapin, D.S.: "Gynecologic and Obstetric Emergencies," in *MGH Textbook of Emergency Medicine*, 2nd ed. Edited by Wilkins, E.W. Baltimore: Williams & Wilkins Co., 1983.

Colapinto, V. "Trauma to the Pelvis: Urethral Injury," *Clinical Orthopaedics and Related Research* 151:46-55, September 1980.

Cook, L.S. "Genitourinary Trauma," in *Trauma Nursing*. Edited by Cardona, V.D. Oradell, N.J.: Medical Economics Books, 1985.

Cucco, C.D., and Moawad, A.H. "Obstetric and Gynecologic Emergencies," *Emergency Medicine*, 1983.

O'Boyle, C.M., et al, eds. *Emergency Care: The First 24 Hours.* East Norwalk, Conn.: Appleton-Century-Crofts, 1985.

Papper, S., and Williams, G. Rainey. *Manual of Medical Care of the Surgical Patient*, 2nd ed. Boston: Little, Brown & Co., 1981.

Shires, G.T. *Care of the Trauma Patient*, 2nd ed. New York: McGraw-Hill Book Co., 1979.

Weems, W.L. "Management of Genitourinary Injuries in Patients with Pelvic Fractures," *Annals of Surgery* 189(6), June 1979.

Musculoskeletal

Adelman, R., and Sarant, G. "Hand Injuries," in *Emergency Department Orthopedics*. Edited by Chipman, C. Rockville, Md.: Aspen Systems Corp., 1982.

Ayella, R.A., et al. "Transcatheter Embolization of Autologous Clot in the Management of Bleeding Associated with Fractures of the Pelvis," *Surgery, Gynecology and Obstetrics* 147(6):849-52, 1978.

Brotman, S., et al. "Management of Severe Bleeding in Fractures of the Pelvis," *Surgery, Gynecology and Obstetrics* 153(6): 823-26, 1981.

Bunkis, J., and Walton, R.L. "Wound Management," in *Current Therapy of Trauma 1984-1985*. Edited by Trunkey, D.D., and Lewis, F.R. Philadelphia: B.C. Decker, 1984.

Burgess, A.R., and Poka, A. "Musculoskeletal Trauma," *Emergency Medicine Clinics of North America* 2(4):871-81, 1984.

Cardona, V.D., ed. *Trauma Nursing*. Oradell, N.J.: Medical Economics Books, 1985.

Carter, P.R. *Common Hand Injuries and Infections*. Philadelphia: W.B. Saunders Co., 1983.

Cavanaugh, C.E. "Digital Replantation," *Critical Care Update* 5-17, August 1981.

Chapman, M.W., and Hansen, S.T. "Part II: Current Concepts in the Management of Open Fractures," in *Fractures in Adults*. Edited by Rockwood, C.A., and Green, D.P. Philadelphia: J.B. Lippincott Co., 1984.

Chipman, C., ed. *Emergency Department Orthopedics*. Rockville, Md.: Aspen Systems Corp., 1982.

Cowley, R A., and Dunham, C.M. *Shock Trauma/Critical Care Manual*. Baltimore: University Park Press, 1982.

Eron, L.J. "Prevention of Infection Following Orthopedic Surgery," *Antibiotics and Chemotherapy* 33:140-60, 1985.

Faddis, D., et al. "Tissue Toxicity of Antiseptic Solutions," *Journal of Trauma* 17(12):895-97, 1977.

Flint, L.M., et al. "Definitive Control of Bleeding from Severe Pelvic Fractures," *Annals of Surgery* 189(6): 709-16, 1979.

Gordon, L., et al. "From Amputation to Replantation," *Emergency Medicine* 15(10):94-100, 1983.

Harkess, J.W., et al. "Principles of Fractures and Dislocations," in *Fractures in Adults*. Edited by Rockwood, C. A., and Green, D.P. Philadelphia: J.B. Lippincott Co., 1984.

Hilt, N.E. "Emergency Care," in *Manual of Orthopedics*. Edited by Hilt, N.E., and Cogburn, S.B. St. Louis: C.V. Mosby Co., 1980.

Hohl, M., et al. "Fractures and Dislocations of the Knee," in *Fractures in Adults*. Edited by Rockwood, C.A., and Green, D.P. Philadelphia: J.B. Lippincott Co., 1984.

London, P.S. "The Management of Multiple Injuries," *Nursing Mirror* 145:17-19, 1977.

Looser, K.G., and Crombie, H.D. "Pelvic Fractures: An Anatomic Guide to Severity of Injury," *American Journal of Surgery* 132(5): 638-42, 1976.

Markison, R.E. "Trauma to the Extremities," in *Current Therapy of Trauma 1984-1985*. Edited by Trunkey, D.D., and Lewis, F.R. Philadelphia: B.C. Decker, 1984.

Mears, D.C., and Fu, F. "External Fixation in Pelvic Fractures," *Orthopedic Clinics of North America* 11(3), July 1980.

Naam, N.H., et al. "Major Pelvic Fractures," *Archives of Surgery* 118(5):610-15, May 1983.

Neer, C.S., and Rockwood, C.A., "Fractures and Dislocations of the Shoulder," in *Fractures in Adults*. Edited by Rockwood, C.A., and Green, D.P. Philadelphia: J.B. Lippincott Co., 1984.

Newmeyer, W.L. *Primary Care of Hand Injuries*. Philadelphia: Lea & Febiger, 1979.

Pennal, G.F., et al. "Assessment and Classification," *Clinical Orthopaedics and Related Research* 151:12, September 1980.

Rockwood, C.A., and Green, D.P., eds. "Fractures and Dislocations of the Elbow," in *Fractures in Adults*. Philadelphia: J.B. Lippincott Co., 1984.

Rockwood, C.A., and Green, D.P., eds. "Fractures and Dislocations of the Hip," in *Fractures in Adults*. Philadelphia: J.B. Lippincott Co., 1984.

Shires, G.T. *Principles of Trauma Care*, 3rd ed. New York: McGraw-Hill Book Co., 1984.

Smoot, E.C., and Robson, M.C. "Acute Management of Foreign Body Injuries of the Hand," *Annals of Emergency Medicine* 434-36, July 1983.

Soderstrom, C.A. "Severe Pelvic Fractures: Problems and Possible Solutions," *American Surgeon* 48(9):441-46, 1982.

Tile, M. *Fractures of the Pelvis and Acetabulum*. Baltimore: Williams & Wilkins Co., 1984.

Vanderbeck, K.A. "Getting the Facts: A Guide to Orthopedic Assessment," *Orthopedic Nursing* 3(5):31-34, 1984.

Wassel, A. "Nursing Assessment of the Lower Extremity," *Nursing Clinics of North America* 16(4):739-48, 1981.

Williams, D.N., and Gustillo, R.B. "The Use of Antibiotics in Orthopaedic Surgery," *Clinical Orthopaedics and Related Research* 190:84-88, 1984.

Wilson, F.C. "Fractures and Dislocations of the Ankle," in *Fractures in Adults*. Edited by Rockwood, C.A., and Green, D.P. Philadelphia: J.B. Lippincott Co., 1984.

Yap, S.N.L. "The Management of Traumatic Pelvic Retroperitoneal Hemorrhage," *Surgical Rounds* 34-39, 42, 44, 1980.

ADDITIONAL
EMERGENCIES

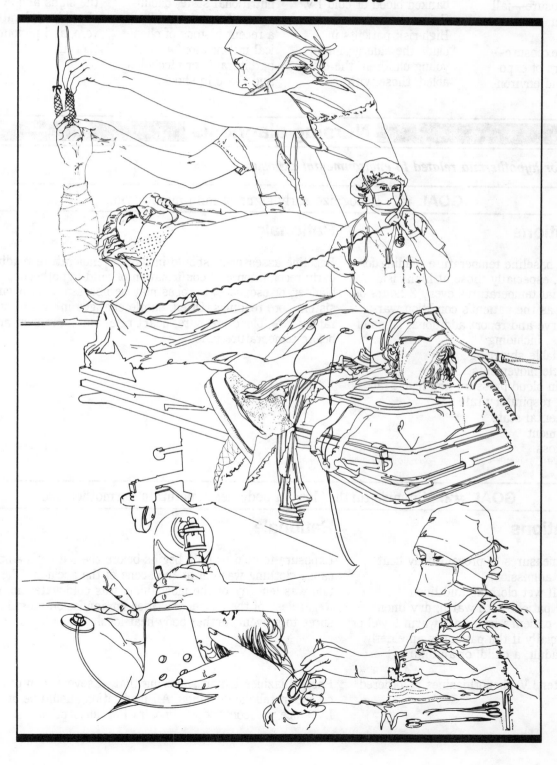

Medical diagnosis

HYPOTHERMIA

Assessment

Mechanism of injury/ etiology:
• acute exposure—fall in cold water, near drowning
• subacute exposure— several hours of exposure to a cold environ-

ment
• rapid infusion of banked blood or cold I.V. fluids
High-risk patients include the elderly; infants; young children; the disabled; those with dia-

betes, hypothyroidism, arteriosclerosis, a poor nutritional state, chemical or thermal burns, or a recent history of chemical intoxication with barbiturates or alcohol; and those in shock.

Physical findings:
Table 3.1 summarizes the signs and symptoms of mild, moderate, severe, and profound hypothermia.

Nursing diagnosis

Potential for hypothermia related to environmental exposure.

| **GOAL #1:** Recognize early signs of mild hypothermia. |

Interventions

1. Obtain a baseline temperature reading for all patients, especially those at high risk. Monitor serial temperatures every 2 hours or more often, as the patient's condition warrants. Observe and report additional signs of hypothermia, including:
• uncontrollable shivering
• stiff muscle movements
• changes in blood pressure and heart rate
• increased respiratory rate
• altered mental state
• poor judgment
• memory loss.

Rationale

Baseline assessment should include a temperature reading for early recognition and confirmation of mild hypothermia. Rectal, bladder, or esophageal probes may be necessary for accurate, consistent core readings. Often, subtle changes in mental state, respiratory rate, blood pressure, heart rate, and movement appear before temperature falls.

| **GOAL #2:** Minimize further loss of body heat; maintain normothermia. |

Interventions

1. Initiate measures to prevent body heat loss during admission:
• remove all wet clothing and linen
• cover the patient with warm, dry linen
• wrap the patient's head in a warm towel or sheet, especially if the patient is an elderly or balding adult, a child, or an infant.

2. Administer I.V. phenothiazines as ordered.

Rationale

Exposure to cold usually begins before the patient's admission, because clothing was cut at the scene of the accident, the extrication was lengthy, or the mechanism was cold-water immersion. Regardless of the cause, priorities on admission must include measures to prevent further body heat loss.

Phenothiazines inhibit shivering that, if severe, can drastically increase metabolic demands. All medication should be administered I.V. since vasoconstriction impairs I.M. absorption.

Table 3.1 Hypothermia: Findings

Core temperatures	Mild 98.6° to 89.6° F. (37° to 32° C.)	Moderate 89.6° to 82.4° F. (32° to 28° C.)	Severe 82.4° to 68° F. (28° to 20° C.)	Profound < 68° F. (< 20° C.)
Metabolic signs	None	Metabolic acidosis: ↑ potassium, calcium ↑ lactic acid ↓ hemolysis ↑ blood sugar ↓ detoxification and metabolism	Acidosis	Acidosis
Heart rate	↑ or ↓	↓ by 50%	Absent	Cardiac standstill
Cardiovascular, ECG	None	Bradycardia, atrial fibrillation, atrioventricular blocks, premature ventricular contractions, ventricular tachycardia ↑ capillary permeability = edema ↓ cardiac output	J wave; all ECG intervals prolonged, T wave inverted, ↑ risk for ventricular fibrillation, *highly irritable heart*	Asystole
Blood pressure	↑ or ↓	Prolonged diastole ↑ compensation often inaudible	Cardiac arrest	Cardiac arrest
Respiratory rate	↑	↓ rate ↓ carbon dioxide production ↑ carbon dioxide retention ↓ cough reflex airway obstruction	Apnea	Apnea
Neurologic status	Conscious, alert or altered level of consciousness, withdrawn behavior, pupils begin to dilate, poor judgment, memory loss	Glassy stare; markedly obtunded, impaired vision and hearing; pupils dilated, nonreactive	Pupils nonreactive, no response to deep pain	Pupils nonreactive, no response to deep pain
Muscle activity	Uncontrollable shivering, stiff movements	No shivering, rigid muscles	Areflexic, no muscle tone	Areflexic, no muscle tone

3. Initiate passive rewarming measures for a patient with mild hypothermia, including:
- heated linens
- warming lights
- a hyperthermia blanket
- warm I.V. bags in both the groin and axilla and around the neck.

Passive rewarming may suffice to normalize temperature in the mildly hypothermic patient.

Nursing diagnosis

Potential for decreased tissue perfusion, carbon dioxide retention, life-threatening dysrhythmias, and metabolic acidosis related to hypothermia.

GOAL #1: Restore core temperature to at least 85° F.

Note: *The priority for a patient with moderate-to-profound hypothermia, after the ABCs, is rapid yet cautious temperature restoration to at least 85° F. Most therapy for the problems already listed will be ineffective, if not detrimental, if the patient's core temperature is < 85° F.*

Interventions

1. Ensure accurate and consistent core temperature measurement.

2. Warm all I.V. fluids before infusion, using either a warming machine or a warming coil.

3. Use heated nebulizers for supplemental oxygen delivery and warming cascades for patients on mechanical ventilators.

4. Warm blood before transfusion either with a blood-warming coil or by mixing with warm normal saline solution (NSS).

5. Use warm NSS or lactated Ringer's solution for peritoneal lavage, which may be performed as either a diagnostic or solely a warming technique.

6. Lavage the stomach with warm NSS via a gastric decompression tube.

7. Restrict movement and unnecessary manipulation while the patient is hypothermic and during rewarming.

Rationale

Continuous monitoring of core temperature is essential to evaluate progress, direct therapy, and prevent overwarming.

Core rewarming is essential to prevent cold-induced shock. This problem occurs when external rewarming is done without regard to the patient's core temperature. Peripheral vasculature dilation causes cold blood to shift from the periphery to the core; the heart, which is still cold, cannot provide adequate output. This influx of blood to the cold heart can increase the shock state and trigger ventricular fibrillation. The stagnant blood begins to move, carrying with it high amounts of metabolic wastes. This development can cause a profound acidosis. The interventions listed represent core rewarming techniques.

Movement can precipitate severe muscle cramps and increase the translocation of cold blood from the extremity to the core, increasing shock.

GOAL #2: Recognize actual or potential hypothermia-induced respiratory problems; initiate prompt therapy when core temperature is at least 85° F.

Interventions

1. Continuously monitor the patient's respiratory status. Establish an airway or assist with airway management and provide venti-

Rationale

In moderate hypothermia, respiratory efforts begin to fail as metabolism slows. This leads to carbon dioxide retention, a decline in carbon dioxide production, and a shift of the oxygen dissociation

latory support as indicated and ordered. (See "Endotracheal Intubation" in Section VII.)
Note: *Intubation may cause ventricular fibrillation. Limit tracheal suctioning unless absolutely needed for this reason. Also be aware that the patient is at risk for pulmonary thromboembolus due to the blood's increased viscosity. Refer to "Pulmonary Thromboembolus" in Section IV.*

curve to the left; all three mechanisms result in impaired tissue oxygenation. As warming occurs, acid metabolites mobilize and may cause profound acidosis.

GOAL #3: Recognize actual or potential cardiovascular problems caused by hypothermia; initiate prompt therapy when core temperature is at least 85° F.

Interventions

1. Monitor the patient's cardiovascular status continuously, including central venous pressure. Maintain the patient on an ECG monitor. Perform cardiopulmonary resuscitation (CPR) as needed but avoid defibrillation until the patient is warm. Administer warm emergency cardiac drugs for dysrhythmias as ordered.

2. Monitor trends in laboratory data closely during rewarming. Avoid administering drugs to correct abnormal laboratory results until the patient's temperature is normalized.

Rationale

Cardiac irritability begins in moderate hypothermia and can increase to asystole in severe hypothermia. CPR must be performed until core temperature rises to at least 85° F. Defibrillation is ineffective on the cold heart and may cause further cardiac damage when the core temperature is < 85° F. Dysrhythmias, which usually disappear when the patient is warmed, may be aggravated by attempts at pacing or insertion of pulmonary artery catheters. The cold heart does not usually respond to drugs like atropine. Warming the drugs before administering them, however, may be beneficial. Close evaluation and trend analysis of hemodynamic parameters aid in proper fluid management to avoid fluid overload. Increased capillary permeability in hypothermia raises the risk of interstitial edema.

Decreased insulin release and response in hypothermia elevate serum glucose levels. Administering insulin before rewarming will cause later hypoglycemia. If drugs are given before establishing a warmer core temperature, decreased circulation and peripheral absorption as well as impaired hepatic detoxification and metabolism can cause additional adverse effects. For example, cumulative effects may cause a drug overdose when temperature is restored.

GOAL #4: Recognize actual or potential hypothermia-induced neurologic problems; initiate prompt therapy when core temperature is at least 85° F.

Interventions

1. Monitor the patient's neurologic status closely. Protect the patient from potential harm during decreased mentation.

Rationale

Mild-to-moderate hypothermia causes progressive deterioration in mental, visual, and auditory acuity. Memory loss and impaired judgment mandate close attention to the patient's safety. Permanent brain damage is unusual because of slowed cerebral metabolism during deeper hypothermia. But residual psychiatric problems may develop after severe hypothermia.

Associated care plans

Near Drowning: Freshwater/Saltwater
Chemical Burns
Thermal Burns
Hemorrhagic Shock
Pulmonary Thromboembolus

Associated procedures

Endotracheal Intubation
Diagnostic Peritoneal Lavage

Medical diagnosis

NEAR DROWNING: Freshwater/Saltwater

Assessment

Mechanism of injury/ etiology:
- aspiration of fresh water or salt water

Physical findings:
Respiratory
- normal respirations (may be normal initially, then deteriorate)
- dyspnea
- tachypnea
- apnea
- bronchospasm
- laryngospasm

- rales and rhonchi
- wheezes
- frothy sputum
- substernal burning
- pleuritic chest pain
- coughing
- cyanosis

Cardiovascular
- hypo- or hypervolemia
- dysrhythmias (brady-cardia, tachycardia, atrial fibrillation, prema-ture ventricular contrac-tions)

- peripheral vasocon-striction
- hypothermia
- fever

Neurologic
- lethargy
- decortication (abnor-mal flexion)
- hyporeflexia
- flaccidity
- alertness
- restlessness
- confusion
- seizure activity

Genitourinary
- oliguria
- azotemia

Gastrointestinal
- abdominal distention

Associated injuries:
- cervical spine fracture and closed head injury—when aspiration follows a diving injury
- hypothermia

Diagnostic studies

- lateral cervical spine radiography—to rule out diving injury fracture
- serial chest radiography—initial chest radiographs do not always show pulmonary changes; serial films are needed for complete assessment
- pulmonary artery thermodilution catheterization—to monitor hemodynamic parameters, intrapulmonary shunt
- ECG—indicates myocardial ischemia

- laboratory data:
  - ☐ ABG levels—reflect degree of hypoxia, intrapul-monary shunt, acid-base imbalance
  - ☐ plasma hemoglobin, CBC—determine hemolysis
  - ☐ serum electrolytes—monitor electrolyte imbalance
  - ☐ blood urea nitrogen (BUN) and serum creatinine levels, urine creatinine clearance, and urinalysis—evaluate renal function

Nursing diagnosis

Potential for ineffective airway clearance and impaired gas exchange related to aspiration of foreign material, for example, mud, sand, algae, gastric contents.

GOAL #1: Establish and maintain a patent airway.

Interventions

1. Ensure equipment availability and proper functioning to provide supplemental humidi-fied oxygen, endotracheal suction and intuba-tion, and mechanical ventilation. (See "Endotracheal Intubation" in Section VII.)

2. Establish an airway if needed and provide supplemental oxygen.

3. Anticipate the need for bronchoscopy. (See "Bronchoscopy" in Section VII.)

Rationale

The near-drowning victim may develop respiratory distress, rang-ing from mild dyspnea to apnea. Establishing an effective airway, if needed, must not be delayed to gather equipment or repair mal-functioning equipment.

Aspirating algae, mud, and sand can obstruct the tracheobron-chial tree and impair gas exchange. Foreign matter removal im-proves gas exchange.

GOAL #2: Minimize the risk of further aspiration.

Interventions

1. Ensure the placement of a gastric tube connected to gastric suction.

Rationale

Near-drowning victims commonly swallow large volumes of water. During resuscitation, air may also be introduced into the stomach. Emptying the stomach is necessary to prevent vomiting and aspiration.

Nursing diagnosis

Potential for fluid volume excess and electrolyte imbalance related to aspirated fresh water.

GOAL: Recognize early signs of hypervolemia; restore and maintain electrolyte balance.

Interventions

1. Monitor hemodynamic parameters, including blood pressure and central venous pressure, for hypervolemia. Administer fluids as ordered.

2. Obtain baseline and serial serum electrolyte levels and analyze trends. Administer an electrolyte supplement as ordered.

Rationale

Aspirated fresh water is absorbed directly into the pulmonary circulation from the lungs, causing a transient hypervolemia. Fluid restriction may be needed.

Severe electrolyte imbalance usually occurs when the victim has aspirated large volumes of fresh water (22 cc/kg). This occurs in less than 15% of near-drowning cases. Aspirating smaller volumes of water causes a milder imbalance and is easily corrected. Trend analysis of serum electrolytes is necessary to evaluate the effectiveness of replacement therapy.

Nursing diagnosis

Potential for impaired gas exchange related to intrapulmonary shunting secondary to aspirated fresh or salt water and late pulmonary edema.

GOAL #1: Optimize gas exchange.

Interventions

1. Administer supplemental oxygen as ordered. Assess the patient closely for signs of hypoxia and hypercapnia.

Rationale

Hypoxia and hypercapnia can develop when a significant intrapulmonary shunt prevents adequate oxygen uptake and carbon dioxide elimination. One of two mechanisms causes shunt increase (an increase in the percentage of unoxygenated blood in cardiac output). In *saltwater* near drowning, aspirated water draws fluid and proteins from the plasma into the alveoli. Although the fluid-filled alveoli continue to be perfused, gas exchange is markedly impaired. In *freshwater* near drowning, the pulmonary circulation quickly pulls aspirated water from the alveoli, but not before altering alveolar surface tension so that the alveoli collapse and atelectasis develops. The perfused alveoli are either poorly ventilated or not ventilated at all. Fresh water, drawn into the pulmonary circulation, causes hemolysis. The resulting damage to the pulmonary capillaries increases the extent of pulmonary edema. As an increased intrapulmonary shunt develops, the $PaCO_2$ increases and a higher inspired oxygen concentration (FiO_2) is needed to maintain an adequate PaO_2.

*Supplemental nursing diagnosis

2. Assess breath sounds frequently for wheezing. Administer bronchodilators as ordered.

Near-drowning victims often develop bronchospasms. Bronchodilators can control these spasms and improve ventilation.

3. Monitor and analyze trends in ABG levels. Anticipate the need for ventilatory assistance, including controlled intermittent mandatory ventilation, continuous positive airway pressure (CPAP), and positive end-expiratory pressure (PEEP).

As the intrapulmonary shunt rises above 20%, ventilatory assistance becomes necessary. The shunt can be estimated from the ratio of PaO_2 to FiO_2. The normal ratio of 500:1 (PaO_2 of 100 and an inspired FiO_2 of 0.2 [room air]) is equivalent to a normal pulmonary shunt of 5% to 6%. The lower the ratio, the higher the shunt value. A patient receiving supplemental oxygen whose $PaO_2:FiO_2$ is 200:1 has a pulmonary shunt of about 20%. Mechanical ventilation is needed for a patient unable to clear carbon dioxide and maintain an adequate PaO_2. When an FiO_2 greater than 50% is needed to maintain an adequate PaO_2, the patient will require PEEP or CPAP.

4. Monitor $PaO_2:FiO_2$. Anticipate the need for pulmonary artery thermodilution catheterization. (See "Pulmonary Artery Catheterization" in Section VII.)

Ventilating with CPAP or PEEP should improve the $PaO_2:FiO_2$ by decreasing the intrapulmonary shunt. PEEP or CPAP is adjusted to reduce the shunt to about 15% (a $PaO_2:FiO_2$ of 300:1). Although PEEP improves gas exchange, it also reduces cardiac output. A patient needing a PEEP greater than 8 to 10 cm H_2O will need a pulmonary artery thermodilution catheter for measurement of hemodynamic parameters.

5. Severely limit suctioning frequency in the patient receiving high PEEP or CPAP ventilation levels. Each institution's critical care medicine department should establish the rationale for frequency of suctioning.

A sudden fall in or discontinuation of PEEP or CPAP can cause the intrapulmonary shunt to rise significantly, the PaO_2 to fall, and pulmonary edema fluids to increase.

GOAL #2: Correct acid-base imbalance.

Interventions

1. Monitor ABG levels and hemodynamic parameters. Administer fluids and bicarbonate as required to correct metabolic acidosis.

Rationale

Metabolic acidosis, a frequent finding in the near-drowning victim, is the result of anaerobic metabolism secondary to hypoxia and fluid volume deficit. Restoring normal PaO_2 and normovolemia often corrects metabolic acidosis. Occasionally, bicarbonate administration is needed in addition to fluid replacement and pulmonary resuscitation.

Nursing diagnosis

Potential for hypothermia related to heat loss secondary to submersion.

GOAL: Restore and maintain normal body temperature.

Interventions

1. Record the baseline temperature of all patients. Initiate rewarming procedures as necessary. (See "Hypothermia" in Section III.)

Rationale

Body heat can be lost 25 to 30 times faster in water than in air at the same temperature. Hypothermia also develops faster in children because they have a larger body surface relative to their small amounts of subcutaneous fat. Children also tend to be more active when submerged. Core temperature must be raised to above 85° F. for therapy to be effective.

Nursing diagnosis

Potential for decreased cardiac output and dysrhythmias related to myocardial ischemia secondary to aspiration-induced hypoxia.

GOAL: Minimize the effect of myocardial ischemia.

Interventions

1. Monitor ECG changes, ABG levels, and hemodynamic parameters. Administer antidysrhythmic drugs as ordered. (See "Acute Myocardial Infarction" in Section II.)

Rationale

Myocardial ischemia is evident from ECG changes and dysrhythmias. Myocardial ischemia is treated by maintaining an adequate PaO_2, correcting acid-base imbalances, and administering antidysrhythmic drugs to the patient. Inotropic therapy may be required if cardiac output is reduced because of myocardial depression.

Nursing diagnosis

Potential for decreased cerebral perfusion related to cerebral edema secondary to hypoxia.

GOAL: Recognize early signs of cerebral edema; optimize cerebral perfusion.

Interventions

1. Monitor the patient's neurologic status closely and continuously. Elevate the head of the bed unless contraindicated.

2. Anticipate placing an intracranial pressure monitor. Monitor intracranial pressure, cerebral perfusion pressure, and ABG levels. Administer steroids as ordered. (See "Intracranial Pressure Monitoring" in Section VII.)

Rationale

Posthypoxic cerebral edema is first reflected by decreased consciousness. Cerebral function changes after a near drowning can occur rapidly. Elevating the patient's head helps reduce cerebral edema by increasing venous return.

Placement of an intracranial monitoring device allows measurement of the patient's cerebral perfusion pressure and evaluation of treatment efficacy. Controlled hyperventilation, $PaCO_2$ of 25 to 30 mm Hg, constricts cerebral vessels, reducing intracranial pressure. Steroids may be used to treat cerebral edema.

Nursing diagnosis

Potential for decreased cardiac output related to increased intrathoracic pressures secondary to the use of PEEP.

GOAL: Restore and maintain normal cardiac output.

Interventions

1. Anticipate and, if required, assist in insertion of a pulmonary artery thermodilution catheter. Monitor hemodynamic parameters: cardiac output, pulmonary arterial wedge pressure (PAWP), central venous pressure (CVP), heart rate, arterial blood pressure, and urine output. Administer fluids and inotropic agents as ordered.

Rationale

Fluids and inotropic agents, administered alone or together, are needed to restore cardiac output. Those parameters measurable by pulmonary artery thermodilution catheterization permit more accurate therapy evaluation.

*Supplemental nursing diagnosis

Nursing diagnosis

Potential for fluid volume deficit related to redistribution of fluids from intravascular spaces to interstitial spaces.

GOAL: Restore and maintain normovolemia.

Interventions

1. Monitor hemodynamic parameters: cardiac output, PAWP, CVP, heart rate, arterial blood pressure, and urine output. Administer fluids as ordered.

Rationale

A relative hypovolemia can develop as intravascular fluids redistribute into the interstitial spaces. Close monitoring and evaluation of fluid therapy will be required to maintain normovolemia and to prevent unnecessary fluid overload.

Nursing diagnosis

Potential for decreased tissue perfusion related to lysis of RBCs secondary to absorption of fresh water into the pulmonary circulation.

GOAL: Recognize early signs of hemolysis; minimize its risk.

Interventions

1. Monitor urine for color changes. Have the patient's blood and urine analyzed for hemoglobin.

2. Monitor urine output and pH. Administer fluids, osmotic diuretics, and bicarbonate as ordered to keep the urine alkaline and its output at 100 cc/hr. Monitor trends in BUN and serum creatinine levels, and urine creatinine clearance. Monitor and maintain adequate cardiac output. (See "Acute Renal Failure" in Section IV.)

3. Obtain baseline and serial RBC counts and analyze trends. Anticipate the need for RBC replacement.

4. Obtain baseline and serial coagulation studies and analyze trends. Monitor venipuncture sites for prolonged bleeding. Anticipate blood product replacement. (See "Disseminated Intravascular Coagulation" in Section IV.)

Rationale

Hypotonic saline solutions or fresh water absorbed by the pulmonary circulation lyse RBCs and liberate hemoglobin into the plasma. Hemoglobin is then eliminated by the kidneys, coloring the urine red. Elevated free hemoglobin levels can be detected in the plasma.

Passing through the kidneys, hemoglobin may crystallize out in the tubules, causing obstruction and possible necrosis and renal shutdown. Maintaining a high urine output and an alkaline urine helps prevent hemoglobin crystallization. Maintaining adequate cardiac output promotes efficient renal blood flow. Serum creatinine and BUN elevations and a urine creatinine clearance decrease reflect reduced renal function.

If lysis is significant, replacing RBCs becomes necessary for adequate tissue perfusion.

Disseminated intravascular coagulation (DIC) is a secondary complication of hemolysis. Prolonged thrombin time, prothrombin time, and partial prothrombin time, together with a decreased platelet count and increased fibrin split products, reflect DIC.

Nursing diagnosis

Potential for infection related to aspiration.

GOAL: Minimize the risk of infection.

Interventions

1. Obtain a sputum sample for culture. Monitor the patient's temperature, and administer antibiotics as ordered.

Rationale

Antibiotics are given if the culture proves positive or a chest radiograph shows lung consolidation. Because a temperature rise is common in near-drowning victims, it is not the sole basis for antibiotic administration.

Associated care plans

Adult Respiratory Distress Syndrome
Pulmonary Edema
Acute Myocardial Infarction
Disseminated Intravascular Coagulation
Acute Renal Failure
Hypothermia

Associated procedures and study

Intracranial Pressure Monitoring
Bronchoscopy
Pulmonary Artery Catheterization
Endotracheal Intubation

| Medical diagnosis |

ACUTE WHOLE-BODY RADIATION EXPOSURE

Assessment

Mechanism of injury/ etiology:
• whole-body exposure to ionizing radiation

Estimated radiation dose received:
The total body injury and the total dose received may be estimated from:
• clinical responses— identified in Table 3.2
Note: *Fear, severe anxiety, and panic can mimic some GI symptoms related to radiation exposure.*
• laboratory values— lymphocyte, granulocyte, and platelet levels
• information from film badge and monitors
• intensity and type of ionizing radiation (alpha or beta particles, gamma rays), distance of patient from radiation source, and length of exposure

Physical findings:
Note: *The patient may be asymptomatic.*

Neurologic
• disorientation
• ataxia
• hyperesthesia
• paresthesia
• delirium
• coma

Gastrointestinal
• bloody diarrhea

• abdominal pain
• anorexia

Cardiovascular
• hypovolemic shock
• bleeding tendencies
• fever
• hypotension

Integumentary
• erythema
• diaphoresis

Table 3.2

Dose	Effect
< 200 rads	Possible nausea with emesis, diarrhea first day, anxiety, tachy-cardia (subclinical syndrome)
200 to 600 rads	Nausea with emesis, diarrhea within 6 to 12 hours, weakness, fatigue (hematopoietic syndrome)
600 to 1,000 rads	Severe nausea with emesis, diarrhea first several hours (gastro-intestinal syndrome)
> 1,000 rads	"Burning sensation" within minutes; nausea with emesis within 10 minutes; confusion, ataxia, and prostration within 1 hour; watery diarrhea within 1 to 2 hours (cerebral syndrome); al-most always fatal

Because exposed individuals' reactions vary, the dose cannot be reliably interpolated on clinical findings alone. Thus, dose is expressed in ranges, for example, 200 to 600 rads. (Also, for this reason, hematology studies are more important as trend indicators than for specific values obtained from an isolated sample.)

Diagnostic study

• absolute lymphocyte count—the most significant drop in lymphocyte concentration occurs in the first 24 to 36 hours after exposure; this early finding is one of the best indicators of exposure severity

Nursing diagnosis

Potential for infection related to diminished leukocyte and granulocyte formation secondary to damage of stem cells in the marrow, spleen, and lymphatic tissue.

GOAL #1: Prevent or minimize the risk of infection.

Interventions

1. Use sterile technique for all invasive procedures, dressing changes, and wound care.

2. Initiate reverse isolation as defined by hospital policy.

3. Schedule laboratory work to minimize the number of venipunctures.

Rationale

Sterile technique minimizes microbial infection.

Microorganisms that are normally nonpathogenic can cause a fatal septic episode in the patient acutely exposed to ionizing radiation.

Any break in skin integrity increases the risk of pathogen entry into the body.

GOAL #2: Recognize the early signs of infection.

Interventions

1. Obtain cultures from the patient's mouth, gums, vagina, infectious skin lesions, blood, urine, sputum, and stool.

2. Monitor and document the patient's vital signs, including temperature; note laboratory data trends, especially in the WBC count.

3. Monitor the patient's stool for frank and occult blood.

Rationale

Preexisting microorganisms require specific antibiotic treatment while granulocyte levels remain near normal. Granulocyte levels bottom out at about 10 days postexposure.

A fatal infectious process can develop rapidly in a severely granulocytopenic patient.

Bleeding may be the only sign of intestinal tract infectious lesions.

Nursing diagnosis

Potential for fluid volume deficit related to blood loss secondary to coagulopathy caused by the hematopoietic syndrome.

GOAL: Recognize the early signs of coagulopathy; minimize complications developing in the hematopoietic syndrome's acute phase.

Interventions

1. Obtain the patient's baseline coagulation studies and monitor profile trends.

2. Prepare for possible human leukocyte Group A antigen typing of the patient and potential donors.

3. Monitor I.V. sites and all wounds, surgical and nonsurgical, for prolonged bleeding. Test the patient's stools for blood and monitor gastric pH.

Rationale

Platelet levels may increase in the first 48 to 72 hours and then decline, bottoming out about 30 days postexposure. Laboratory data trend analysis helps recognize coagulopathy early.

During the latter stage of bone marrow depression caused by stem cell destruction, granulocyte and platelet transfusions may be required as a support measure.

A decreased platelet level prolongs clotting times, promoting increased bleeding. The patient is susceptible to gastric bleeding because of the radiation injury and related stress.

Nursing diagnosis

Potential for fluid volume deficit and electrolyte imbalance related to excessive diarrhea secondary to destruction of the GI tract mucosa.

GOAL: Establish and maintain fluid and electrolyte balance.

Interventions

1. Establish venous access and begin volume replacement as necessary. Closely monitor the patient's intake and output.

2. Record baseline central venous pressure and monitor trends.

3. Obtain baseline and serial serum electrolyte levels and evaluate trends.

Rationale

Current theory suggests that radiation impairs cellular mitosis in the intestinal mucosa (crypts of Lieberkühn). The mucosa loses electrolytes while normal bacterial flora, seeding the GI tract, plant infections. The resulting vomiting and diarrhea cause fluid loss.

CVP measurements help evaluate fluid replacement effectiveness.

Laboratory data trend analysis helps assess electrolyte replacement effectiveness.

Nursing diagnosis

Potential for alteration in sensory perception possibly related to decreased cerebral perfusion secondary to hypotension.

Note: *The neurologic changes are thought to occur because of refractory hypotension developing after high-exposure doses, not from radiation injury to brain tissue.*

GOAL: Recognize the early signs of neurologic deterioration.

Interventions

1. Monitor and document the patient's blood pressure and neurologic status.

Rationale

The patient exposed to very high radiation doses is alert at first. But then his level of consciousness declines. Concomitantly, intractable hypotension can develop.

Nursing diagnosis

Potential for severe anxiety and fear related to knowledge deficit about short- and long-term health effects of radiation exposure.

GOAL: Reduce the patient's fear and anxiety.

Interventions

1. Explain all procedures to the patient in terms he understands. Repeat as necessary.

Rationale

Anxiety can impair a patient's comprehension. Because short-term memory may also be impaired, you may have to repeat explanations.

*Supplemental nursing diagnosis

2. Monitor the bedside conversation of health care personnel.

Misinterpreting conversations can cause the patient needless anxiety.

3. Assist appropriate radiation experts in educating the patient about potential long-term illnesses.

The patient needs accurate information from recognized experts about potential short- and long-term health problems.

4. Procure psychiatric counseling for the patient, if necessary.

Long-term health problems include leukemia, malignant tumors, cataracts, and sterility. The patient may require long-term counseling because of the exposure's traumatic impact.

Associated care plans

Hemorrhagic Shock
Vasogenic Shock
Disseminated Intravascular Coagulation
Psychosocial Support of the Trauma Patient

GENERAL BURN CARE CONSIDERATIONS

Certain components of nursing care apply to all burn patients, regardless of the burn type: chemical, thermal, electrical, or those caused by caustic chemical ingestion. For example, the ABCs (airway, breathing, circulation) are consistent priorities for these patients.

This burn care overview was structured in conjunction with "Thermal Burns" in Section III to provide the cornerstone for burn care. Care plans for specific burn types—such as electrical burns or caustic chemical ingestion—were written to provide rapid access to specific interventions, with the reader then referred to "Thermal Burns" for additional considerations. To avoid overlooking any facet of burn care, first read the specific care plan—such as "Electrical Burns" in Section III—then refer to "Thermal Burns" for general principles and apply the information, as appropriate. "General Burn Care Considerations" supplements and links the various burn care plans.

Associated injuries

Assess all burn patients for signs and symptoms of concomitant toxic inhalation exposure and multiple trauma. (Remember: the burn wound does not bleed.) Associated injuries such as these require immediate recognition and intervention to prevent life-threatening sequelae. Resuscitation and stabilization for traumatic injuries supersede burn wound care. The emergency care nurse must avoid allowing the obvious to take precedence over covert associated injuries.

Assessment factors

Assessment components, essentially the same for all types of burns, should incorporate the nursing process and a systematic approach to evaluate respiratory, cardiovascular, neurologic, gastrointestinal, renal, musculoskeletal, and metabolic status. Laboratory data require close monitoring because changing values aid diagnosis of shock states, adult respiratory distress syndrome, acute renal failure, and other complications commonly associated with burns.

Transfer to the regional burn center

Specific patient criteria necessitating transfer to a regional burn center are outlined in Table 3.6. The burn patient's needs must be weighed against the services available in the initial receiving facility. If the environment, lack of personnel or equipment, and lack of adjunctive services preclude optimal care, transfer to a more appropriate facility must be initiated as soon as the patient is resuscitated and stabilized.

Volume replacement

Calculation of the percentage of total body surface burn area (BSBA) involved and volume replacement are imperative to replenish lost body fluids and electrolytes and to prevent hypovolemia. Various calculation methods exist to determine the BSBA, such as the Lund & Browder chart and the Rule of Nines. (An easy method for calculating BSBA in a patient with irregular burns is to assume that the patient's palm equals 1% of his body surface.) Fluid replacement needs are determined and directed using a preestablished guideline, such as the Baxter (Parkland) formula, the Brooke formula, or the Evans formula. Accurate estimation of the burned area is usually difficult in the patient with chemical or electrical burns. These injuries pose a special challenge in volume replacement. In chemical burns, the total area may not be large, but the depth may produce severe effects. In electrical burns, while external trauma may appear minimal, substantial systemic damage usually occurs along the current's pathway. Vascular and organ damage may result in hemorrhage, requiring blood and component therapy infusion.

Tetanus immunization and analgesic administration

All burn patients require prophylactic tetanus immunization and an effective pain management regimen. The tetanus injection is the only medication administered intramuscularly, preferably not at a burn site. Separate injection sites should be used if immune globulin is required in addition to the tetanus booster. Analgesics should be titrated and administered intravenously to achieve maximum therapeutic effects without incurring untoward side effects. The drug of choice is morphine sulfate, 0.1 mg/kg I.V. **Note:** *The burn victim is at high risk for narcotic addiction due to need for chronic pain management.*

Infection

Infection, which may progress to sepsis, poses a constant threat to the burn victim. Contamination occurs at the time of injury, when the skin integrity is disrupted. Strict adherence to aseptic technique is a priority when caring for burns of any size. The patient with a large BSBA may require multiple I.V. catheters, a total parenteral nutrition (TPN) line, a gastric decompression tube, an indwelling urinary catheter, and an artificial airway and ventilation, all of which provide additional entry routes for contaminants. Despite strict compliance with a protective isolation policy and sterile technique, overwhelming infection may occur secondary to pathogen contamination. Antibiotics are prescribed after cultures identify specific causative organisms. Multiple daily dressing changes and debridement remove necrotic tissue and enable application of fresh layers of local antibiotic ointment on burn surfaces.

Surgical intervention

Surgical intervention may be required for numerous reasons, including escharotomy, debridement, achievement of hemostasis (necessary for associated traumatic injuries), and, when the patient has stabilized, skin grafting and multiple long-term plastic reconstructive procedures.

Additional required care

Daily care of the burn victim must include constant assessment to identify and prevent potential complications, dressing changes, nutritional support (gastric tube feedings, gastrostomy, TPN), and physical therapy. Occupational and physical therapy—including range-of-motion exercises (commonly during hydrotherapy) and proper joint splinting—are integral to prevent contracture formation.

Special needs of pediatric and geriatric burn patients

Emergency care providers may discover burns resulting from child or elderly abuse and are ethically and legally required to report such injuries to the proper authorities. Pediatric and geriatric patients require especially judicious volume administration. Overhydration and fluid overload are common, but preventable, complications with these patients. The threat of infection and subsequent sepsis is even greater in the young and the elderly because they may have immature or impaired antibody and immune responses. An elderly victim with malnutrition, poor skin integrity, and a preexisting disease process (for example, diabetes) is prone to impaired wound healing. The pediatric patient presents inherent problems caused by otherwise healthful aspects of a rapid metabolic and growth rate. For example, greater nutritional and oxygen demands must be met, as rapid healing—seemingly a benefit in the young—can result in excessive scarring and contractures if these needs are not managed optimally. A common complication in the pediatric burn patient is hypertension; although this will resolve when healing is complete, it must be treated in the interim. Also, young burn patients, particularly those under age 1, may become hypoglycemic as a result of decreased glycogen stores in the liver.

Psychosocial aspect

The burn victim may experience an immense change in body image and loss of self-esteem, depending on the burn's extent, severity, and sequelae. This patient is usually alert on admission and will interpret verbal and nonverbal communication he receives from those around him long before he sees himself. Health care providers should monitor all bedside conversations and facial expressions, beginning with emergency medical services field responders and continuing throughout the rehabilitation process. The patient may also have difficulty coping with his family's and friends' responses. Interruption in or failure to perform role functions may develop as the burn patient may miss school or work and be separated from his family, community, and social involvements for many months. Initial hospitalization, rehabilitation, and long-term reconstructive surgeries interrupt his daily routine and life-style. Occupational and vocational training can prepare the patient to reintegrate into the working society in another profession if necessary. The burn patient needs immediate psychosocial care, from crisis intervention at the time of injury to continued counseling through the recovery/rehabilitation process. Referral to a self-help group may be appropriate, when geographically available. Family counseling may also be necessary because the patient's family commonly experiences the loss and grieves in a fashion similar to the patient. Effective patient reintegration requires a total effort, not only by the patient, but also by his support systems. Additionally, the family may be directly involved in his care, and specific family teaching must be planned and instituted early in the hospitalization.

Medical diagnosis

CHEMICAL BURNS

Assessment

Note: *The mechanism and severity of a partial- or full-thickness chemical burn depend on the action and penetrability of the chemical and on the duration of tissue contact. The mechanisms below damage and destroy the skin and continue to penetrate deeper tissues, causing cellular death, until the chemical is completely neutralized. Most chemical burns, like other burns, cause initial vasodilation and hyperemia.*

Initially, superficial vessels are involved, then subcutaneous vessels. As the damage increases, tissue congestion and inflammation result from fluid and WBC infiltration in the injured tissue. In severe chemical burns, tissue necrosis and dissolution may occur.

Mechanism of injury/ etiology:
- tissue damage caused by heat release from acidic or alkaline substances
- cellular dehydration resulting from biochemical reaction
- protoplasmic poisoning resulting from biochemical reaction
- protein coagulation or dissolution of cellular contents from direct biochemical reaction between the chemical and the skin

Physical findings:
Skin
- extent of the burn
- depth of the burn
  - ☐ appears moist, red or mottled white, and blistered; is painful (partial-thickness burn)
  - ☐ appears red, brown, black, or leathery white and waxy; has hard, dry eschar; is painless (full-thickness burn)

Respiratory
- dyspnea
- tachypnea
- stridor

Associated injuries:
- inhalation injuries from toxic chemical fumes
- eye irritation and burns
- multiple trauma (for example, from a chemical explosion or falls into a chemical container)

Diagnostic study

See "Thermal Burns" in Section III.
- radiography—serial chest radiographs reveal the presence of atelectasis, chemical pneumonia, and pulmonary edema

Nursing diagnosis

Potential for additional loss of skin integrity related to continuation of the burning process by ongoing skin exposure to chemical agents.

GOAL: STOP THE BURNING PROCESS.

Interventions

1. Remove contaminated clothing and carefully brush any dried chemical substance from the skin.

Rationale

Removal of chemical-saturated clothing decreases the amount of chemicals on the skin and aids reduction of the burning process. Health care professionals must exert caution when removing clothing to prevent chemical contact with their own skin.

2. *Immediately* begin irrigation to the exposed area with *copious* amounts of tepid tap water.

Copious irrigation with tap water should begin immediately after skin exposure to irritating chemicals. Depending on the chemical agent and its strength, continuous irrigation may be required for from 30 minutes to 12 to 24 hours. Seat the patient in a shower or in a Hubbard tank to facilitate prolonged irrigation. If the chemical agent is not removed and the burning process is not halted, a partial-thickness burn can progress to a full-thickness burn. Ice or cold water should not be used for irrigation because it can result in hypothermia.

3. Assign one team member the responsibility of contacting the hospital's burn referral center for specific information concerning the care of chemical burns.

Some chemicals create heat when united with water, causing a thermal injury in addition to the damage caused by the chemical. This increased tissue damage can convert the burn to a deeper classification. Continuous, copious irrigation with tap water is the initial intervention for all chemical burns. More specific interventions, such as neutralization, are secondary to irrigation and should only be instituted after consultation with medical specialists at a burn center. Consultation is imperative for care of burns from the following chemicals:
- hydrofluoric acid
- elemental phosphorus
- phenol
- sodium, lithium, and other magnesium metals.

4. Immediately begin eye irrigation with a minimum of 2 to 3 liters of normal saline solution at low flow. (See "Eye Injuries" in Section III.)

Patients with chemical burns to the head or neck should also undergo copious irrigation of the eyes and an eye examination by an ophthalmologist. It is not uncommon for these patients to sustain corneal ulcerations and eye infections as a result of chemical burns.

Nursing diagnosis

Potential for impaired gas exchange and infection related to lower airway obstruction secondary to retained secretions and atelectasis.

GOAL: Maintain a patent airway and adequate gas exchange.

Interventions

1. Ensure the availability and proper functioning of equipment for humidified oxygenation, intubation, and mechanical ventilation. (See "Endotracheal Intubation" in Section VII.)

2. Auscultate breath sounds frequently. Provide optimal pulmonary hygiene, including:
- frequent suctioning
- turning every 2 hours
- placement in semi-Fowler's (unless contraindicated)
- chest physiotherapy
- incentive spirometry.

Rationale

Inhalation of chemical fumes may burn and irritate the tracheobronchial tree, producing edema and copious secretions, which can cause airway obstruction. Respiratory injury and complications may not be evident initially but may appear 2 to 72 hours after the burn incident. Depending on the severity of the respiratory involvement, the patient may require supplemental humidified oxygen by face mask or tracheal intubation. Auscultation of rales and wheezes indicates probable lower airway obstruction.

Pulmonary hygiene initiated early in the resuscitation phase optimizes aeration and minimizes the risk of complications from aspirated and retained secretions. These measures mobilize secretions, prevent pooling, and promote full lung expansion. Prompt and consistent removal of pulmonary secretions reduces the risk of infection, pneumonia, and other pulmonary complications.

3. Prepare the patient for bronchoscopy, as indicated. (See "Bronchoscopy" in Section VII.)

Bronchoscopy permits direct evaluation of the extent of injury to the tracheobronchial tree and removal of secretions.

Additional considerations

Please refer to "Thermal Burns" in Section III for the following information:
- *fluid deficit and replacement*
- *hypothermia*
- *vascular disruption*
- *eschar formation*
- *compartment syndrome*
- *wound care*
- *paralytic ileus*
- *alteration in comfort*
- *infection*
- *impaired physical mobility*
- *psychosocial support*
- *Parkland formula for calculation of volume replacement*
- *American Burn Association transfer criteria.*

Systemic absorption of certain chemicals causes problems in addition to those of topical burns. Such chemicals as phenol, chromic acid, formic acid, phosphorus, creosol, and tannic acid absorbed into the circulatory system can result in cardio-vascular failure, hepatic necrosis, nephrotoxicity, methemoglobinemia, and hemolysis. Health care providers must be aware of the properties of all chemicals; the best source for this information is the regional poison control or burn center.

Associated care plans

Thermal Burns
Caustic Chemical Ingestion
Upper Airway Obstruction
Lower Airway Obstruction
Inhalation Injuries
Psychosocial Support of the Trauma Patient
Pulmonary Edema
Eye Injuries
Malnutrition in the Trauma Patient
Adult Respiratory Distress Syndrome

Associated procedures and study

Preparation for Surgery
Endotracheal Intubation
Bronchoscopy

Medical diagnosis

CAUSTIC CHEMICAL INGESTION

Assessment

Mechanism of injury/ etiology:
- accidental or intentional ingestion of industrial or household solutions such as fertilizers, drain cleaners, battery acid

Note: *Determining the type of ingested substance is paramount in the assessment as* *this indicates the presence of an acid or alkali.*

Physical findings:
Gastrointestinal
- burns of the oral mucosa
- increased salivation
- esophageal edema, strictures, perforation, crepitation
- gastric perforation
- nausea, vomiting
- pain
- hypoactive or absent bowel sounds
- abdominal rigidity

Respiratory
- dyspnea
- tachypnea
- stridor
- hoarseness
- bronchospasms
- dysphagia
- soapy white oral mucous membranes
- asphyxia

Cardiovascular
- shock state
- chest pain

Neurologic
- anxiousness/panic

Diagnostic studies

- esophagoscopy—may reveal alkali ingestion
- esophagogastroscopy—may suggest acid ingestion (both studies determine the extent of injury)
- chest radiograph—may reveal evidence of lower airway burns
- ABGs—assist in determination of adequate oxygenation
- barium swallow (10 days to 3 weeks after ingestion)—

may reveal the extent of injury to the upper GI tract
Note: *Many states have poison control or burn center hotlines that provide easy access to specific interventions for specific chemicals. Some chemical containers give the manufacturer's toll-free number to contact for specific care guidelines. Table 3.3 describes the series of events occurring after ingestion of acids and alkalis.*

Table 3.3

Acids such as:
- Battery acid
- Drain cleaners
- Hydrochloric acid

▽

Acids create a coagulative necrosis with a protective eschar that delays caustic damage.

▽

Pyloric spasm causes acid to pool in the stomach, damaging its mucosal lining.

▽

Some acid may pass through the pyloric sphincter before it spasms and may damage the small bowel.

▽

- Hemorrhage
- Gastric perforation
- Pyloric stenosis
- Achlorhydria

Alkalis such as:
- Drain cleaners
- Refrigerants
- Fertilizers
- Photographic developers

▽

Alkalis combine with proteins and fats to produce a rapidly penetrating liquefactive necrosis of the esophagus.

▽

The esophagus is perforated.

▽

Edema develops and obstructs the esophagus.

▽

- Hemorrhage
- Infection
- Respiratory distress
- Esophageal strictures

Nursing diagnosis

Potential for ineffective airway clearance related to structural damage secondary to corrosive effect of ingested chemical substance.

GOAL: Recognize early signs of respiratory distress; restore and maintain a patent airway.

Interventions

1. Observe the patient closely for signs of respiratory distress:
● monitor respiratory rate
● auscultate breath sounds
● evaluate respiratory effort
● assist with chest radiograph
● monitor ABG results.

2. Ensure the availability and proper functioning of airway equipment and a mechanical ventilator. Assist as necessary with:
● endotracheal intubation
● cricothyroidotomy.
(See "Endotracheal Intubation," "Needle Cricothyroidotomy," and "Surgical Cricothyroidotomy" in Section VII.)

3. Initiate pulmonary hygiene using:
● coughing and deep breathing
● incentive spirometry
● suctioning
● frequent turning
● chest physiotherapy, as ordered.
Prepare for the use of positive end-expiratory pressure (PEEP) on ventilated patients.

Rationale

The patient with chemical airway burns may appear asymptomatic initially, and then quickly deteriorate to acute respiratory distress. Vigilant respiratory assessment is imperative because acids cause oral burns and chemical pneumonitis and alkalis can cause epiglottitis, edema, and possibly airway obstruction.

Airway management and respiratory support may range from temporary measures (such as endotracheal intubation or cricothyroidotomy) to long-term, possibly permanent, maintenance with a tracheostomy.

Chemical damage to the lower airways can cause obstruction through pulmonary edema and adult respiratory distress syndrome. These interventions aid aeration, mobilize secretions, and prevent retention of pulmonary secretions. PEEP aids alveolar ventilation and reduces the risk of atelectasis.

Nursing diagnosis

Potential for alteration in nutrition and bowel elimination related to corrosive chemical damage to the GI tract.

GOAL: Reduce the potential for GI tract perforation.

Interventions

1. Administer a diluent such as milk or water, as ordered. **Note:** *DO NOT INDUCE VOMITING.*

Rationale

Coagulation tissue necrosis occurs with acid burns. Mild-to-moderate acid burns affect the oral mucosa and esophagus, whereas more severe burns involve the stomach. Liquefaction necrosis occurs with alkali burns. Crystalline alkalis can cause esophageal and gastric burns without evidence of oral burns. Milk (the diluent of choice) and water aid acid and alkali dilution and help stop the burning process. Use of emetics or a gastric decompression tube may induce vomiting and potentially increase the risk of perforation. Gastric lavage is contraindicated in the patient who has ingested an alkaline agent, and it is controversial in cases of acid ingestion.

2. Administer antibiotics and steroids, as ordered.

Antibiotics are administered to combat infection. Steroids, although controversial, may decrease edema and minimize the inflammatory response.

3. Prepare the patient for surgery. (See "Preparation for Surgery" in Section VII.)

A feeding gastrostomy tube with supplemental feedings or corrective or reconstructive GI surgery may be required for short- or long-term therapy. Total parenteral nutrition may be instituted for adjunctive therapy. **Note:** *If gastric perforation occurs, it may produce a fluid volume deficit resulting in shock. Vigilant assessment facilitates early diagnosis and rapid resuscitation. Surgery may be necessary to achieve hemostasis. (See "Hemorrhagic Shock" and "Acute Upper Gastrointestinal Bleeding" in Section II.)*

Nursing diagnosis

*Potential for fluid and electrolyte imbalance related to acid ingestion.

> **GOAL:** Restore electrolyte balance.

Interventions

1. Monitor the following:
- ABG results
- serum electrolyte, blood urea nitrogen, and creatinine levels
- urine output.

2. Administer sodium bicarbonate, as ordered.

Rationale

Acid ingestion, especially of formaldehyde, can cause metabolic acidosis. If acute renal failure occurs, the acidosis will worsen as the kidneys lose their ability to produce bicarbonate.

Associated care plans	Associated procedures
Adult Respiratory Distress Syndrome	Preparation for Surgery
Hemorrhagic Shock	Endotracheal Intubation
Acute Upper Gastrointestinal Bleeding	Needle Cricothyroidotomy
Chemical Burns	Surgical Cricothyroidotomy
Inhalation Injuries	
Thermal Burns	
Malnutrition in the Trauma Patient	
Upper Airway Obstruction	
Lower Airway Obstruction	
Pulmonary Edema	
Psychosocial Support of the Trauma Patient	
General Burn Care Considerations	

*Supplemental nursing diagnosis

Medical diagnosis

THERMAL BURNS

Assessment

Mechanism of injury/ etiology:
- destruction of skin and underlying tissues from extreme heat or fire

Physical findings:
Skin
- alteration in skin appearance and integrity (see Table 3.4)
- presence of continued burning

Respiratory
- hyperventilation
- tachypnea
- hoarseness
- loud, stridorous, labored respirations
- wheezing
- singed nasal hairs and oral mucous membranes
- blisters around the mouth
- carbonaceous sputum, soot in the oropharynx
- drooling (caused by edematous tongue)

Cardiovascular
- dysrhythmias
- hypotension
- tachycardia
- low cardiac output
- prolonged capillary refill time (CRT)
- weak to absent peripheral pulses
- hypothermia

Neurologic
- anxiety, fear
- confusion
- neurologic deterioration—with associated carbon monoxide inhalation: decreased coordination and/or sensorimotor impairment; can progress to stupor and unresponsiveness

Gastrointestinal
- decreased or absent bowel sounds
- abdominal distention
- nausea and vomiting

Genitourinary
- hematuria
- myoglobinuria
- oliguria to anuria

Associated injuries:
- inhalation injuries related to burned material or closed-space fires
- blunt or penetrating trauma, such as fractures and/or lacerations related to a motor vehicle accident or explosion producing flames or extreme heat, or a fall from a burning structure or explosion

Diagnostic studies

- laboratory data:
  - ☐ ABG analysis—initial results may reveal respiratory alkalosis from hyperventilation; later results may show metabolic acidosis from hypoxia and anaerobic metabolism
  - ☐ hemoglobin/hematocrit levels—increased initial levels from hemoconcentration, then decreased levels as RBCs are damaged or lost and fluid returns to intravascular space
  - ☐ serum sodium level—hyponatremia, initially from plasma volume shift or loss and later from diuresis
  - ☐ serum potassium level—hyperkalemia from cellular trauma releasing potassium into the serum, hemoconcentration, and RBC hemolysis; hypokalemia then develops as potassium shifts from the extracellular fluid into the cells
  - ☐ serum lactate level—elevated from anaerobic metabolism caused by decreased tissue perfusion and hypoxia
  - ☐ blood urea nitrogen level—elevated from increased protein catabolism, especially with oliguria
  - ☐ carboxyhemoglobin level—elevated in smoke inhalation or carbon monoxide poisoning
  - ☐ total protein level—hypoproteinemia from capillary defect and massive gluconeogenesis
- radiography—chest radiographs may be normal initially (up to 48 hours after the injury); serial films later reveal atelectasis, chemical pneumonia, and pulmonary edema

Table 3.4

Classification of Burn Depth

Classification		Formulary	Areas involved	Appearance	Sensitivity	Healing time
Partial thickness	Superficial	First degree to second degree	Epidermis and the papillae of the dermis	Bright red to pink, blanches to touch, serum-filled blisters, glistening and moist	Pain is severe; skin sensitive to air temperature and touch	7 to 14 days—usually no scarring
	Deep	Second degree	Epidermis and ½ to ⅞ of the dermis; appendages (hair follicles, sweat gland, and sebaceous gland) usually present	Possibly blistered, pink to light red to white, soft and pliable, blanching present	Pressure may be painful from exposed nerve endings	14 to 21 days—scarring and discoloration usually occur; can convert to full thickness from infection, exposure to air, or impaired circulation
Full thickness		Third degree to fourth degree	All epidermis and dermis; may include subcutaneous tissue, muscle, bone	In toddlers, may appear bright red and dry due to hemoglobin trapped in tissue; otherwise, snowy white, gray, or brown; firm and leathery in texture; inelastic	No pain, as nerve endings are destroyed	Needs skin grafting to heal and to minimize scarring

Courtesy of Patricia Orr, RN, MBA, CCRN; Janice Fitzgerald, RN, MSN

Nursing diagnosis

Potential for additional loss of skin integrity related to continued burning.

GOAL: STOP THE BURNING PROCESS.

Interventions

1. Assess the patient for active burning. If heat is evident, cool the burn with room temperature normal saline solution or cool water for 10 to 15 minutes. DO NOT USE ICE WATER OR APPLY ICE. Cover the patient with sterile sheets and blankets.

2. Remove all clothing and jewelry from the patient.

Rationale

Reducing skin temperature helps stop the burning. DO NOT USE ICE as it may damage tissue and cause hypothermia. Body heat escapes through the open wounds.

Clothing, coins, belts, and jewelry can retain heat and prolong the burning process.

Nursing diagnosis

Potential for impaired gas exchange related to airway burns and carbon monoxide inhalation.

GOAL: Promote and maintain optimal gas exchange.

Interventions

1. Assess the patient's respiratory status and maintain a patent airway. If signs of upper airway edema are present, prepare for emergency airway management. (See "Endotracheal Intubation," "Needle Cricothyroidotomy," and "Surgical Cricothyroidotomy" in Section VII.)

2. Assess the patient for signs of smoke inhalation, including:
- complaint or report of inhalation
- facial or neck burns
- soot or edema in the mouth
- carbonaceous sputum
- blisters around the mouth
- singed nasal or facial hairs.

3. Administer 100% humidified oxygen via a nonrebreathing mask, as ordered.

4. Monitor ABG and carbon monoxide levels and evaluate chest radiograph results.

Rationale

Smoke inhalation can cause airway burns, laryngospasms, and progressive edema resulting in partial or complete airway obstruction. Upper airway edema is the most rapidly progressive pulmonary injury and can totally occlude the larynx in less than 8 hours after the burn.

The half-life of carbon monoxide decreases as fractional inspired oxygen is increased. For example, the half-life of carbon monoxide is 40 to 90 minutes on 100% oxygen or 360 minutes on 21% oxygen, or room air.

Carbon monoxide binds to hemoglobin and inhibits oxygen transport and utilization. Carbon monoxide poisoning or smoke inhalation elevates carboxyhemoglobin levels. Initially, ABG and chest radiograph results may not reveal changes indicative of smoke inhalation, but later radiographs show signs consistent with deterioration as pulmonary inflammation and edema develop (may not become evident for 12 to 24 hours).

*Supplemental nursing diagnosis

5. Anticipate the need for endotracheal intubation and mechanical ventilation. Suction the patient as needed. (See "Endotracheal Intubation" in Section VII.)

Early intubation before laryngeal edema and spasms develop may prevent a later tracheostomy. Tracheostomy-related infections increase the morbidity and mortality for burn patients. Tracheostomy ties (twill tape) are recommended to secure an endotracheal tube if the patient has facial burns and edema. Frequent suctioning is usually needed to clear copious mucus and debris from the smoke inhalation victim; however, judicious suctioning is required with pulmonary edema. (See "Pulmonary Edema" in Section IV.)

6. Assess chest wall movement and chest compliance during ventilation, and prepare for an escharotomy if the patient has circumferential chest burns.

Anterior or circumferential eschar formation restricts chest wall expansion and impedes ventilation, usually requiring an escharotomy.

Nursing diagnosis

Potential for decreased tissue perfusion and fluid volume deficit secondary to loss of skin barrier and redistribution of fluid into interstitial space.

GOAL: Optimize tissue perfusion by restoring normovolemia.

Interventions

1. Monitor vital signs, ECG, and central venous pressure and pulmonary arterial pressure (if available) every 5 to 15 minutes or as the patient's condition warrants. Closely monitor urine output.

2. Assess the patient for signs of hypovolemia, including:
- hypotension
- tachypnea
- tachycardia
- excessive thirst.

3. Insert two large-bore I.V. lines and draw baseline laboratory samples, as ordered. Monitor ongoing laboratory data. Assemble equipment and assist with arterial line insertion.

4. Calculate the extent of the burns using the Rule of Nines or the Lund & Browder chart. Calculate volume replacement using the Parkland formula.

5. Administer calculated fluid volume replacement as follows:
- ½ amount of fluid in first 8 hours
- ¼ amount of fluid in second 8 hours
- ¼ amount of fluid in third 8 hours.
Monitor urine output and specific gravity.
Note: *Fluid resuscitation refers to postinjury and not postadmission to the hospital.*

Rationale

The stratum corneum is the skin's water barrier. Damage to this layer causes a massive fluid loss. Stasis and increased capillary permeability cause redistribution of existing volume. The resultant hypovolemia can reduce cardiac output by as much as 50%. Dysrhythmias may result from electrolyte imbalance, fluid volume deficit, decreased cardiac output, and hypothermia.

Large-bore catheters permit rapid infusion of substantial fluid volumes. Baseline laboratory data help assess hemodynamic status and enable later trend analysis. Frequent blood sampling provides a guide to fluid, blood, electrolyte, and clotting factor replacement. Baseline blood cultures aid monitoring and treatment of infection. Arterial line accessibility minimizes percutaneous punctures and facilitates frequent blood sampling.

Determination of the percentage of body surface burn area (BSBA) provides a basis for calculating fluid volume replacement. The American College of Surgeons recommends using the Rule of Nines and the Parkland formula.

Although the Parkland formula permits calculation of replacement volume, urine output and specific gravity most accurately reflect the adequacy of therapy and hydration. If the calculated volume replacement does not furnish adequate tissue perfusion, reassess the percentage of BSBA and the volume replacement calculations and reevaluate the patient for concomitant injuries.

6. Monitor serum pH and administer sodium bicarbonate, as ordered.

Compensatory vasoconstriction and blood flow shunted from the periphery cause metabolic acidosis and lactic acid accumulation. Sodium bicarbonate supplements aid acid neutralization.

7. Insert an indwelling urinary catheter and monitor output for volume and character. Maintain fluid replacement as ordered to achieve a urine output of 50 to 100 cc/hour for an adult and 0.5 cc/kg body weight/hour for a child. Anticipate the need for diuretics.

Urine output is the most effective measurement of tissue perfusion. Muscle tissue destruction and RBC damage release myoglobin and hemoglobin into the circulation. These by-products clog the renal tubules. This, combined with decreased renal perfusion, can cause acute renal failure. Aggressive fluid replacement promotes clear renal tubules by flushing the kidneys. Pigmented urine usually warrants an increased output of approximately 100 cc/hour and may require diuretics.

Figure 3.1 Using the Rule of Nines

You can quickly estimate the extent of an adult patient's burn by using the Rule of Nines. This method divides an adult's body surface area into percentages that, when totaled, equal 100%. To use this method, mentally transfer your patient's burns to the body chart shown here, then add up the corresponding percentages for each burned body section. The total, a rough estimate of the extent of your patient's burn, enters into the formula to determine his initial fluid replacement needs.

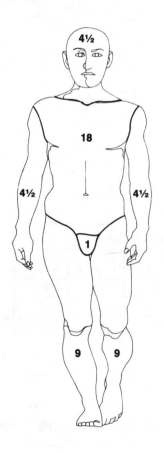
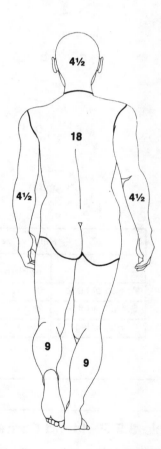

Figure 3.2 Using the Lund & Browder Chart

The Rule of Nines is a quick way to roughly estimate the percentage of your patient's body surface that has been burned. But you cannot use it for infants and children. Why? Because their body section percentages differ from those of adults. (For example, an infant's head accounts for about 19% of his total body surface area, compared to 9% for an adult.) To determine the extent of an infant's or child's burns, use the Lund & Browder chart shown here. This chart, unlike the Rule of Nines, takes proportional age-size differences into account.

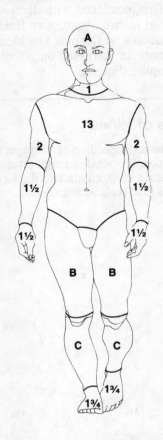
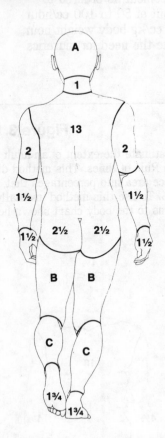

Relative percentages of areas affected by growth						
	At birth	1 year	5 years	10 years	15 years	Adult
A: Half of head	9½%	8½%	6½%	5½%	4½%	3½%
B: Half of thigh	2¾%	3¼%	4%	4¼%	4½%	4¾%
C: Half of leg	2½%	2½%	2¾%	3%	3¼%	3½%

Table 3.5 Parkland Formula for Calculation of Volume Replacement

Adult: 2 to 4 cc of Ringer's lactate × kg of body weight × % body surface burn area (BSBA) in first 24 hours after injury.

Child: 3 cc of Ringer's lactate × kg of body weight × % BSBA in first 24 hours after injury.

Nursing diagnosis

Potential for hypothermia related to heat loss secondary to loss of the skin barrier.

> **GOAL:** Prevent or minimize the risk of hypothermia.

Interventions

1. Monitor the patient's core temperature by using an esophageal, bladder, or rectal probe (or pulmonary artery catheter, if available).

2. Prevent further heat loss and shivering by:
- maintaining an ambient room temperature of at least 86° F. (30° C.)
- using warmed intravenous fluids for volume replacement
- covering the patient with sterile burn sheets
- cautiously using warming lights, when appropriate.

Note: *Never use ice on a burned area of significant size as it promotes hypothermia and can convert a burn to a deeper classification.*

Rationale

Severe hypothermia can precipitate dysrhythmias and cardiac arrest as the sinoatrial node cools. These probes most accurately measure the core temperature. Heat is lost through burned areas, massive volume replacement with room temperature fluids, and a cool environmental temperature. Shivering increases metabolic demands. Sterile burn sheets shield the patient from air currents (which increase heat loss and pain), reduce the risk of infection, and prevent inadvertent debridement of burns. Warm room temperatures decrease total energy expenditure. Warming lamps provide thermal continuity during burn care and dressing application. Survival blankets can also maintain body heat and moisture by preventing evaporation.

Nursing diagnosis

Potential for decreased peripheral perfusion related to vascular disruption, eschar formation, and compartment syndrome.

> **GOAL:** Recognize early signs of decreased peripheral perfusion; maximize tissue perfusion.

Interventions

1. Assess for alteration in quality of pulses, CRT, or skin color; sensory/motor impairment; circumferential burns; and degree of pain.

2. Ensure availability of equipment for measuring intracompartment pressures. (See "Intracompartment Pressure Measurement" in Section VII.)

3. Elevate the patient's extremities, but not higher than the level of the heart.

4. Anticipate the need for fasciotomy and escharotomy.

Rationale

These signs indicate severe circulatory impairment and inadequate deep-tissue perfusion. Pain disproportionate to burns may indicate impending compartment syndrome.

Elevation promotes venous return and minimizes swelling.

These procedures release constrictive burned areas, thereby improving capillary and tissue perfusion.

Nursing diagnosis

Potential for paralytic ileus related to splanchnic constriction secondary to hypovolemia.

GOAL: Prevent or minimize the risk of paralytic ileus.

Interventions

1. Assess the abdomen by:
- observing for nausea or vomiting
- auscultating bowel sounds
- palpating the abdomen.

2. Insert a gastric decompression tube. Maintain patency and proper suction levels. (See "Paralytic Ileus" in Section IV.)

3. Monitor gastric pH every 1 to 2 hours initially. Administer antacids, as ordered.

Rationale

Absent bowel sounds in the presence of nausea and vomiting and abdominal distention indicate a need for gastric decompression.

Burn victims with > 20% to 25% BSBA require a gastric tube because paralytic ileus and stress ulcers may occur. Antacids help neutralize gastric secretions and prevent or minimize the effects of a gastric or intestinal ulcer. Gastric pH should be > 5.

Nursing diagnosis

Potential for alteration in comfort related to burned nerve endings.

GOAL: Maximize the patient's comfort level.

Interventions

1. Administer I.V. analgesia and sedation, as ordered. Schedule dressing changes and debridements 10 to 15 minutes after analgesia administration. Reassess pain after administration of analgesia. **Note:** *Repeat half of the first I.V. narcotic dose after 20 minutes for severe pain, as ordered.*

Rationale

Edema in burned areas combined with inadequate tissue perfusion precludes the even absorption of medication when administered I.M. Patient assessment helps determine if the pain and anxiety are due to burns, associated injuries, hypoxia, or hypovolemia. The degree of pain is directly related to the percentage of second- and third-degree burns; second-degree burns are painful because of injury and exposure of nerve endings. Pain disproportionate to the injury should be suspect: compartment syndrome may be developing. Medicating the burn patient before therapeutic but painful procedures reduces unnecessary pain and strengthens the patient's ability to cooperate.

Nursing diagnosis

Potential for infection related to loss of skin barrier, inadequate tissue perfusion, and depressed immunologic response.

GOAL: Prevent or minimize the risk of infection.

Interventions

1. Use sterile technique when caring for the burn wound, including the use of gloves, mask, gowns, and sheets.

Rationale

Damaged, avascularized tissue destroys the skin's normal defense response and promotes bacterial growth. Infection can extend the degree of the burn; for example, it can convert a partial-thickness to a full-thickness burn.

2. Cleanse burns with mild soap and sterile water or normal saline solution. Apply topical antibiotics and dressings, as ordered.

Topical antibiotics are indicated because decreased tissue perfusion reduces the peripheral efficacy of systemic antibiotics.

3. Maintain the patient in protective isolation, if indicated.

Any patient with second-degree burns of > 25% BSBA or third-degree burns > 10% BSBA requires protective isolation. Frequent colony counts, wound cultures (preferably three times a week), and clinical assessments facilitate rapid infection recognition and treatment.

4. Inspect burned areas for signs of infection at each dressing change and debridement. Culture burns three times a week.

5. Obtain the patient's allergy and tetanus immunization history. Administer systemic antibiotics and tetanus immunization as ordered. (See Appendix 6, "Tetanus Prophylaxis.") Monitor the patient's temperature, sensorium, and bowel sounds. Culture all body areas including blood and burn wounds if signs of infection develop.

Antibiotics are rarely prescribed prophylactically; they are more commonly initiated after a positive culture has been obtained. Devitalized, burned tissue provides an optimal medium for growth of anaerobic tetanus organisms.

6. Monitor chest radiographs. Obtain a sputum sample for culture and sensitivity, as ordered.

Bacterial invasion, inadequate pulmonary circulation, and chemical irritation from toxic product inhalation can lead to chemical pneumonitis, bronchopneumonia, and atelectasis. These circumstances also increase the risk of pulmonary emboli.

7. Monitor laboratory data for results indicating infection.

An increased or decreased WBC count, decreased platelet count, and positive cultures signal infection.

Nursing diagnosis

Potential for impaired physical mobility related to contractures secondary to loss of elasticity of burn tissue.

GOAL: Prevent or minimize contracture formation.

Interventions

1. Position the patient properly using specialized beds or turning frames, egg-crate mattresses, and nonadherent burn sheets and pillows. Ensure that burned skin surfaces do not touch each other or bed surfaces, if possible.

2. Maintain position of function:
- neck—slight hyperextension
- axilla/shoulder—60° abduction
- arm—90° angle with 30° to 40° flexion
- wrist/hand—25° to 30° dorsiflexion with hands slightly flexed
- hips—15° to 20° abduction
- knees—extended with slight flexion
- ankles—90° flexion.

Rationale

Rehabilitation begins immediately in the emergency department or acute resuscitation area. Proper positioning promotes full range-of-motion capacity for each joint by preventing contractures and promoting healing.

3. Do not use pillows if the patient has ear or neck burns.

This avoids direct pressure on burned areas and prevents contracture formation.

4. Assess burn wounds frequently for exposed tendons, banding, or contracture formation. Position and splint as previously indicated.

Exposed tendons need to be identified and require special care to preserve function. Contracture or banding of the burn wound can develop within 8 hours without proper positioning. Splints maintain functional positions, especially of the hands and feet.

Additional considerations

Rehabilitation of the burn victim and psychosocial support for him and his family begin immediately. Body image is severely affected because the physical and emotional changes are often overwhelming. Many burn victims require months to years of reconstructive surgery and rehabilitation. The patient's injury and needs must be considered in conjunction with services available at the initial receiving facility. Burn patients usually require transfer to a major burn facility. Transfer criteria according to the American Burn Association are summarized in Table 3.6.

Table 3.6
American Burn Association Transfer Criteria

- > 25% BSBA
- > 20% BSBA in children under 10 years, adults over 40 years
- Full-thickness burns involving more than 10% BSBA
- All burns involving face, eyes, ears, hands, feet, perineum
- Burns associated with significant fractures or other major injury
- High-voltage electrical burns
- Inhalation injury and significant facial burns
- Lesser burns in patients with significant preexisting disease
- Suspected abuse of pediatric or elderly patients

Associated care plans

Upper Airway Obstruction
Lower Airway Obstruction
Inhalation Injuries
Psychosocial Support of the Trauma Patient
Pulmonary Edema
Paralytic Ileus
Eye Injuries
Vasogenic Shock
Malnutrition in the Trauma Patient
Substance Abuse in the Trauma Patient
Adult Respiratory Distress Syndrome

Associated procedures

Preparation for Surgery
Endotracheal Intubation
Needle Cricothyroidotomy
Surgical Cricothyroidotomy
Intracompartment Pressure Measurement

ELECTRICAL BURNS

Assessment

Mechanism of injury/ etiology:
- contact with a source of electrical current (mechanically generated or from lightning, by arc or direct contact)

Physical findings:
Skin
- exit wounds (round or oval gray lesions surrounded by inflammation)

- entry wounds (black or charred areas of necrosis with ischemia, cyanosis, or edema formation)

Respiratory
- respiratory arrest

Cardiovascular
- shock state
- hemorrhage
- dysrhythmias or cardiac standstill

- signs of circulatory impairment (such as weak or absent peripheral pulses, pallor, prolonged capillary refill time [CRT])
- chest pain

Neurologic
- loss of consciousness or altered level of consciousness
- headache

- focal nervous irritability

Genitourinary
- myoglobinuria (resulting from muscle breakdown)

Musculoskeletal
- long-bone fractures
- spinal column fractures

Diagnostic studies

- patient history and physical examination diagnose the injury
- studies such as 12-lead ECG, radiographs, DPL, laboratory data, and measurement of intracompartmental pressure are utilized to confirm or rule out injuries associated with the electrical burn

Nursing diagnosis

Potential for ineffective breathing patterns related to respiratory paralysis secondary to nervous system damage from electrical current.

GOAL: Establish and maintain a patent airway and optimize gas exchange.

Interventions

1. Monitor the patient's respiratory status closely.

2. Ensure the availability and proper functioning of equipment for supplemental oxygenation, intubation, and mechanical ventilation. (See "Endotracheal Intubation" in Section VII.)

Rationale

Electrical shock victims may initially lack signs of respiratory dysfunction but then rapidly deteriorate to respiratory failure as respiratory muscles develop tetanic contractions or become paralyzed. Artificial airway insertion and mechanical ventilation combat respiratory insufficiency until spontaneous respiratory function can be restored.

Nursing diagnosis

Potential for decreased tissue perfusion related to decreased circulating blood volume from capillary leakage and/or hemorrhage and myocardial dysfunction secondary to circulatory damage resulting from severe systemic electrical shock.

GOAL: Restore and maintain normovolemia.

Interventions

1. Assess the patient's cardiovascular status, including:
- baseline ECG
- vital signs
- hemoglobin/hematocrit levels
- cardiac status (continuous cardiac monitoring).

2. Ensure immediate availability of emergency drugs and equipment for cardiac defibrillation.

3. Observe for signs and symptoms of shock and internal and external hemorrhage.

4. Obtain serial cardiac enzymes, as ordered.

5. Ensure fluid administration through large-bore I.V.s. Monitor urine output and urine myoglobin. Administer osmotic diuretics, as ordered.

6. Monitor ABG results. Administer sodium bicarbonate, as ordered.

Rationale

Electrical current passing through the chest may cause myocardial damage or disruption in conduction resulting in dysrhythmias, such as ventricular fibrillation or cardiac standstill. Shock secondary to capillary leakage and/or hemorrhage from vessels, organs, intestines, or concomitant injuries may develop rapidly or subtly over time. Cardiopulmonary resuscitation and defibrillation may be required to correct myocardial irritability or asystole. Cardiac enzymes aid assessment of structural myocardial damage and infarction.

It is more difficult to calculate volume replacement for patients sustaining electrical burns than for patients with thermal burns (because this assessment is based on the percentage of total body surface area). The most accurate hydration indicator is urine output, which should be approximately 100 cc per hour in the adult. Hydration also promotes myoglobin clearance, if present. If myoglobin persists after achieving optimal hydration, osmotic diuretics are recommended.

ABG analysis may reveal metabolic acidosis secondary to anaerobic metabolism. Hypovolemia, acidosis, and myoglobin predispose the patient to acute renal failure (ARF). Proper volume replacement and the alkalinizing properties of sodium bicarbonate aid correction of serum and urine acidosis, thereby decreasing the risk of ARF.

Nursing diagnosis

Potential for altered level of consciousness, sensation, and motor function related to injury to the central nervous system secondary to the effects of electrical shock.

> **GOAL:** Identify early signs of central nervous system involvement; prevent further injury during episodes of altered sensorium or seizure activities.

Interventions

1. Assess neurologic signs every hour after admission for the first 24 hours. Report any deterioration. (Refer to "Head Injury" in Section II.)

2. Institute seizure precautions according to hospital protocol.

Rationale

Electrical current may cause brain stem shock or contusion, epidural or subdural hematoma, brain tissue burns, intraventricular hemorrhage, seizures, and loss of consciousness. Manifestation of neurologic damage may be as severe as above or evidenced by irritability and amnesia. Seizure precautions, for example, bed rest and padded side rails, can aid in the prevention of additional injury.

*Supplemental nursing diagnosis

Nursing diagnosis

Potential for impaired physical mobility related to fractures.

> **GOAL:** Recognize actual or potential associated injury; prevent secondary disability.

Interventions

1. Ensure proper spinal immobilization. Assist with vertebral and extremity immobilization and radiographs as necessary. (See "Cervical Spine Injury," "Thoracic, Lumbar, and Sacral Spine Injury," and "Fractures: Open/Closed" in Section II.)

Rationale

Tetanic contractions or falls caused by the electrical current may produce vertebral and long-bone fractures. Assume spinal cord injury until proven otherwise.

Nursing diagnosis

Potential for impaired tissue perfusion related to venous thrombosis secondary to denaturing of protein caused by heat produced by electrical current.

> **GOAL:** Maximize tissue perfusion.

Interventions

1. Assess the patient's extremities for:
- presence, quality, and equality of peripheral pulses
- skin color and integrity
- CRT
- neuromuscular function
- pain.

2. Ensure availability of equipment for intracompartment pressure measurement. (See "Intracompartment Pressure Measurement" in Section VII.) Prepare the patient for surgery. (See "Preparation for Surgery" in Section VII.)

Rationale

Electrical energy conversion to thermal heat causes denaturing of tissue protein, resulting in damage from tissue coagulation. This is manifested by vessel thrombosis and muscle, bone, tendon, and nerve necrosis, commonly resulting in compartment syndrome. This patient may require surgical exploration and debridement of entry and exit wounds, fasciotomy, or amputation.

Additional considerations

Burn wounds resulting from electrical current require the same resuscitation methods as thermal burns. (See "Thermal Burns" in Section III for specific wound care information.) Locating the current's entry and exit sites is imperative and may require a comprehensive physical examination. Assessment of the current's tract helps evaluate underlying tissue and structural damage. Skin damage and external signs of injury may appear minimal on early examination, causing the inexperienced health care provider to overlook life-threatening pathology. Total manifestation of burn injury may take 7 to 10 days to become apparent. The patient should remain in the hospital for monitoring and observation if he has experienced a loss of consciousness, dysrhythmias, or concomitant injuries such as thoracic, abdominal, eye, ear, neurologic, and orthopedic damage. The patient may arrive at the hospital in cardiopulmonary arrest secondary to electrical current striking the heart or brain stem and halting cardiovascular or neurologic function.

Associated care plans

Hemorrhagic Shock
Compartment Syndrome
Fractures: Open/Closed
Thermal Burns
Acute Myocardial Infarction
Head Injury
Cervical Spine Injury
Thoracic, Lumbar, and Sacral Spine Injury
External Genitalia Injury
Psychosocial Support of the Trauma Patient

Associated procedures

Preparation for Surgery
Endotracheal Intubation
Intracompartment Pressure Measurement

Medical diagnosis

INHALATION INJURIES: Smoke, Carbon Monoxide, Cyanide/Hydrogen Cyanide, Polyvinyl Chloride

Assessment

Note: *Toxic inhalation may cause thermal and chemical burns in the airway and lung parenchyma and systemic toxic chemical effects. Clinical manifestations may reflect one, all, or any combination of these three types of injuries.*

Note: *Examine all inhalation victims for concomitant thermal or chemical burns and institute appropriate measures to stop the burning process as necessary. Eliciting accurate and comprehensive information from the patient, family, and prehospital care providers is critical in determining the type, severity, and potential complications of the inhalation exposure. Ask about:*
- *the mechanism of exposure, for example, fire, industrial machinery, exhaust*
- *the type of fire, for example, closed or open space*
- *the duration of the patient's exposure*
- *the type of materials found smoldering or burning*
- *the distance the patient was found from the fire*
- *the patient's condition when found: conscious or unconscious.*

Mechanism of injury/ etiology:
- smoke inhalation: exposure to forced hot air, smoke, steam, or the toxic chemical or gaseous products of combustion, including carbon monoxide, nitrogen oxide, benzenes, aldehydes, ammonia, hydrogen cyanide, or hydrochloric acid; can cause thermal respiratory injury
- carbon monoxide: component of all fires; exposure to products of incomplete combustion of gasoline, oil, wood, coal; present in automobile exhaust and a by-product of combustion in faulty or improperly maintained or ventilated furnaces or heating systems, water heaters, indoor barbecue grills, fireplaces; industrial exposure can occur in mills and mines and from locomotive gases and blast furnaces; causes systemic effects
- cyanide/hydrogen cyanide: inhalation exposure to combustion products of silk, wool, polyurethane, and nylon; cyanide-containing ingredients are found in silver polish, fumigants, and metal cleaners; causes systemic effects
- polyvinyl chloride: inhalation exposure in the form of hydrochloric acid upon combustion of electrical or telephone wires; wall or floor coverings; synthetic fibers in furniture, carpet, draperies, appliances, records, toys, shower curtains, office equipment or furniture, and raincoats; causes chemical burn in the lungs

Physical findings: Table 3.7 in Section III summarizes the clinical manifestations of smoke, carbon monoxide, hydrogen cyanide, and hydrochloric acid inhalation.

Diagnostic studies

- smoke—chest radiograph may later reveal a clinical picture of adult respiratory distress syndrome (ARDS); ABG results may reflect hypoxia or hyperventilation; bronchoscopy may confirm thermal or chemical burns, presence of soot
- carbon monoxide—actual carboxyhemoglobin percentage can be calculated from an arterial or venous blood sample; a venous blood sample placed in a purple-top blood tube should be obtained at the exposure site; expired air concentration can be determined with a carbon monoxide analyzer; psychometric testing should be done to assess the patient's cognitive and psychomotor skills
- hydrogen cyanide—serum thiocyanate or direct cyanide levels will be higher than normal
- hydrochloric acid—ABGs will reflect decreased PaO_2; chest radiograph may be normal initially but later reveal a clinical picture of ARDS; bronchoscopy may confirm airway edema and mucosal damage

Nursing diagnosis

Ineffective airway clearance related to complete or partial airway obstruction by laryngeal spasms or edema of the vocal cords, epiglottis, and upper trachea secondary to inhalation of heated, toxic agents.

GOAL: Restore and maintain a patent airway.

Interventions

1. Assess the patient rapidly for signs of airway obstruction:
- dyspnea, tachypnea
- retractions on inspiration
- stridor, snoring
- decreased or absent breath sounds
- anxious expression, restlessness.

2. Assess the patient for indications of inhalation of heated steam or smoke-filled air:
- dyspnea
- hoarse, raspy voice; laryngitis
- hacking cough
- burning sensation in mucous membranes and chest on inspiration
- singed nasal or facial hair
- soot in mucosa and sputum
- rhinitis, conjunctivitis
- altered mental state.

3. Ensure immediate availability and proper functioning of endotracheal intubation and cricothyroidotomy equipment. Assist with airway establishment as necessary. (See "Endotracheal Intubation," "Needle Cricothyroidotomy," and "Surgical Cricothyroidotomy" in Section VII.)

4. Ensure availability of equipment necessary for bronchoscopy; assist as necessary. (See "Bronchoscopy" in Section VII.)

5. Administer bronchodilators, as ordered.

Rationale

Inhaled carbon particles deposited in the upper and lower airways cause severe mucosal irritation. Heated air or steam may cause respiratory burns followed by progressive edema. On admission, the smoke inhalation patient may exhibit severe respiratory distress, necessitating rapid airway management. However, he may have, on admission, a patent natural airway, which later becomes obstructed as pulmonary inflammation and edema develop. Overt signs of pulmonary inflammation may not develop for as long as 12 to 24 hours after the exposure. Expect a patient showing obvious signs of soot and smoke inhalation to develop secondary pulmonary complications. **Note:** *Assume that any patient who has inhaled smoke has also inhaled toxic gases. Anticipate pulmonary and systemic complications.*

The patient with respiratory irritation or burns who rapidly develops airway obstruction requires an artificial airway—possibly a cricothyroidotomy, if edema is excessive.

Early bronchoscopic examination helps determine the severity of respiratory burns, mucosal injury, and edema and permits deep pulmonary suctioning.

Bronchodilators, administered parenterally or by inhalation, reduce bronchospasms caused by the inflammatory reaction and aid restoration of airway patency.

Nursing diagnosis

Potential for impaired gas exchange related to decreased transport, release, and utilization of oxygen secondary to toxic levels of carbon monoxide, hydrogen cyanide, and hydrochloric acid.

GOAL #1: Rapidly identify the inhaled toxin.

Interventions

1. Ensure that the prehospital blood sample is analyzed for carboxyhemoglobin level. Send admission blood samples for an ABG study as well as for carboxyhemoglobin, thiocyanate, and direct cyanide levels as ordered. Additional studies may include those for CBC, cardiac enzymes, and electrolyte levels.

Rationale

Prehospital carbon monoxide levels generally reflect the degree of toxic exposure. Early confirmation of the specific toxic chemical inhaled and current levels in the circulation help determine the severity of exposure and direct further care. Other laboratory studies may be requested based on preexisting disease and associated injuries.

GOAL #2: Restore normal gas exchange.

Interventions

1. Administer 100% oxygen at 10 to 15 liters via a tight-fitting, nonrebreathing mask to the conscious patient immediately after exposure.

2. Administer 100% oxygen via an endotracheal or cricothyroidotomy tube to the unconscious patient; assist respirations with a mechanical ventilator and positive end-expiratory pressure (PEEP) as ordered.

Rationale

Hypoxia is the most common insult regardless of the toxic inhalant. Carbon monoxide rapidly combines with hemoglobin, displaces oxygen, and forms carboxyhemoglobin. The remaining oxygen clings to the hemoglobin and cannot be released or utilized in cellular respiration. The impaired cellular gas exchange causes decreased circulating $PaCO_2$ and tissue hypoxia. Hydrogen cyanide also causes tissue asphyxia. It interrupts electron transfer, decreasing the tissues' ability to use oxygen and thus impairing cellular respiration. Finally, pulmonary mucosal and capillary damage from heated air and hydrochloric acid causes clinical manifestations of pulmonary edema, hemorrhage, and ARDS. Early administration of 100% oxygen begins the carbon monoxide washout process and increases capillary oxygen availability. Although oxygen may be beneficial in hydrogen cyanide poisoning, hydrogen cyanide inhalation is virtually fatal. Supplemental 100% oxygen must be administered early to all patients with known or suspected toxic chemical inhalation, whether or not they have symptoms, to minimize secondary pulmonary complications. Early use of PEEP promotes patency of the smaller airways and alveoli.

3. Minimize patient exertion and stimulation.

Any activities that increase metabolism and oxygen consumption accelerate hypoxia.

4. Prepare the patient for hyperbaric oxygen (HBO) therapy if available. Ensure completion of chest radiograph and ECG before HBO therapy. Assist with myringotomies as necessary. Follow institutional or referral center guidelines for preparation for HBO therapy.

Carbon monoxide's affinity to hemoglobin enables it to cling strongly and resist displacement. HBO therapy, providing high oxygen concentrations at increased atmospheric pressure, speeds the carbon monoxide washout. It reduces the half-life of carbon monoxide to 23 minutes, whereas 100% oxygen via a nonrebreathing mask only reduces it to 90 minutes. The half-life of carbon monoxide in room air is 5 to 6 hours.

GOAL #3: Maintain optimal gas exchange.

Interventions

1. Monitor the patient continuously for deterioration in respiratory status as evidenced by changes or trends in chest radiographs, vital signs, ABGs, breath sounds, secretions.

Rationale

Serial laboratory studies, radiographs, and constant monitoring of the overall clinical picture aid early detection of pulmonary complications. Patients should remain under constant observation for 18 to 24 hours after inhalation exposure because of the risk of delayed pulmonary complications.

2. Measure carbon monoxide levels every 2 to 4 hours while continuing oxygen therapy.

Oxygen therapy is usually discontinued when the carboxyhemoglobin level falls below 10%. Patients who do not respond to surface therapy with 100% oxygen may require transfer to the nearest HBO center.

3. Provide scrupulous pulmonary hygiene, including:
- frequent suctioning
- patient repositioning
- chest physiotherapy
- incentive spirometry.

Early initiation of pulmonary hygiene optimizes aeration and minimizes complications from retained secretions. These measures mobilize secretions, prevent pooling, and promote full lung expansion.

Nursing diagnosis

Potential for decreased cardiac output related to dysrhythmias secondary to myocardial toxicity.

GOAL: Recognize early signs of myocardial compromise.

Note: *Patients with preexisting cardiac disease have an increased sensitivity to toxic inhalants.*

Interventions

1. Maintain the patient on a continuous ECG monitor for at least 18 to 24 hours or as his condition warrants.

2. Assess serial ECGs for:
- atrial fibrillation
- atrioventricular blocks
- a prolonged PR interval
- bundle branch blocks
- premature ventricular contractions.

3. Obtain baseline lactate dehydrogenase, serum glutamic-oxaloacetic transaminase, and creatine phosphokinase levels; monitor trends in serial studies.

4. Ensure availability of emergency cardiac drugs.

Rationale

Myocardial hypoxia can cause potentially life-threatening dysrhythmias. Hypoxia-related ischemic changes can be detected on serial 12-lead ECGs and via serial cardiac enzyme evaluation. Drug therapy may be ineffective unless accompanied by measures to correct the hypoxia.

Nursing diagnosis

*Potential for ineffective breathing patterns and impaired sensorimotor and cognitive functions related to anoxia secondary to disruption in cerebral and medullary cellular respiration by carbon monoxide and hydrogen cyanide.

GOAL #1: Optimize respiratory function.

Interventions

1. Ensure availability and proper functioning of equipment needed for endotracheal intubation and mechanical ventilation. Assist as needed. (See "Endotracheal Intubation" in Section VII.)

Rationale

Medulla-regulated respirations cease as the nerve cells are deprived of the oxygen required for their respiration.

*Supplemental nursing diagnosis

> **GOAL #2:** Recognize impaired mentation and mobility; support the patient during period of impairment.

Interventions

1. Assess the patient's baseline neurologic status and monitor trends every hour or more often, as his condition warrants.

2. Provide for the patient's safety during impairment.

3. Assist with psychomotor testing as necessary.

Rationale

Impaired oxygenation causes cerebral changes ranging from disorientation to unconsciousness. Cerebral anoxia from smoke or toxic chemical inhalation is the major cause of fire-related deaths. Mentation, coordination, and cognitive function should improve with oxygen therapy.

Changes in vision, hearing, motor coordination, and judgment occur with toxic inhalation anoxia.

Subtle changes in mentation and cognitive function are not easily identified in routine neurologic examinations. Psychometric evaluations identify patient difficulty with such activities as visual discrimination, fine motor coordination, time estimation, memory, and concentration.

Additional considerations

Patients suspected of inhaling or known to have inhaled toxic agents should undergo a thorough history taking and physical examination and be admitted for observation for at least 18 to 24 hours after exposure. They should also be scheduled for follow-up appointments for repeated psychometric, laboratory, and possibly radiographic evaluation 24 to 36 hours after discharge. Psychiatric evaluation may be indicated for inhalation injuries of suspicious origin. Carbon monoxide poisoning is a common route for attempted suicide. Patient education with appropriate referrals may be necessary for victims of smoke and toxic chemical inhalation from house fires, faulty ventilation, or automobile exhaust.

Associated care plans

Upper Airway Obstruction
Lower Airway Obstruction
Thermal Burns
Chemical Burns
Adult Respiratory Distress Syndrome
Pulmonary Edema

Associated procedure and study

Bronchoscopy
Endotracheal Intubation

Table 3.7
Physical Findings in Inhalation Injuries

Heated or burning air or smoke:
Symptoms usually evident immediately after exposure:
- dyspnea
- chest pain or tightness
- burning sensation in mucous membranes, especially on inspiration
- stridor
- hoarse, raspy voice/laryngitis
- hacking cough
- wheezing
- conjunctivitis
- rhinitis
- carbonaceous sputum
- singed nasal or facial hair
- neurologic deterioration[1]

Carbon monoxide:
Symptoms usually evident immediately after exposure:[2]

10% to 20% carbon monoxide level:
- headache/tightness in forehead
- slight breathlessness
- decreased visual acuity
- decreased cerebral function
- cognitive and psychometric changes, possibly subtle

20% to 40% carbon monoxide level:[3]
- severe headache with throbbing temples
- generalized weakness, aching limbs
- dizziness, syncope
- dim vision
- nausea/vomiting
- tinnitus
- confusion, irritability
- hyperreflexia
- yawning
- dilated pupils
- hypotension, tachycardia
- atrial and ventricular dysrhythmias, ST-segment depression

40% to 60% carbon monoxide level:
- tachycardia
- tachypnea
- dysrhythmias
- cardiopulmonary instability
- unresponsiveness
- seizures

60% to 80% carbon monoxide level:
- severely depressed cardiopulmonary and neurologic functions (usually fatal)

Hydrogen cyanide:[4]
- almond odor to breath and blood (classic finding)
- giddiness
- headache
- palpitations
- dyspnea
- unconsciousness
Hydrogen cyanide is toxic and potentially fatal at 2 to 10 mg/liter; a fatal level, usually > 10 mg/liter, can be reached within a few seconds.

Hydrochloric acid:[5]
- respiratory distress
- cerebral dysfunction
- pulmonary edema, hemorrhage
- airway obstruction with bronchospasms, mucous membrane irritation
- premature ventricular contractions, potentially fatal dysrhythmias
- chest pain
- eye irritation, increased tearing

[1]Neurologic deterioration results from simultaneous inhalation of carbon monoxide, hydrogen cyanide, polyvinyl chloride, and other highly toxic chemicals.

[2]Symptoms may be associated with either pure carbon monoxide poisoning or the physical findings of smoke inhalation.

[3]The patient may seem inebriated owing to cognitive/psychomotor changes.

[4]Symptoms usually develop within seconds of inhalation.

[5]Symptoms may not develop for as long as 6 to 24 hours after exposure.

MAXILLOFACIAL INJURIES

Assessment

Note: *Suspect all maxillofacial-injured patients of having a cervical spine injury until proven otherwise. Ensure proper spine alignment, immobilization, and stabilization with a hard cervical collar.*

Mechanism of injury/ etiology:
- blunt or penetrating facial trauma

Physical findings:
Soft tissue/Maxillofacial

- abrasions, contusions, lacerations
- hematoma, discoloration
- asymmetry
- crepitus
- bleeding, epistaxis
- pain, tenderness on palpation
- malocclusion
- trismus—tonic contractions of the masticatory muscles

- fractures (see Table 3.8, "Facial Fractures.")

Table 3.8
Facial Fractures

Upper one third of face:
- Frontal bone
- Frontal sinuses
- Supraorbital ridge

Middle one third of face:
- Nasal bones
- Zygoma and zygomatic arch
- Orbital bones
- Maxilla

Lower one third of face:
- Mandible

- enophthalmos
- diplopia
- facial anesthesia

Respiratory

- restlessness, anxiety
- air hunger
- coughing, gagging
- nasal flaring
- stridor
- retraction—intercostal, supraclavicular
- foreign object(s) blocking the airway—tongue, dentures, broken teeth, blood, mucus, vomitus, tobacco, food, gum, displaced bone fragments

Neurologic

- loss of sensation and movement due to cranial nerve damage
- Cerebrospinal fluid (CSF) leak, rhinorrhea, otorrhea

Cardiovascular

- tachycardia from blood loss and fear
- hypotension from blood loss

Gastrointestinal

- nausea and vomiting from swallowed blood

Diagnostic studies

- physical craniofacial examination—palpation of maxillofacial area pinpoints suspect areas that require further diagnostic studies
- radiography—facial bone series, tomograms, Towne's and Water's views may confirm facial fractures; cervical spine and chest radiographs help locate lodged foreign bodies
- imaging—computerized tomography of the face can help diagnose or confirm fractures and soft tissue, sinus, and craniocerebral injuries

Ineffective airway clearance related to obstruction by soft tissue edema, foreign body, or the tongue.

GOAL #1: Restore a patent airway.

Interventions

1. Manually remove any obvious obstruction from the nose or mouth; gently suction the oropharynx with a tonsillar-tip catheter.

Rationale

Blood, mucus, or foreign matter can obstruct the airway and predispose the patient to aspiration. Suctioning or manual removal of debris may alone open the airway. All attempts should be made to avoid pushing debris farther into the airway.

2. Perform the jaw-thrust or chin-lift maneuver. **Note:** *Never turn the patient's head to one side or hyperextend the head and neck.*

These maneuvers open the airway by elevating the mandible, which in turn lifts the tongue away from the pharyngeal wall. They also maintain head and neck alignment, which is essential since an undiagnosed cervical spine fracture may be present. Depending on the location and severity, patients with mandibular fractures may not respond to these maneuvers.

3. Insert an artificial oral or nasal airway.

Soft tissue relaxation often permits the tongue to fall against the posterior pharyngeal wall. This represents the most common cause of upper airway obstruction. Artificial airways reposition the tongue and may temporarily relieve the obstruction by allowing air passage around or through the airway. However, great care must be taken when inserting an artificial airway in the presence of facial fractures to minimize further injury.

4. Anticipate the need for supplemental oxygen.

Supplemental oxygen therapy may improve tissue perfusion by increasing available oxygen at the alveolar/capillary membrane.

5. Ensure availability of oral and nasal intubation equipment; assist as needed. (See "Endotracheal Intubation" in Section VII.)

The previous interventions can successfully restore a patent airway and obviate intubation. The maxillofacially injured patient usually requires emergency intubation because he is unable to maintain a patent airway. This inability results from rapidly increasing edema, difficulty in swallowing, and anatomic derangement. Intubation routes—oral, nasal, or tracheal—are determined by the access needed for operative repair. Nasal intubation is contraindicated in nasal fractures and CSF leaks.

6. Ensure availability of emergency cricothyroidotomy equipment, including surgical instruments and tracheostomy tubes in various sizes; assist as needed. (See "Needle Cricothyroidotomy" and "Surgical Cricothyroidotomy" in Section VII.)

Extensive maxillofacial injuries may impede endotracheal intubation. Upper airway obstruction is life-threatening; therefore, advanced preparation of an airway tray saves valuable time in this emergency.

7. Ensure the availability of manual and mechanical ventilation devices.

Respiratory deterioration usually requires mechanical ventilatory support.

GOAL #2: Maintain a patent airway.

Interventions

Rationale

1. Monitor the patient closely for signs of respiratory distress, including:
- air hunger
- retractions
- tachypnea
- stridor.

Ensure availability and proper functioning of intubation equipment. (See "Endotracheal Intubation" in Section VII.)

Maxillofacially injured patients who can initially protect their airways may later suffer respiratory difficulty from either progressive soft tissue edema or neurologic deterioration from an associated head injury.

2. Ensure the availability and proper functioning of appropriate suction apparatus; suction the patient as needed and document the secretions obtained.

Continued bleeding and mucus accumulation can obstruct the artificial airway. Because they provide an excellent medium for bacterial growth, retained secretions can cause lower airway complications.

Nursing diagnosis

Potential for fluid volume deficit related to hemorrhage secondary to facial trauma.

GOAL #1: Restore hemostasis and minimize fluid volume loss.

Interventions

1. Control bleeding by applying pressure; elevating the head of the bed to semi- or high-Fowler's position, unless contraindicated; and applying a cool pack.

2. Monitor the patient for signs of hemorrhagic shock. (See "Hemorrhagic Shock" in Section II.)

Rationale

Applying direct pressure stops bleeding. Caution must be exercised, however, when applying pressure to prevent injury to underlying structures. In massive hemorrhage from facial trauma, temporary presurgical hemostatic measures include anteroposterior nasal packing, insertion of large urinary catheters into the nasopharynx, clamping or ligation of bleeders, and electrocoagulation.

Maxillofacial injuries can precipitate hemorrhagic shock. The multitrauma patient can also lose blood from associated injuries.

GOAL #2: Restore and maintain normovolemia.

Interventions

1. Ensure volume replacement with at least two large-bore peripheral I.V.s.

2. Obtain baseline and serial laboratory data (hemoglobin/hematocrit levels, coagulation profile); ensure that typing and cross matching are done.

3. Administer I.V. fluids, blood, and blood products as ordered.

4. Continually monitor the patient for signs of persistent hemorrhagic shock.

Rationale

Multiple large-bore I.V. catheters permit rapid volume infusion and blood administration.

Trend analysis of laboratory results provides necessary information for evaluating replacement-therapy efficacy. Early typing and cross matching ensure readily available blood for transfusion.

I.V. fluids, blood, and component therapy together replace lost volume.

Signs and symptoms of unrelenting or progressive shock may reflect associated injuries or inadequate hemostasis or volume replacement.

Nursing diagnosis

*Potential for altered sensory and motor function related to possible associated head injury.

GOAL: Recognize those patients at risk for concomitant neurologic injury.

Interventions

1. Assess the patient for signs of neurologic deficit, including:
• decreased level of consciousness
• impaired pupil reaction, conjugate movements, and vision
• impaired sensation and movement
• basilar skull fracture (otorrhea with CSF and blood, and mastoid bruising).

Rationale

Presence of craniocerebral injury must be ascertained. Positive neurologic findings help differentiate among focal facial nerve trauma, ocular trauma, and central nervous system deficit.

*Supplemental nursing diagnosis

Nursing diagnosis

Potential for infection related to introduction of pathogens secondary to disruption of dura, bone, or skin.

> **GOAL #1:** Minimize the risk of infection.

Interventions

1. Cleanse and irrigate wounds; avoid iodine products.

2. Shave all facial hair except the eyebrows.

3. Apply sterile dressing to open wounds until surgical repair is performed.

4. Obtain the patient's tetanus immunization history; administer tetanus toxoid as ordered. (See Appendix 6, "Tetanus Prophylaxis.")

5. Monitor the patient for CSF leak, rhinorrhea, otorrhea; cover the nose or ear(s) with a loose, sterile drip pad. Test for nuchal rigidity unless contraindicated.

6. Obtain the patient's drug allergy history; administer antibiotics if ordered.

Rationale

Early removal of blood, dirt, and foreign matter minimizes the risk of infection and facial scarring and optimizes final results of surgical repair. Normal sterile saline solution is preferred to iodine-based products because iodine not only damages the cells responsible for tissue repair and local antimicrobial defense but also may contribute to facial scarring.

Hair is an excellent medium for bacterial growth. Eyebrows are left intact because they provide landmarks during facial reconstruction and may, if shaved, not grow back normally.

Dressings provide a mechanical barrier to environmental contamination, reducing the further introduction of microorganisms.

Clostridium tetani can contaminate open wounds and cause traumatic tetanus.

A CSF leak indicates a dural tear. This provides pathogens with direct entry to the brain, promoting the risk of meningitis. A loose, sterile drip pad absorbs draining CSF without impeding its outward flow. All nasal tubes are contraindicated in CSF rhinorrhea.

Allergies to specific medications alter the choice of antibiotic agents. Antibiotic therapy remains a controversial issue, especially in the presence of a CSF leak.

> **GOAL #2:** Recognize the signs of infection.

Interventions

1. Closely monitor the patient for signs of infection, including:
- swelling disproportionate to the injury
- foul-smelling, purulent drainage
- fever and chills
- elevated WBC count
- delayed or abnormal healing
- ischemic skin, muscle, tissue
- altered mentation.

Rationale

Early recognition of signs of an infectious process, such as cellulitis or osteomyelitis, can minimize morbidity.

Nursing diagnosis

Potential for fear related to change in body image secondary to facial disfigurement.

GOAL: Decrease fear of body image change.

Interventions

1. Explain all procedures, using terms the patient understands. Repeat as often as necessary.

2. Monitor and limit inappropriate bedside conversation (verbal and nonverbal).

3. Promote and maintain the patient's established support systems by allowing telephone calls or visits from family and friends.

4. Furnish the patient with an alternative to verbal communication.

Rationale

Fear of pain, disfigurement, and corrective surgery heightens the patient's anxiety, impairing his ability to understand and retain information.

Misinterpreting conversation may increase the patient's anxiety and alienation.

The patient needs reestablishment of his existing support systems as soon as possible. Be sure to warn visitors about the changes in the patient's appearance to minimize negative and inappropriate reactions.

An artificial airway will prevent the patient from speaking, so written and other forms of communication (for example, pencil and paper, or chalkboard) will be necessary.

Additional considerations

Facial injuries can be severely disfiguring and require frequent hospitalization for multiple-stage reconstructive surgery. This patient can experience serious disturbances in self-concept related to changes in body image and role performance. Both the patient and the family can benefit from crisis intervention and follow-up family counseling. Aspects of rehabilitation should begin in the emergency resuscitation area.

Associated care plans

Hemorrhagic Shock
Eye Injuries
Upper Airway Obstruction
Lower Airway Obstruction
Cervical Spine Injury
Head Injury
Psychosocial Support of the Trauma Patient

Associated procedures

Preparation for Surgery
Intrahospital Transport of the Shock Trauma Patient
Needle Cricothyroidotomy
Surgical Cricothyroidotomy
Endotracheal Intubation

SUBSTANCE ABUSE IN THE TRAUMA PATIENT

Note: *Substance abuse, particularly of alcohol, may be a precipitating factor in the patient's traumatic incident. Also, acute drug intoxication can confound and complicate diagnosis and treatment.*

Drug-screening protocols vary according to institution. But, at a minimum, all patients with an altered level of consciousness should receive a general drug screening as part of their initial evaluation. Any patient with a positive drug or alcohol screen should be assessed for referral to a drug and alcohol counselor.

It is important to note that most patients with a history of substance abuse also have a very high potential for abuse of prescribed pain medications. While pain medications should never be withheld because of a history of abuse, pain medication use should be monitored very carefully and the patient detoxified if necessary.

Information in Table 3.9 includes signs and symptoms of intoxication, medical treatment, and nursing interventions for the major classifications of substances of abuse. The mediconursing management of substance abuse must be incorporated into the management of traumatic injuries; this procedure may mandate alterations in the care provided to the patient with isolated substance abuse.

Table 3.9

Signs/symptoms	Medical treatment	Nursing interventions
Opioids		
• coma • hypotension • tachycardia • constricted pupils • needle track marks • skin abscesses • thrombophlebitis • respiratory depression	• prevent or reverse shock • maintain respirations and ventilation • reverse central nervous system depression with naloxone (Narcan)	• continually monitor respiratory status • restrain before administering naloxone • assess for cardiac dysrhythmias and signs of withdrawal (gooseflesh, frequent yawning, tachycardia, hypertension, vomiting, abdominal cramps)
Amphetamines		
• anxiety • hyperactivity • irritability • insomnia • muscle tension • compulsive movement • teeth grinding • aggression or violence • paranoid or schizophrenic-like behavior • fever • hypertension • dilated pupils • tachycardia • convulsions • hallucinations • needle track marks • skin abscesses • thrombophlebitis	• perform gastric lavage, give activated charcoal and cathartics for ingestion • provide antihypertensives, barbiturates for seizure activity • give haloperidol for agitation	• apply therapeutic restraints to protect the patient and others • monitor for and report cardiac dysrhythmias • treat hyperthermia • provide a quiet environment • initiate suicide precautions • monitor neurologic status (primarily for seizures)
Cocaine		
• tremors • seizures • delirium • cardiovascular or respiratory failure • hallucinations • dilated pupils • tachycardia • twitching • violence • perforated nasal septum • paranoid behavior with prolonged use	• induce vomiting • perform gastric lavage • give activated charcoal • give cathartics • provide antipyretics for fever • provide anticonvulsants for treatment or prevention of seizure activity • treat tachycardia	• monitor respiratory and cardiovascular status • provide a quiet environment • monitor for seizures and protect from injury

Signs/symptoms	Medical treatment	Nursing interventions
Barbiturates		
• Central nervous system and respiratory depression • slurred speech • diminished coordination, mental alertness, and attention span • memory losses • hypotension • aggressive or suicidal behavior	• prevent or reverse shock • maintain ventilatory status • perform gastric lavage • give vasopressors (for phenobarbital overdose) • perform dialysis for extreme intoxication	• monitor neurologic, cardiac, and respiratory systems • monitor for signs of withdrawal and seizure activity • protect from injury
Phencyclidine		
• apnea • status epilepticus • coma • paralysis • paresthesias • hallucinations • anxiety • dissociative reaction • paranoia • violence • rage	• perform gastric lavage • monitor for acidic diuresis • provide diazepam or haloperidol for agitation or psychotic behavior • give diazepam for seizures • control hypertension and tachycardia	• provide a quiet environment • maintain hydration and acidic urine • initiate suicide precautions as appropriate
Hallucinogens		
• anxiety • hallucinations • depression	• perform gastric lavage • give activated charcoal • give cathartics • give diazepam for seizure control	• frequent reorientation attempts • apply restraints to protect the patient and others, as ordered • provide a quiet environment
Alcohol		
• alcohol odor on breath • slurred speech • impaired coordination • sedation • respiratory depression • agitation • vomiting	• maintain respiratory status • give haloperidol for severe agitation • give diazepam for seizure activity • provide thiamine • promote hydration	• closely monitor respiratory status • monitor for seizures • protect the airway if the patient is vomiting • monitor closely for signs and symptoms of delirium tremens (early—tremors, tachycardia, hypertension; late—hallucinations)
Cannabis		
• euphoria • relaxation • impaired depth perception and ability to estimate time • impaired immediate memory and thought continuity • dry mouth • conjunctival irritation • ataxia • tremors • agitation • hallucinations • psychotic or panic reactions • paranoia	• provide reassurance • "talk down" • give diazepam for agitation	• provide a quiet environment • protect the patient from injury • reassure him

Medical diagnosis

VENOMOUS SNAKEBITES

Assessment

Note: *Venomous snakes native to the United States belong for the most part to two families, Elapidae and Viperidae. Elapids native to the United States are the coral snakes, of which three species (Eastern, Texas, and Sonoran) are recognized. The native pit vipers are copperheads, cottonmouths, massasauga, pygmy rattlesnakes, and rattlesnakes. Together, these five species contain 40 recognized subspecies of snake. The pit vipers are distributed most widely, accounting for most snake envenomations in the United States. Venoms are usually classified as either neurotoxic or hemotoxic, which may be helpful as a general, simplified guide. Physical findings differ, depending on the species. A significant number of bites even by venomous snakes do not result in envenomation.*

Mechanism of injury/ etiology:
- snakebite with introduction of venom

Physical findings:
Coral snakes (about 2% of all snakebites in the United States)
- fang marks (may be difficult to locate)
- mild local reaction
- euphoria

- drowsiness
- nausea or vomiting
- excessive salivation (caused by dysphagia, not by excessive saliva production)
- paresthesia at the bite
- headaches
- bulbar paralysis—ptosis, myosis, blurred vision, dyspnea, dysphoria
- abnormal reflexes
- generalized paralysis

Pit vipers (95% of all venomous snakebites in the United States)
- puncture wound(s)— usually oozing blood
- pain (sometimes numbness) at the bite—may radiate up the extremity
- edema—early onset, rapidly progressive
- hypotension—nausea, diaphoresis, dizziness, weakness

- ecchymosis at the bite
- hemorrhagic blebs
- lymphangitis and lymphadenitis
- paresthesias
- muscle fasciculations
- clinical evidence of coagulopathy—persistent hypotension, petechiae, conjunctival hemorrhage, bleeding
- disseminated intravascular coagulation (DIC)— rare

Diagnostic studies

Coral snakes:
- ABG determination in severe cases—to monitor respiratory compromise

Pit vipers:
- baseline laboratory data:
  - ☐ CBC

- ☐ coagulation profile
- ☐ urinalysis
- ☐ blood type and screen (should blood be needed later to treat coagulopathy)
- ☐ repetition of the above as indicated

Nursing diagnosis

Potential for alteration in neurologic function related to coral snake neurotoxic envenomation.

> **GOAL #1:** Determine coral snake envenomation.

Interventions

1. Identify the species responsible for the bite from:
- patient description of size, coloration, and head shape
- examination of the snake.

Rationale

Treating bites is predicated on the species inflicting the bite. The coral snake has round pupils, a black nose, and red, black, and yellow stripes. Coral snakes can be differentiated from similarly colored snakes by their color-band pattern. The coral snake always has yellow and black bands bordering each other. This contrasts with similar-looking snakes that have the red and black stripes next to each other. Also, coral snakes' bands completely encircle the body; those of look-alikes do not. Finally, the nonvenomous mimics may lack the coral snake's characteristic black nasal coloring.

GOAL #2: Recognize early signs of systemic reactions to venom; initiate appropriate interventions before the respiratory system is compromised.

Interventions

1. Establish adequate I.V. access.

2. Administer antivenin as ordered.

3. Have epinephrine at the patient's bedside during the skin test.

4. Administer antivenin slowly for the first 15 to 30 minutes. If no reaction occurs, increase the rate to 15 to 20 minutes per vial. Closely observe the patient for allergic reaction, including:
- anxiety
- pruritus
- lethargy
- dyspnea
- tachycardia.

5. Administer antivenin I.V. by pump.

6. Assess the patient every 30 to 60 minutes for:
- drowsiness
- nausea or vomiting
- paresthesia at the bite
- blurred vision
- ptosis, myosis
- weakness
- dysphagia
- dyspnea
- peripheral paralysis.

7. Report signs and symptoms to the physician. Administer additional antivenin as ordered.

Rationale

I.V. lines provide a route to administer maintenance fluids (the patient may have difficulty swallowing) and antivenin.

Usually, a patient with a confirmed bite is treated with 3 to 5 vials of *Micrurus fulvius* antivenin. A skin test is generally done to elicit his sensitivity to this serum.

Epinephrine is kept immediately available for use in the event of an anaphylactic reaction.

Even when a skin test is negative, an allergic reaction can occur. With I.V. administration, a reaction usually occurs within 15 minutes.

The I.V. route is generally preferred because it is more effective and rapid-acting than other routes.

Systemic reactions to coral snake envenomation may not develop for 5 to 10 hours after the bite. But once they appear, they usually progress quickly. Drowsiness, nausea, and vomiting may develop. Without rapid intervention, the patient develops complete peripheral paralysis and respiratory arrest. Frequent assessments will uncover systemic reactions at an early stage before respiratory involvement.

A patient with systemic symptoms usually receives another dose of 3 to 5 vials of antivenin. The skin test is not usually repeated, but other precautions already mentioned apply.

Nursing diagnosis

Alteration in skin integrity related to soft tissue injury secondary to snakebite.

> **GOAL:** Prevent or minimize the risk of infection; promote healing.

Interventions

1. Determine the patient's tetanus immunization status. Administer prophylaxis as ordered.

2. Clean the wound and apply a dry, sterile dressing. Observe and document the wound condition at dressing changes. Obtain cultures and administer antibiotics as ordered.

Rationale

Active tetanus immunization prevents traumatic tetanus.

The wound from a coral snake's bite is generally small and local reaction is either absent or mild. Standard wound care usually gives the patient ample protection. Occasionally, a wound may become infected. If it does, standard principles of infection management are used.

Nursing diagnosis

Potential for fluid volume deficit related to coagulopathy secondary to pit viper envenomation.

> **GOAL #1:** Determine envenomation by pit viper species.

Interventions

1. Identify the species of snake responsible for the bite from:
● patient description of size, coloration, head shape, pit between eyes and nose, and rattle sounds
● examination of the snake
● examination of the wound.

Rationale

Pit vipers have triangular heads and vertically slit pupils. Rattlesnakes make a distinctive rattle sound with their tail when alarmed, although this tail may be missing. The bite characteristically consists of one or two fang marks, but there may be more due to reserve fangs or multiple strikes. The fang marks usually ooze a small amount of blood.

> **GOAL #2:** Maintain a normovolemic state.

Interventions

1. Draw blood samples for baseline analysis, including:
● CBC
● coagulation profile
● type and screen.
Obtain a urine specimen for urinalysis.

2. Establish I.V. access with the number and type of lines appropriate to the patient's condition; consider:
● the time since the bite
● degree of envenomation
● presence of hypotension, shock, coagulopathy.

Rationale

Baseline analysis is the starting point from which to measure developing coagulopathy. The studies are repeated as necessary to monitor symptoms and therapeutic effectiveness.

I.V. lines provide an access route to replace fluid volume deficits and administer antivenin. A patient with mild envenomation without coagulopathy needs less aggressive I.V. therapy than one with massive envenomation.

3. Administer antivenin as ordered.

A patient with confirmed pit viper envenomation receives Crotalidae antivenin, polyvalent. The dosage is determined by the extent of envenomation, not the patient's weight, as follows:
• minimal—3 to 5 vials (local tissue reaction at bite, no systemic symptoms or laboratory changes)
• moderate—6 to 12 vials (tissue reaction beyond bite area, significant systemic symptoms and moderate laboratory changes)
• severe—13 to 30+ vials (tissue reactions involve entire extremity, severe symptoms and pronounced laboratory changes).
The precautions about skin testing, allergic reactions, and administration already mentioned under coral snake bites should be followed for patients bitten by vipers.

4. Administer I.V. fluids as ordered.

Fluid therapy is indicated to treat blood loss, shock, and fluid or electrolyte losses from vomiting. Guidelines on fluid type and volume are not significantly different for snakebite victims than for any other shocked or bleeding patient.

Nursing diagnosis

Potential for decreased tissue perfusion related to vascular compression by edema secondary to envenomation.

> **GOAL:** Recognize early signs of vascular compromise in the affected extremity; intervene appropriately.

Interventions

1. Assess the patient for signs of vascular compromise in the affected extremity, including:
• prolonged capillary refill time
• extremity pallor or cyanosis (difficult to assess due to ecchymosis)
• paresthesias (may be the primary effect of venom unrelated to vascular compromise)
• lowered skin temperature
• absent pulses (by palpation or Doppler).

2. Monitor edema. Measure the extremity just proximal to the bite and at 10- and 20-cm intervals above it. Document measurements every 15 minutes while giving antivenin and every 4 hours thereafter.

3. Assist with intracompartment pressure measurements as needed. (See "Intracompartment Pressure Measurement" in Section VII.) Prepare the patient for surgery if indicated.

Rationale

The edema from pit viper bites can be dramatic. Bites of the hand can easily cause edema extending throughout the entire arm and into the chest wall. Despite this fact, vascular compromise of the extremity is rare. But if it occurs, the extremity may be lost unless interventions are prompt. Repeated, careful assessments aid prompt recognition of deterioration.

The main treatment for snakebite-related edema is antivenin. Measuring the extremity aids evaluation of therapy.

Fasciotomy is indicated if compartment syndrome develops.

███████████████████████████████ **Nursing diagnosis** ████████████████

Alteration in skin integrity related to edema, hemorrhagic blebs, and possible tissue necrosis secondary to snakebite.

> **GOAL:** Promote wound healing; prevent or minimize infection.

Interventions

1. Assess the patient's tetanus immunization status; administer prophylaxis as ordered.

2. Administer antibiotics and obtain samples for culture and sensitivity tests as ordered.

Rationale

Active tetanus immunization prevents traumatic tetanus.

Prophylactic antibiotics may be prescribed for severe bites. Usually, a broad-spectrum antibiotic is given to prevent infection. If infection occurs, culture and sensitivity tests are done to identify the causative organism. Culture results may mandate a change in antibiotic therapy.

Note: *Medical/surgical wound management of the snakebite victim is highly individualized. It may range from no treatment to skin grafting. The wound itself may be managed simply with dry, sterile dressings. Nursing care of surgical wounds in snakebite patients is similar to that for surgical wounds in other types of patients.*

Additional considerations

Many treatment aspects for snakebites remain controversial, and sources are often in direct conflict with each other. Historically, treatment included ice, tourniquets, and incision and suction. But recent sources argue that these modalities may be dangerous. Controversy also surrounds administering platelets for a decreasing platelet count. Many authorities feel that this is inadvisable: the venom will only destroy infused platelets. Agreement is broader that heparin is contraindicated in managing the rare occurrence of DIC after snakebite. Recommended treatment is administering both blood to replace losses and appropriate amounts of antivenin. Local and regional poison control centers maintain information on the latest therapy for snakebites. We recommend that you contact the poison control center nearest you for this information. These centers can not only answer questions about managing snakebites but also identify bites by uncommon or exotic species.

Associated care plans	Associated procedures
Psychosocial Support of the Trauma Patient	Intracompartment Pressure Measurement
Compartment Syndrome	Preparation for Surgery
Vasogenic Shock	
Soft Tissue Injuries	

Medical diagnosis

EYE INJURIES

Assessment

Mechanism of injury/ etiology:
- nonpenetrating blunt trauma
- penetrating globe injury
- superficial foreign body
- corneal abrasion
- burns—chemical or thermal

- radiation exposure—ultraviolet or infrared

Physical findings:
(See Table 3.10 for additional assessment findings.)

Neurologic
- loss of vision or visual field

- visual perception changes
- ptosis
- asymmetric pupils
- asymmetric eye movement
- pain
- nausea or vomiting
- eye wounds—abrasion, laceration, burn, contusion

Musculoskeletal
- periorbital hematoma or edema
- articular crepitus
- palpable defects

Diagnostic studies

- radiography—identifies location of foreign body
- computed tomography (CT)—identifies location of radiopaque and nonradiopaque substances
- tonometry—measures intraocular pressure

Nursing diagnosis

Potential for alteration in comfort related to irritation secondary to a foreign body.

GOAL #1: Determine the presence of a foreign body.

Note: *If a penetrating globe injury is suspected, no attempt should be made to examine the eye. Both eyes should be shielded and patched immediately. All patients with suspected penetrating globe injuries require consultation with an ophthalmologist.*

Interventions

1. Carefully inspect the eyelid and periorbital area.

2. Obtain information about the mechanism of injury.

Rationale

Superficial lacerations or soft tissue wounds may be the only visible indications of penetrating trauma. Suspect a penetrating injury until diagnosis proves otherwise.

A history of an explosion or metal striking metal before the patient became injured should make you suspect a penetrating injury. A patient complaining of having "something in my eye" and with a history of ultraviolet radiation exposure 4 to 6 hours prior to the symptom onset may need treatment for radiation burns.

3. Carefully examine the eye under a bright light:
• evert the lower lid by pressing against the lower orbital rim and sliding the skin while asking the patient to look up
• evert the upper lid by first asking the patient to look down. Then, grasp the lashes of the upper lid while pushing down and inward with a finger or cotton-tipped applicator and evert the upper lid. Reposition the lid by gently pulling the lashes out and down while the patient looks up.

Everting the lower lid exposes the lower conjunctival sac. Having the patient look up protects the cornea from manipulation.

Having the patient look down protects the sensitive cornea from stimulation by upper lid manipulation. This maneuver also relaxes the levator muscle, which is attached to the tarsal plate. Above it, use pressure with a cotton-tipped applicator to flip the lid. When returning the lid to its normal position, having the patient look up pulls on the levator muscle, which eases the tarsus back into position. Gently pulling the lashes out and down also helps flip the tarsus back into position.

GOAL #2: Remove any superficial foreign body.

Interventions

1. Irrigate the eye; attempt to flush out the foreign object.

2. Promote patient cooperation by:
• administering topical analgesics as ordered
• having the patient gaze steadily at a stationary object.

Rationale

Irrigating the eye is a nontraumatic way of removing a superficial foreign body.

Topical analgesics relieve pain and facilitate the patient's cooperation. Having the patient gaze at an immobile object helps keep the eye open and stationary while extracting a foreign body.

GOAL #3: Promote healing.

Interventions

1. Administer topical antibiotics as ordered (avoid ointments).

2. Patch the eye as ordered for the patient's comfort.

Rationale

Topical antibiotics help prevent corneal ulcers—a likely complication of contaminated foreign bodies. Ointments tend to delay healing; generally, drops are preferable.

Patching the eye for 24 hours helps the eye rest and promotes healing. Patching an *infected* eye is contraindicated, since it retains contaminated secretions.

Nursing diagnosis

Potential for alteration in comfort and visual perception related to corneal abrasion.

GOAL #1: Determine corneal epithelial defects.

Interventions

1. Remove contact lenses, if applicable; if no penetrating injury exists, stain the eye with fluorescein; use separate strips for each eye.

Rationale

Staining is performed *only* if no penetrating injury is present. Otherwise, staining can disseminate dye into the wound. Bottled fluorescein drops are contraindicated because they are easily contaminated with and are excellent cultures for *Pseudomonas* microorganisms. Contact lenses cover the cornea and must be removed before examination. Soft contact lenses, because of their high water content, absorb dye and will be permanently stained.

2. After staining, examine the eye under a blue light, such as a Wood's light. A plain reflected light can also be used and sometimes provides better visualization than a Wood's light. **Note:** *If a dendritic, or branching, staining pattern develops in conjunction with decreased corneal sensitivity, suspect herpes simplex keratitis.*

Corneal epithelial defects, such as abrasions or ulcers, are detectable because green fluorescein dye adheres only to damaged epithelial layers, interrupting the mirrorlike corneal surface.

GOAL #2: Promote healing.

Interventions

1. Irrigate the eye with sterile normal saline solution.

2. Administer antibiotics as ordered.

3. Patch the eye for comfort.

Rationale

Irrigation minimizes infection by helping to flush away bacteria that may have been introduced by the abrading substance.

Corneal ulcers can sometimes be prevented by early antibiotic administration.

Eyelid movement tends to irritate the corneal epithelium, which usually heals 24 to 48 hours after treatment.

GOAL #3: Promote the patient's comfort.

Interventions

1. Administer oral analgesics as ordered.

Rationale

Analgesics relieve the pain typically caused by corneal abrasions. Oral medications are recommended over topical ones; the latter tend to retard regeneration. But they will probably be needed for the initial examination.

GOAL #4: Protect corneal integrity and prevent ulcers.

Interventions

1. Tape the eyelids closed if the patient is unconscious.

2. Administer artificial tears as ordered.

3. Provide a pneumatic seal for eyes that either must remain open or have severely damaged eyelids by:
• first applying a thin layer of petroleum jelly or mineral oil to the periorbital skin
• then applying a rectangular sterile plastic wrap to the periorbital area. (These wraps can be individually packaged and gas sterilized.)

Rationale

Taping the lids closed prevents corneal exposure and drying.

Artificial tears lubricate the eye surface.

Petroleum jelly or mineral oil blocks air passage, creating a pneumatic seal. The plastic adheres to the skin through static charge and surface tension. The resulting pneumatic seal retains moisture and prevents air from drying the exposed cornea.

Nursing diagnosis

Potential for further injury related to further disruption of tissue secondary to movement of the eyes or penetrating object.

GOAL #1: Protect the eye from further injury.

Interventions

1. Immediately refer eye examination of a patient with a penetrating injury to an ophthalmologist.

2. Avoid wiping an eye with suspected or confirmed intraocular injury.

3. Cover both eyes. Apply a metal shield or paper cup to the injured eye.

4. Explain all procedures to the patient and provide reassurance.

Rationale

Manipulating the eye can cause extrusion of ocular contents.

Material near the eye may be attached to prolapsed contents; wiping can cause extrusion.

Covering both eyes decreases movement and possible damage to adjacent structures. Applying a shield or paper cup helps immobilize the impaled object and alerts other team members to the patient's injury.

These steps facilitate the patient's cooperation and ease his anxiety.

GOAL #2: Determine the type and exact location of the penetrating object.

Interventions

1. Assist with the radiographic procedures as needed.

2. Assist with obtaining a CT scan as needed.

Rationale

Radiographic visualization confirms a foreign body's location in the globe. The Water's view is usually ordered for bone-free visualization.

A CT scan can pinpoint the location of both radiopaque and nonradiopaque substances. Radiating lines on a CT scan can be caused by diffraction of light from metallic intraocular foreign bodies. Remember that rust and iron diffuse rapidly through the eye, causing permanent blindness, and copper can produce rapid toxic endophthalmitis.

GOAL #3: Prevent infection.

Interventions

1. Administer antibiotics as ordered.

2. Obtain the patient's tetanus immunization history, and administer medications as ordered.

Rationale

All penetrating foreign bodies are considered to be contaminated; antibiotic therapy should be initiated as soon as possible.

Immunization must be active to prevent traumatic tetanus.

Nursing diagnosis

Potential for loss of visual perception related to burning mechanism.

GOAL #1: Establish the presence of a burn injury.

Interventions

1. Obtain information about the patient's history and the events leading up to the eye complaint(s).

Rationale

Thermal burns rarely involve the cornea and globe because of the lid closure reflex and Bell's phenomenon of upward eye rotation. But the eyelids are commonly involved. From 6 to 10 hours elapse between exposure to ultraviolet rays generated by the sun, sun lamps, welding arcs, snow, and ice reflection and the onset of symptoms. Glassblowers and metal-furnace stokers who receive prolonged exposure to infrared radiation and its intense heat risk developing heat cataracts if their eyes are not properly protected. The eye's lens has a minimal blood supply, making it particularly vulnerable because heat is not rapidly removed and injured cells are not replaced. Either alkaline or acidic substances can cause chemical burns, with alkaline substances causing the more extensive damage.

GOAL #2: Protect the eye from further injury; restore a normal pH.

Interventions

1. Irrigate the burn with copious volumes of water as soon as possible. Make an initial determination of the eye's pH to discover whether the chemical was acidic or alkaline; then recheck after irrigation to confirm that normal pH is restored.

2. Administer cycloplegics as ordered.

3. If the eyelids are injured, apply artificial tears and a pneumatic seal to the eye as ordered to protect the cornea while the eyelids heal.

Rationale

Immediate, copious irrigation is the best treatment to remove chemical substances. Acid burns cause damage within the first few hours. Acid damage is self-limiting since the denatured tissue tends to neutralize the acid and thereby protect itself from greater penetration. Injury from alkali burns, although more destructive, usually is not evident for 3 or 4 days. Alkaline substances combine with cellular membrane lipids, totally disrupting cells, softening the tissue, and allowing progressive penetration for days. Unless copious irrigation is started within minutes of the accident, the eye may be lost.

Cycloplegics paralyze the ciliary body, which allows the eye to accommodate to light and dilate the pupil. Dilation minimizes iris adhesions to the lens, a complication of ocular chemical burns.

Preventing corneal ulcers is easier than treating them.

GOAL #3: Promote wound healing and the patient's comfort.

Interventions

1. Administer topical anesthetics as ordered for examination.

Rationale

Administering anesthetics facilitates the patient's cooperation during the examination.

2. Administer oral analgesics as ordered.

Oral analgesics relieve pain and promote comfort. Topical analgesics are not advocated for prolonged use because they delay healing.

3. Patch the eye(s) as ordered.

Eye patching restricts blinking and promotes corneal epithelial healing. It also promotes resting of the eyes, increasing comfort.

Nursing diagnosis

Potential for loss of vision related to increased intraocular pressure secondary to blunt trauma.

GOAL #1: Identify increased intraocular pressure.

Interventions

1. Assist with intraocular pressure measurement as needed.

Rationale

A tonometer supplies a precise measurement. Normal intraocular pressure is 11 to 22 mm Hg. Intraocular pressure information is important because nerve fibers are progressively destroyed when pressure remains high. A 7% incidence of late-onset glaucoma is associated with a history of traumatic hyphema.

GOAL #2: Maintain intraocular pressure within the normal range.

Interventions

1. Elevate the head of the bed unless contraindicated.

2. Administer medications as ordered.

Rationale

Elevation minimizes venous congestion, decreasing intraocular pressure.

Oral carbonic anhydrase inhibitors, such as acetazolamide, decrease intraocular pressure.

GOAL #3: Anticipate potential complications and their treatment.

Interventions

1. Assist with corneal staining assessment.

Rationale

Corneal bloody pigment, caused by hemorrhage that has not reabsorbed, stains the cornea rust brown and can be detected by slit-lamp examination. Corneal staining tends to increase intraocular pressure, the intensity of which determines the extent of subsequent visual loss. Secondary hemorrhage occurs most commonly 3 to 5 days after blunt trauma and original hyphema. Rebleeding puts the patient at risk for corneal staining and visual disability.

Associated care plans

Fractures: Open/Closed
Soft Tissue Injuries
Head Injury
Acute Whole-Body Radiation Exposure

Chemical Burns
Thermal Burns
Maxillofacial Injuries

Table 3.10
Examining the Eye

Test: Visual acuity

Procedure	Normal findings	Abnormal findings	Possible causes
Determine preinjury level of acuity for comparison.			
Have the patient wear corrective lenses, if possible.			
Provide adequate illumination.			
Assess acuity using a Snellen's chart, pocket vision screener, newsprint.	Normal visual acuity, 20/20 for both eyes	Visual acuity of 20/200, legal blindness	Corneal damage, retinal detachment, glaucoma, hyphema
If these are unavailable or not visualized by the patient, proceed with the following until successful: count fingers shown (CF), hand movement perceived (HM), light perception (LP).		Recorded as CF/distance, HM/distance, LP/NLP (no light perception)	No light perception: total blindness
		Complaints of double vision (diplopia)	Extraocular muscle injury, orbital fracture, cranial nerve palsy (III, IV, and, and VI), macula impairment
		Flashes of light, floating spots, or a veil-like coating over the eye	Retinal detachment
		Halos seen around artificial lights	Glaucoma

Test: Extraocular movement

Procedure	Normal findings	Abnormal findings	Possible causes
Have the patient stare straight ahead while shining a light onto his cornea from 12″ to 15″.	Symmetrical reflection of light off each cornea	Asymmetric reflection due to deviating eye	Weak or paralyzed extraocular muscle
Have the patient rotate his eyes to the six cardinal positions of gaze by following movement of an object.	Smooth and parallel movement of both eyes	Altered movement ability: • Medial • Lateral • Diagonally up and lateral • Diagonally down and medial • Diagonally down and lateral • Diagonally up and medial	Muscle impairment: • Medial rectus • Lateral rectus • Superior rectus • Superior oblique • Inferior rectus[1] • Inferior oblique[1]

[1]Commonly involved in orbital floor blowout fractures

Examining the Eye (continued)

Test: Visual field

Procedure	Normal findings	Abnormal findings	Possible causes
Test each eye separately with the examiner and patient facing each other; slowly bring an object into the field of vision midway between patient and examiner, checking all four quadrants; compare the point at which examiner and patient first visualize.	Patient and examiner see objects entering field of vision at same time	Delayed or absent object visualization	Optic nerve damage, retinal disorder

Test: Sensorimotor

Procedure	Normal findings	Abnormal findings	Possible causes
Ask the patient to raise his eyebrows.	Symmetrical movement	Absent eyebrow movement	Facial nerve impairment
Check periorbital sensation.	Sensation intact	Loss of sensation above eyebrow, over cheek, and around teeth and gums	Trigeminal nerve impairment
Examine the patient's eyelids in normal gazing position.	Pupils not covered by upper eyelids at all, iris covered only slightly, and sclera totally	Drooping lid (ptosis)	Oculomotor nerve lesion, congenital disorder
		High lid margin (sclera visible)	Thyroid disease

Test: Pupillary light reflex

Procedure	Normal findings	Abnormal findings	Possible causes
Shine a light directly onto one pupil at a time.	Pupils round and equal in size and constrict quickly to light with only minimal redilation	Marked redilation when affected eye illuminated (Marcus Gunn's syndrome)	Conduction defect due to optic nerve lesion
		Pupil(s) dilated (mydriasis)	Oculomotor nerve injury, iris sphincter injury, administration of mydriatic drugs
		Pupil(s) constricted (miosis)	Impaired cervical sympathetic nerve innervation (Horner's syndrome), blunt or penetrating global injury, narcotic use, administration of miotic drugs

REFERENCES

ADDITIONAL EMERGENCIES

Hypothermia

Besdine, P.W. "Accidental Hypothermia: The Body's Energy Crisis," *Geriatrics* 34(12):51-59, 1979.

Clochesy, J.M. "Profound Hypothermia," *Focus on Critical Care* 11(1):19-21, February 1984.

Kinney, M.R., et al., eds. *AACN'S Clinical Reference for Critical Care Nurses.* New York: McGraw-Hill Book Co., 1981.

LaVoy, K. "Dealing with Hypothermia and Frostbite," *RN* 48(1):53-56, January 1985.

MIEMSS Trauma Resuscitation Area Standardized Care Plan: Hypothermia—Mild, Moderate, Severe. Baltimore, 1983.

Near Drowning: Freshwater/Saltwater

Cowley, R A., and Dunham, C. M. *Shock Trauma/Critical Care Manual.* Baltimore: University Park Press, 1982.

Glennon, S.A., et al. "Respiratory Disorders," in *AACN'S Clinical Reference for Critical-Care Nursing.* Edited by Kinney, M.R. New York: McGraw-Hill Book Co., 1981.

Kizer, K.W. "Resuscitation of Submersion Casualties," *Emergency Medicine Clinics of North America* 1(3):643-51, 1983.

Modell, J.H., and Boysen, P.G. "Drowning and Near-Drowning," in *Textbook of Critical Care.* Edited by Shoemaker, W.C., et al. Philadelphia: W.B. Saunders Co., 1984.

Molyneux-Luick, M. "Water-Sport Injuries: The Old and the New," *Nursing78* 8(8):50-55, 1978.

Spyker, D.A. "Submersion Injury, Epidemiology, Prevention, and Management," *Pediatric Clinics of North America* 32(1):113-25, 1985.

Acute Whole-Body Radiation Exposure

Andrews, G.A. "Medical Management of Accidental Total-Body Irradiation," in *The Medical Basis for Radiation Accident Preparedness.* Edited by Hubner, K.F., and Fry, S.A. New York: Elsevier/North-Holland, 1980.

Moses, D.G. "The Hematopoietic System," in *AACN'S Clinical Reference for Critical-Care Nursing.* Edited by Kinney, M.R. New York: McGraw-Hill Book Co., 1981.

Rados, B. "Primer on Radiation," *FDA Consumer.* Washington, D.C.: U.S. Government Printing Office, July/August 1979.

Burns

American College of Surgeons—Committee on Trauma. *Advanced Life Support Student Manual,* 1984.

Auerback, P.S. "Disorders Due to Physical and Environmental Agents," *Current Emergency Diagnosis and Treatment.* Edited by Mills, J., et al. Los Altos, Calif.: Lange Medical Pubns., 1985.

Emergencies. Nurse's Reference Library. Springhouse, Pa.: Springhouse Corp., 1985.

Jacoby, F.G. *Nursing Care of the Patient with Burns.* St. Louis: C.V. Mosby Co., 1976.

Kenner, C., and Manning, S. "Emergency Care of the Burn Patient," *Critical Care Update* 7:24-33, 1980.

Meyer, A.A., and Salber, P.R. "Burns and Smoke Inhalation," *Current Emergency Diagnosis and Treatment.* Edited by Mills, J., et al. Los Altos, Calif.: Lange Medical Pubns., 1985.

O'Boyle, C.M., et al., eds. *Emergency Care—The First 24 Hours.* East Norwalk, Conn.: Appleton-Century-Crofts, 1985.

Parker, J.G. "A Burn Injury," in *Emergency Nursing—A Guide to Comprehensive Care.* New York: John Wiley & Sons, 1984.

Robertson, K., et al. "Burn Care—The Crucial First Days," *American Journal of Nursing* 85(1):29-50, January 1981.

Woolridge-King, M. "Nursing Considerations of the Burned Patient During the Emergent Period," *Heart & Lung* 11(4):353-61, July/August 1982.

Inhalation Injuries

Brandeburg, J. "Inhalation Injury: Carbon Monoxide Poisoning," *American Journal of Nursing* 98: January 1980.

Caroline, N.L. *Emergency Care in the Streets.* Boston: Little, Brown & Co., 1979.

Grant, H.D., and Murray, R.H. *Emergency Care.* Bowie, Md.: Robert J. Brady Co., 1978.

Meyer, A.A., and Salber, P.R. "Burns and Smoke Inhalation," chapter 27 in *Current Emergency Diagnosis and Treatment.* Edited by Mills, J., et al. Los Altos, Calif.: Lange Medical Pubns., 1985.

Myers, R.A.M., et al. "14 Years Experience with Hyperbaric Oxygen Therapy at MIEMSS," *Maryland State Medical Journal,* May 1981.

Maxillofacial Injuries

Cowley, R A., and Dunham, C.M. *Shock Trauma/Critical Care Manual.* Baltimore: University Park Press, 1982.

Dingman, R. *Surgery of Facial Fractures.* Philadelphia: W.B. Saunders Co., 1978.

Emergencies. Nurse's Reference Library. Springhouse, Pa.: Springhouse Corp., 1985.

Grabb, W. "Injuries of the Face," in *Initial Management of the Trauma Patient.* Edited by Frey, C.F. Philadelphia: Lea & Febiger, 1976.

O'Boyle, C.M., et al., eds. *Emergency Care—The First 24 Hours.* East Norwalk, Conn.: Appleton-Century-Crofts, 1985.

Parker, J.G. *Emergency Nursing—A Guide to Comprehensive Care.* New York: John Wiley & Sons, 1984.

Schultz, R., and Oldham, R. "An Overview of Facial Injuries," *Surgical Clinics of North America* 57(5):987, 1977.

Schultz, R.C. *Facial Injuries,* 2nd ed. Chicago: Year Book Medical Pubns., 1977.

Whitlock, R.I. "Maxillofacial Injuries," in *Trauma Care.* Edited by Odling-Sme, W., and Crockard, A. New York: Grune & Stratton, 1981.

Substance Abuse in the Trauma Patient

O'Brien, J.O. "Behavioral Problems Due to Substance Abuse," *Topics in Emergency Medicine* 4(4):30-41, January 1983.

Yearbook86/87. Nurse's Reference Library. Springhouse, Pa.: Springhouse Corp., 1986.

Venomous Snakebites

Auerbach, P.S. "Disorders Due to Physical and Environmental Agents," *Current Emergency Diagnosis and Treatment.* Edited by Mills, J., et al. Los Altos, Calif.: Lange Medical Pubns., 1985.

Kunkel, D.B. "Bites of Venomous Reptiles," *Emergency Medicine Clinics of North America* 2(3):563-77, August 1984.

Thompson, S.W., and Verbeek, D. "When a Snake Bites," *American Journal of Nursing* 620-23, May 1984.

Eye Injuries

Paton, D., and Goldberg, M.F. *Management of Ocular Injuries.* Philadelphia: W.B. Saunders Co., 1976.

Sheehy, S. Budassi, and Barber, J. *Emergency Nursing Principles and Practice.* St. Louis: C.V. Mosby Co., 1985.

Shires, G.T. *Care of the Trauma Patient.* New York: McGraw-Hill Book Co., 1979.

Walt, A.J., and Wilson, R.F. *Management of Trauma: Pitfalls and Practice.* Philadelphia: Lea & Febiger, 1975.

COMPLICATIONS

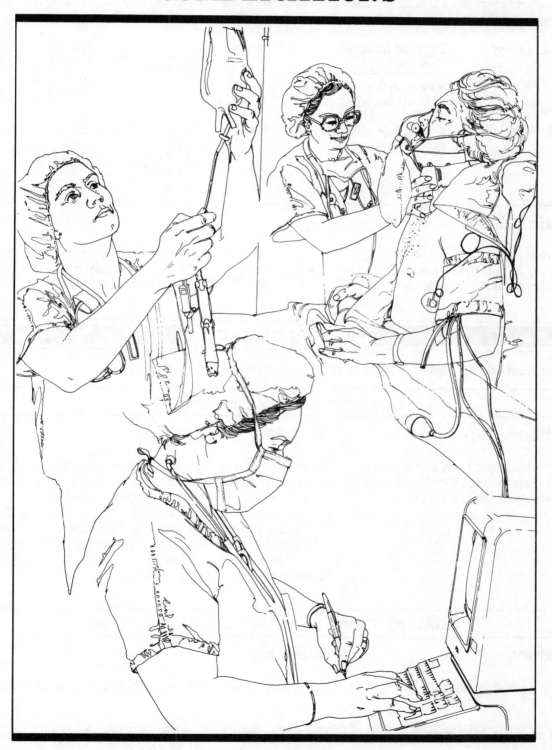

Medical diagnosis

DIABETES INSIPIDUS (D.I.)

Assessment

Note: *When DI develops secondary to head injury, it results from either direct trauma to the hypothalamus or the neural hypophysis or indirect trauma to these two structures secondary to increasing intracranial pressure. These events hinder secretion of antidiuretic hormone (ADH). DI resulting from head injury may be either self-limiting (resolving spontaneously in about 72 hours) or permanent.*

Mechanism of injury/ etiology:
- history of polyuria or polydipsia
- head injury
- recent intracranial surgery

Physical findings:
Genitourinary
- increased urine output (5 to 10 liters/day or more)
- low urine specific gravity (1.000–1.005)

Neurologic
- fatigue, weakness
- dizziness
- anxiety

Metabolic
- increased serum sodium concentration and

osmolality
- decreased urine sodium concentration and osmolality

Skin
- dry skin and mucous membranes

Diagnostic studies

- 24-hour urine volume
- urine and serum osmolality and sodium concentration
- water deprivation test—patient given no water for 8

hours, urine output remains greater than 30 cc/minute; urine osmolality remains greater than 200 mOsm/liter; specific gravity remains 1.000–1.005

Nursing diagnosis

Potential for fluid volume deficit related to increased urine output.

GOAL #1: Recognize the onset of DI.

Interventions

1. Monitor intake/output from admission on, especially in patients with significant head trauma or symptoms suggesting DI.

Rationale

Failure to recognize DI onset may permit hypovolemic shock to develop. The kidneys are unable to concentrate urine because of inadequate ADH levels. This triggers a rapid loss of large volumes of water during metabolic waste product elimination. If this lost fluid is not replaced, hypovolemic shock develops. Because DI may not become apparent in the head-injured patient for several hours, monitoring urine output from admission on establishes a baseline by which to determine DI onset.

GOAL #2: Restore and maintain a normovolemic state.

Interventions

1. Assess the patient for signs of hypovolemic shock.

2. Establish adequate I.V. access.

Rationale

Hypovolemic shock reflects inadequate volume replacement.

The patient may need multiple I.V. lines to replenish a large fluid loss, which may amount to more than 1 liter/hour.

3. Strictly monitor intake/output, together with serial specific gravity measurements.

Maintain an accurate record of the fluid volume deficit to help plan replacement. Urine output in DI has a low specific gravity, usually between 1.000 and 1.005. Monitoring these parameters helps assess the disease course.

4. Provide for adequate P.O. or I.V. intake.

Depending on the patient's condition and urine output, oral intake may suffice. If not, I.V. replacement will be needed. Urine output is usually replaced hourly, "cc for cc."

5. Anticipate the use of vasopressin (Pitressin) in an I.V. drip.

If the urine output rate exceeds the rate at which fluids can be replaced—because of the body's physical limits or inadequate I.V. access—fluid volume deficit increases. Vasopressin is titrated to maintain urine output at a manageable level (about 200 cc/hr).

6. Monitor urine and serum osmolality levels.

Decreasing urine osmolality and sodium concentration and increasing serum osmolality and sodium concentration indicate DI. Evaluate these parameters to assess therapeutic effectiveness. Oral or I.V. fluid replacement to match urine output usually keeps serum osmolality and sodium concentrations within normal ranges. A continued rise in serum values indicates inadequate fluid replacement.

Nursing diagnosis

Alteration in urinary elimination patterns related to excessive urine output.

GOAL #1: Provide for elimination of large volumes of urine.

Interventions

1. Anticipate the need for an indwelling urinary catheter.

2. Insert the urinary catheter, using strict sterile technique.

Rationale

The catheter enables accurate measurement of urine output and promotes patient comfort by decreasing urinary frequency.

A break in sterile technique during catheter insertion can introduce bacteria into the patient's urinary tract and cause infection.

GOAL #2: Maintain an accurate measurement of urine output.

Interventions

1. Empty the entire drainage system hourly.

Rationale

The urimeter on the drainage bag usually overflows when large volumes of urine drain. One way to maintain accurate output measurement is to let the urimeter overflow and empty the entire drainage system hourly. As an alternative, measure output more frequently, perhaps every 15 minutes; however, this may interfere with other aspects of nursing care.

Additional considerations

Patients with chronic DI are usually managed at home with desmopressin acetate. A synthetic substitute for naturally occurring ADH, this drug is administered intranasally. Anticipate the need to teach chronic DI patients about this medication and about proper home management of DI.

PULMONARY THROMBOEMBOLUS (P.T.E.)

Assessment

Mechanism of injury/etiology:
- history of fractures of long bones or pelvis
- prolonged bed rest and/or surgical procedure
- age (risk increases with age)
- obesity
- sedentary life-style
- history of deep vein thrombosis

Physical findings:
Respiratory
- hypoxia, hypocarbia, respiratory alkalosis, increased alveolar-arterial PO_2 difference
- bronchial breath sounds
- pleural friction rub
- high fever with pulmo- nary infarct (rare)
- sudden onset of dyspnea

Cardiovascular
- dusky, pale, or cyanotic skin
- diaphoretic or cool skin
- hypotension
- tachycardia
- substernal chest pain

Neurologic
- decreased level of consciousness

Psychosocial
- anxiety (manifested by facial expression or behavior)

Diagnostic studies

- stat and serial ABGs—may reflect respiratory alkalosis, hypoxemia, hypocarbia, increased alveolar-arterial PO_2 difference
- erect chest radiograph—usually clear initially but may show atelectatic areas after several days; examination rules out other causes of dyspnea/pain
- ECG—commonly reveals a sinus tachycardia; with massive PTE or profound hypoxemia, the ECG also may indicate signs of ischemia
- ventilation/perfusion scan—commonly shows normal ventilation in the absence of atelectatic lung tissue and reveals areas of decreased or absent perfusion
- pulmonary angiography—a definitive diagnostic study for PTE, it clearly delineates areas of decreased perfusion

Nursing diagnosis

Impaired gas exchange related to decreased pulmonary perfusion secondary to PTE.

GOAL: Maximize pulmonary ventilation and oxygen uptake.

Interventions

1. Provide supplemental oxygen.

2. Encourage the patient to cough and deep-breathe. Perform chest physiotherapy every 2 to 4 hours or as ordered and suction patients who are intubated hourly.

3. Turn the immobilized patient at least every 2 hours.

Rationale

In PTE, serotonin-induced alveolar constriction causes atelectatic areas. This process results in hypoxemia. Also, alveoli served by the blocked vessel(s), although ventilated, are not perfused, and so are unavailable for gas exchange. Providing the patient with supplemental oxygen permits greater oxygen uptake by perfused, ventilated alveoli.

Atelectatic lung tissue and mucus decrease the alveolar tissue available for gas exchange. These interventions assist in opening atelectatic areas and in removing secretions, thereby increasing the alveoli available for gas exchange.

4. Maintain the patient in semi-Fowler's position, unless contraindicated.

Atelectasis and bronchiolar-alveolar spasm raise airway resistance. Breathing becomes labored. Placing the patient in semi-Fowler's eases breathing efforts because gravity helps depress the diaphragm on inspiration.

5. Medicate the patient for pain, as prescribed.

Pulmonary ventilation decreases as the patient splints secondary to pain. Pain may also inhibit coughing and deep breathing. Appropriate relief allows the patient to breathe more deeply and freely.

Nursing diagnosis

Decreased pulmonary tissue perfusion related to blockage in pulmonary circulation by thromboembolus.

GOAL: PTE will resolve. Minimize the risk of additional emboli.

Interventions

1. Anticipate streptokinase and/or urokinase administration.

2. Anticipate I.V. administration of heparin to anticoagulate the patient's blood.

3. Monitor trends in stat and serial coagulation profiles.

Rationale

These agents lyse existing emboli and may prevent others from developing. I.V. administration of heparin is generally accepted as the treatment of choice for anticoagulation. Continuous I.V. infusion causes less peak and valley effect than does intermittent injection.

Coagulation times should be approximately 2 to 2½ times normal. Monitoring these trends helps to evaluate therapeutic effect. Values below this range reflect ineffective therapy; values above it reflect increased bleeding risk. Monitoring of these times should continue as long as the patient is on anticoagulant therapy, usually 7 to 10 days, or as long as he is on bed rest.

Nursing diagnosis

Potential for decreased cardiac output related to increased pressure in pulmonary vasculature and release of vasoactive substances secondary to PTE.

GOAL: Recognize and treat hypotension/shock at an early stage.

Interventions

1. Assess the patient frequently for signs and symptoms of hypotension/shock. Assessment frequency depends on the patient's condition and institutional standards.

2. Ensure adequate I.V. access.

Rationale

Hypotension/shock develops in PTE as a result of right ventricular failure secondary to the thromboembolus increasing pulmonary vascular resistance.

The patient may need hemodynamic support with fluid or vasopressor therapy.

Nursing diagnosis

*Potential for minor blood loss related to anticoagulant therapy.

**Supplemental nursing diagnosis

> **GOAL:** Prevent/minimize additional bleeding secondary to nursing care.

Interventions

1. Limit or exclude I.M. injections.

2. Apply manual pressure to all venipuncture sites for 10 minutes.

3. Avoid aggressive brushing of teeth and gums.

4. If serial ABGs are required, consider having an arterial line inserted to minimize arterial punctures.

Rationale

Increased coagulation time caused by anticoagulant therapy increases the patient's risk of bleeding episodes. These actions are designed to eliminate or minimize this risk.

Nursing diagnosis

Potential for fluid volume deficit related to occult blood loss secondary to anticoagulant therapy.

> **GOAL:** Prevent shock secondary to occult blood loss.

Interventions

1. Monitor trends in laboratory data, particularly hemoglobin/hematocrit levels and coagulation profile.

2. Screen stools, urine, and gastric contents for blood at least once daily.

Rationale

Anticoagulant therapy may result in occult blood loss from the GI and genitourinary tracts. These measures are designed to detect occult loss before it becomes severe enough to result in shock.

Nursing diagnosis

Potential for activity intolerance related to hypoxemia secondary to PTE.

> **GOAL:** Minimize patient fatigue.

Interventions

1. Observe the patient closely for signs of fatigue and limit activities of daily living as needed.

2. Block patient care activities.

3. Allow the patient adequate resting time between periods of activity.

Rationale

Hypoxemia results in less oxygen being available to muscle tissue, thus increasing oxygen demand. Usually, respiratory and heart rates increase to compensate for an increased oxygen demand. However, secondary to PTE and atelectasis, the oxygen demand exceeds compensatory capacities. With this insufficiency of available oxygen, the patient fatigues rapidly.

Associated care plans

Hemorrhagic Shock
Deep Vein Thrombosis

Medical diagnosis

PULMONARY EDEMA

Assessment

Mechanism of injury/ etiology:
- blunt trauma to the myocardium
- excessive I.V. fluid administration
- myocardial infarction (MI), hypertension, val-

vular heart disease, or diabetes

Physical findings:
Respiratory
- air hunger
- dyspnea
- labored breathing
- tachypnea

- foamy and/or blood-tinged sputum
- diffuse rales
- wheezing

Cardiovascular
- cyanosis
- tachycardia

- elevated central venous pressure (CVP)
- diaphoresis

Neurologic
- decreased mentation
- restlessness and combativeness

Diagnostic studies

- ABG analysis—demonstrates hypoxemia, hypocarbia, and respiratory alkalosis
- chest radiograph—shows atelectasis, consolidation, and a "ground-glass" appearance of the lung fields

- ECG—reveals tachycardia and conduction changes consistent with myocardial ischemia (if MI or contusion is the causative factor)

Nursing diagnosis

Impaired gas exchange related to accumulation of fluid in alveoli and pulmonary interstitium.

> **GOAL:** Maximize pulmonary ventilation.

Interventions

1. Anticipate the use of supplemental oxygen. Ensure availability of equipment needed for intubation and mechanical ventilation with positive end-expiratory pressure (PEEP). (See "Endotracheal Intubation" in Section VII.)

2. Place the patient in semi-Fowler's position.

3. Perform chest physiotherapy and suctioning (if the patient is intubated), or have the patient cough and deep-breathe at least every 4 hours.

4. Auscultate breath sounds at least every 2 hours or as dictated by the patient's condition, and after each of the above nursing interventions.

Rationale

Ventilation/perfusion mismatch occurs when a portion of the alveoli is blocked by edema and is therefore unavailable for gas exchange. Increasing fraction of inspired oxygen (FiO_2) permits greater uptake of oxygen by the available alveoli. If an adequate PaO_2 (> 60 mm Hg) cannot be maintained with the patient breathing spontaneously, the patient will require intubation and mechanical ventilation. PEEP increases functional residual capacity and helps keep distal airways open throughout the ventilatory cycle. PEEP distends alveoli and forms a layer around them of pooled fluid, thereby increasing alveolar gas diffusion.

This position eases respiratory effort by utilizing gravity to aid depression of the diaphragm during inspiration.

These measures help clear the airway of fluid, increasing the number of alveoli available for gas exchange. **Note:** *Suctioning may be contraindicated in intubated patients on high levels of PEEP.* (See "Adult Respiratory Distress Syndrome" in Section IV.)

Frequent respiratory assessment evaluates the patient's progress and the effectiveness of nursing therapy and indicates the need for possible further intervention.

Nursing diagnosis

Potential for decreased cardiac output related to diminished cardiac efficiency secondary to myocardial contusion, myocardial infarction, or use of high levels of PEEP.

GOAL: Support myocardial action.

Interventions

1. Administer vasoactive drugs, such as digitalis preparations, dobutamine, or dopamine, as ordered.

2. Monitor vital signs at least every hour, or as the patient's condition warrants; prepare for insertion of CVP, arterial, and/or pulmonary artery catheters. (See "Pulmonary Artery Catheterization" in Section VII.)

3. Provide a quiet environment and keep patient activity to a minimum.

Rationale

These drugs, while differing in precise effects, increase cardiac contractility and efficiency of cardiac stroke work.

Invasive monitoring lines, in conjunction with vital sign measurement, assist in effective adjustment of I.V. drug therapy and in monitoring trends in the patient's condition.

Mental and physical activity increase cardiac work load. Tachycardia greater than 120 beats per minute decreases left ventricular filling time, which in turn reduces cardiac output.

Nursing diagnosis

Fluid volume excess related to overhydration.

GOAL: Restore and maintain a normovolemic state.

Interventions

1. Administer morphine to dilate the peripheral vasculature, as ordered.

2. Administer I.V. diuretics (usually a furosemide dose of 40 to 80 mg), as ordered.

3. Anticipate the use of rotating tourniquets.

Rationale

In addition to its sedative and analgesic effects, morphine is a potent vasodilator that increases the size and capacity of the peripheral vascular compartment. This creates a relative decrease in fluid overload by decreasing venous return to the heart.

Diuretics increase urine output and decrease fluid overload through the elimination of free water.

Rotating tourniquets sequester a portion of the peripheral blood supply in the extremities, decreasing venous return and lessening cardiac work load, and thereby increase cardiac efficiency. **Note:** *Rotating tourniquets are rarely used today due to the usual effectiveness of drug therapy and the accumulation of lactic acid caused by the tourniquets.*

Additional considerations

After the patient has experienced an episode of pulmonary edema, he requires continuing assessment of fluid volume status, including accurate monitoring and recording of intake and output, assessment of general cardiovascular status, and monitoring of vital signs and cardiac parameters. If pulmonary edema resulted from a myocardial contusion or infarction, the risk of recurrence is high. Therefore, this patient will need continued fluid restriction and/or cardiopulmonary support until the myocardium has recovered.

ADULT RESPIRATORY DISTRESS SYNDROME (A.R.D.S.)

Assessment

Mechanism of injury/ etiology:
- history of shock (hemorrhagic, cardiogenic, or vasogenic)
- pulmonary infection
- aspiration
- fat embolus
- air embolus
- oxygen toxicity
- head injury
- sepsis

Physical findings:
Respiratory
- dyspnea
- restlessness
- cough
- increased peak inspiratory pressure
- rales, rhonchi, bronchial breath sounds

Cardiovascular
- tachycardia
- diaphoresis
- cyanosis

Neurologic
- decreased mentation

Diagnostic studies

- chest radiograph—may show microatelectasis, blurred bronchial margins, consolidation (late finding)
- ABGs—reveal decreased PaO_2 that does not respond to increases in fraction of inspired oxygen (FiO_2), hypercarbia with respiratory alkalemia
- alveolar-arterial oxygen difference [$D(A-a)O_2$]—is increased because of impaired oxygen diffusion across the alveolar-capillary membrane
- arteriovenous oxygen difference [$D(a-v)O_2$]—increases as tissues increase oxygen extraction rate, secondary to hypoxemia
- intrapulmonary shunt (QS/QT)—reveals increased shunting because of interstitial fluid
- functional residual capacity—decreases as pulmonary compliance falls because of pulmonary congestion

Nursing diagnosis

Potential for impaired gas exchange, related to accumulation of interstitial pulmonary fluid.

GOAL #1: Recognize physical changes that signal ARDS onset.

Interventions

1. Assess the patient's respiratory system at least every 4 hours if he is at risk for ARDS.

2. Draw (or have drawn) blood for ABGs, as ordered—department protocol usually determines frequency. At a minimum, ABGs should be analyzed after a change in the patient's condition or in ventilator settings.

Rationale

ARDS results from a pulmonary hypoperfusion episode. For 24 to 48 hours after the initial insult, pulmonary ventilation usually remains within the normal range. Frequent assessments aid early recognition of ARDS.

As ARDS develops, PaO_2 decreases and a compensatory mechanism increases respiration rate and depth. Thus, as the patient's PaO_2 falls, his $PaCO_2$ decreases, too. Furthermore, the falling PaO_2 resists increases in FiO_2.

GOAL #2: Maximize pulmonary ventilation.

Interventions

1. Anticipate the need for intubation and mechanical ventilation.

2. Maximize patient compliance with the ventilatory regimen, using:
• emotional support
• sedatives and/or hypnotics, as ordered
• neuromuscular blocking agents, as ordered.

3. Severely limit suctioning frequency for the patient receiving high levels (above 15 cm) of PEEP. The Department of Critical Care Medicine should establish protocols governing frequency and reasons for suctioning.

Rationale

ARDS is best managed by early intubation and positive end-expiratory pressure (PEEP).

Fear of the unknown, related to mechanical ventilation, may cause patient noncompliance, reducing the therapeutic effect. Thus an intermittent minute ventilation or synchronized intermittent minute ventilation mode is best because both allow the patient to breathe spontaneously from a gas reservoir and lessen his anxiety. If this proves ineffective, small doses of narcotics (usually morphine or fentanyl) may be prescribed to sedate the patient and keep his respirations in phase with the ventilator. As a final alternative, neuromuscular blocking agents (such as pancuronium bromide) may be ordered in conjunction with sedatives to block spontaneous respirations.

One of the major problems in ARDS is surfactant destruction. This substance decreases friction within the pulmonary system and allows the airways to remain open. High levels of PEEP yield many benefits, especially keeping distal airways open. Thus, if you discontinue PEEP to suction the patient, these small airways will collapse; then an even greater pressure may be required to reopen them.

Nursing diagnosis

Potential for decreased gas exchange related to barotrauma secondary to use of high levels of PEEP.

GOAL: Recognize signs of pneumothorax and intervene immediately.

Interventions

1. Assess the respiratory system of patients on high levels of PEEP at least every hour.

2. Notify the physician immediately if you note any of the above signs. Make sure equipment is immediately available for chest radiography and chest tube insertion and maintenance.

Rationale

PEEP above 15 cm may rupture pulmonary blebs or parenchyma and result in a spontaneous pneumothorax. The following suggest pneumothorax:
• sudden airway pressure increase
• absent or diminished breath sounds on affected side
• sudden PaO_2 decrease
• tracheal shift toward side contralateral to injury.
Frequent assessments aid prompt recognition and permit rapid treatment.

Suspected spontaneous pneumothorax requires verification by chest radiography and chest tube insertion.

Nursing diagnosis

Potential for decreased cardiac output related to increased pulmonary vascular resistance and increased intrapulmonary pressure secondary to high levels of PEEP.

GOAL: Maintain cardiac output within an acceptable range.

Interventions

1. Anticipate pulmonary artery (PA) catheter insertion.

2. Assess the cardiovascular system at least every hour. Include blood pressure, central venous pressure, PAP, and PAWP measurements. **Note:** *Under most circumstances pulmonary artery diastolic pressure is monitored instead of PAWP because inflating the PA catheter balloon risks pulmonary infarction. If a patient is receiving high levels of PEEP, pulmonary artery diastolic pressure may not accurately reflect PAWP. Although PEEP results in increased pulmonary vascular resistance (PVR) (which, in turn, increases PA pressure), PAWP may remain relatively unchanged. Therefore, in these patients, PAWP should be used for left ventricular evaluation.*

3. Administer vasoactive drugs, such as digitalis preparations, dobutamine, or dopamine, as ordered.

Rationale

PA catheterization permits monitoring of pulmonary arterial pressure (PAP) and pulmonary arterial wedge pressure (PAWP) and measurement of cardiac output.

PEEP decreases cardiac output by distending alveoli, which increases PVR. Also, increased intrapulmonary pressure impairs blood return to the heart, thereby decreasing cardiac output. Trend analysis of these parameters helps detect falling cardiac output.

These drugs, while differing in precise effects, increase cardiac contractility and efficiency of cardiac stroke work.

Associated care plans

Tension Pneumothorax
Use of Neuromuscular Blocking Agents

Associated procedure

Pulmonary Artery Catheterization

DEEP VEIN THROMBOSIS (D.V.T.)

Assessment

**Mechanism of injury/
etiology:**
Venous stasis

- immobility/bed rest
- surgical procedures
- shock states
- spinal cord injuries
producing paralysis or
venous dilitation (neuro-
genic shock)

Injury to venous intima

- vessel trauma during
surgery
- multiple needle punc-
tures
- infusion of irritating
fluids/drugs
- soft tissue injuries

*Increased blood
coagulability*

- trauma
- surgery

Other risk factors

- age (> 40 years)
- obesity
- history of acute myo-
cardial infarction, con-
gestive heart failure

Physical findings:
Musculoskeletal

- swelling
- tenderness
- positive Homan's sign
(calf pain on rapid dorsiflexion)

Respiratory

- signs of pulmonary
thromboembolus (PTE)

Note: *An estimated 50% (or more) of all patients undergoing general or orthopedic surgery develop DVT. Of these, more than one half may exhibit no signs/symptoms of this disorder. PTE may be the first indication of DVT. Homan's sign, although considered a classic finding in DVT, is not diagnostic. A positive Homan's sign may be elicited in almost any condition producing calf pain and is absent in many DVT patients.*

Diagnostic studies

- venography—conclusively diagnoses DVT with 90% to 95% accuracy
- ^{125}I labeled fibrinogen study (based on the concentration of fibrinogen in a forming clot)—indicates DVT by increased radioisotope presence in a given area
- Doppler flow study—ultrasonically indicates absence of blood flow or altered flow velocity in response to compression to delineate the DVT area
- venous pressure measurement—may be increased in early DVT development but returns to normal levels after sufficient collateral circulation develops
- electrical plethysmography—uses electrical impedance to indirectly indicate DVT

Potential for alteration in peripheral tissue perfusion related to formation of DVT.

GOAL: Prevent or minimize the risk for DVT.

Interventions

1. Identify patients at risk for developing DVT.

2. Eliminate pressure points along legs:
- keep the patient's knees straight while on bed rest
- remove constrictive clothing.

Rationale

Clearly a majority of trauma patients are at risk for DVT as indicated by the items under "Mechanism of Injury/Etiology." Most trauma patients will fall into one, if not more, of these categories. Many DVTs seem to be triggered during surgery. Early identification of patients at risk allows planning of early interventions to prevent DVT.

Point pressure may result in venous occlusion and the formation of a thrombus. Keeping the patient's knees straight (with no supports under the knees; knee gatch flat) prevents occlusion of the veins in the popliteal space. Elevating the foot of the bed provides uniform support to the entire leg and prevents pressure on the calf or popliteal area. Restrictive clothing may have a tourniquet effect and should be avoided to permit free venous return.

3. Elevate the patient's legs, unless contraindicated.

Leg elevation promotes venous return. Trendelenburg, unless contraindicated by other injuries, is an excellent position.

4. Ensure proper fit and application of graded elastic stockings:
• measure the patient's legs accurately, according to manufacturer's directions
• eliminate all wrinkles and rolled-down tops from stockings
• recheck the fit of stockings frequently and readjust; educate the patient and enlist his aid in maintaining proper fit.

Graded elastic stockings compress the legs, which increases blood flow velocity and volume and thus reduces pooling. Compression by the stocking gradually decreases proximally from the ankle, creating a pressure gradient to increase venous return. Proper functioning of the stockings depends on proper fit and use. A tourniquet effect may result from wrinkles or rolled stockings and must be avoided.

5. Ensure proper functioning of pneumatic pressure devices, including:
• cuffs and hoses
• electrical supply
• alarm system
• inflation pressure/cycle.
Ensure proper application of cuffs.

Pneumatic cuffs are used in the early treatment of the trauma patient when the use of heparin is contraindicated. These devices can be either sequential or nonsequential, are generally used continuously while the patient is in bed, and may be used in conjunction with elastic stockings. As with stockings, their effectiveness depends on proper use and equipment function.

6. Teach the patient his prescribed exercise program and promote compliance.

Active leg exercises increase venous return by muscular compression of the veins. The effect of these exercises has a limited duration and, therefore, they should be repeated at frequent intervals. The patient requires education about the purpose and performance of the exercises and may need encouragement to perform them consistently.

7. Administer prophylactic anticoagulants as ordered. Monitor coagulation studies.

High-risk patients may be treated prophylactically with anticoagulants to prevent DVT. In trauma patients, prophylaxis is delayed until all sources of hemorrhage are controlled and postoperative hemostasis is confirmed. Coagulation studies (prothrombin time [PT], partial thromboplastin time [PTT]) monitor the effectiveness of the low-dose heparin therapy. Anticoagulation therapy usually continues until the patient is fully ambulatory.

Nursing diagnosis

Alteration in peripheral tissue perfusion related to the presence of DVT.

GOAL #1: Recognize the onset of DVT.

Interventions

Rationale

1. Assess patients at risk for DVT as their conditions warrant; check for:
• pain on palpation of the calf or thigh
• edema of the calf or thigh.

DVT onset is usually marked by subtle changes in the patient's condition. Careful, repeated assessments will provide the best clues to the presence of DVT.

2. Palpate gently with the fingertips from the ankle proximally to the groin (concentrate on the posterior calf and medial thigh) for tenderness.

Only gentle pressure is needed to elicit the pain associated with DVT. More pressure than this may obscure findings. Most DVTs occur in the calf veins. DVTs may also occur in the femoral vein, iliac vein, and pelvic veins. Thrombosis may be limited to one area or occur in almost any combination. Palpation along the stated areas will detect any tenderness.

3. Assess for edema by comparing measurements of opposing ankles, calves, and thighs.

Swelling resulting from DVT is usually subtle, except in cases of iliofemoral DVT, when edema may be marked. Usually calf measurements will only differ by 1 to 1.5 cm and will not be visibly discernible.

GOAL #2: Prevent or minimize the risk of PTE from fragmentation of DVT, extension of current clot, or formation of new thrombi.

Interventions

1. Place the patient on bed rest with his legs elevated, unless contraindicated.

2. Administer anticoagulants and thrombolytics as ordered.

3. Consult the physician concerning the need for stool softeners; administer them as ordered.

Rationale

Patients with DVT are usually placed on bed rest until the DVT has organized, which may lower the risk of thrombus fragmentation. This organization may be indicated by the resolution of inflammatory signs. Elevation of the legs increases venous return and may prevent clot extension and new clot formation.

Anticoagulant therapy aims to prevent clot extension and new clot formation. The initial treatment usually consists of heparin administered by continuous infusion for a minimum of 7 days. The patient then continues on an oral anticoagulant for long-term therapy. Thrombolytics, such as streptokinase or urokinase, may be ordered to hasten the lysis of thrombi. **Note:** *Keep in mind aspirin's anticoagulant effects. Patients on anticoagulants requesting a mild analgesic should be given a nonsalicylate medication.*

The Valsalva maneuver, performed while straining at defecation, significantly elevates deep venous pressure. Stool softeners may be ordered to lessen the need for this maneuver.

Nursing diagnosis

Potential for fluid volume deficit related to bleeding secondary to anticoagulant therapy.

GOAL: Prevent or minimize bleeding. Detect blood loss immediately and institute appropriate interventions.

Interventions

1. Assess the patient on anticoagulants for bleeding; check for
● occult blood in stools
● hematuria
● hemoptysis/hematemesis
● bleeding from the gums
● bleeding from surgical or traumatic wounds
● petechiae.

Rationale

Patients receiving heparin or Coumadin-type drugs are at risk for bleeding. Frequent assessment of these factors promotes early detection of blood loss and allows prompt intervention.

2. Monitor the coagulation studies and platelet counts of patients receiving anticoagulant therapy.

Anticoagulants exert a therapeutic effect in DVT when PT/PTT are maintained at approximately twice normal. Values exceeding this increase the patient's risk for bleeding without additional therapeutic effect. Thrombocytopenia is a complication of heparin therapy.

3. Prevent bleeding triggered by patient activities or nursing care measures by:
- using a soft toothbrush and performing oral hygiene gently
- suctioning endotracheal tubes gently
- padding side rails for restless/agitated patients (such as head-injured patients)
- applying pressure to needle puncture sites for at least 10 minutes
- minimizing or completely avoiding intramuscular injections.

The anticoagulated patient may incur bleeding from overly aggressive self-care or nursing care measures. Agitated patients may hit side rails and cause bruising. These precautions help prevent bleeding.

Additional considerations

In some circumstances, DVT treatment may include surgical intervention. This is generally most effective early in the clot development course, before the clot is securely anchored in the vein.

Although not discussed in this plan, it is possible to develop a DVT of the upper extremities. This generally occurs in patients with advanced cancer or congestive heart failure, but it may occur in otherwise healthy individuals. Upper extremity DVT in healthy persons usually occurs after some unusual muscular activity of the arms and generally develops in the subclavian vein between the clavicle and first rib. Diagnosis and treatment of upper extremity DVT is substantially the same as for DVT of the legs.

Associated care plan

Pulmonary Thromboembolus

Medical diagnosis

USE OF NEUROMUSCULAR BLOCKING AGENTS

A neuromuscular blocking agent may be required to treat the multisystem trauma patient effectively. These agents may be used to:
- gain rapid airway control and facilitate endotracheal intubation
- decrease chest wall resistance, permitting efficient mechanical ventilation
- permit the use of therapeutic interventions, such as high levels of positive end-expiratory pressure or independent lung ventilation
- create complete muscle relaxation for the reduction of severely comminuted fractures or dislocated joints.

The use of these agents, however, causes a number of problems that require nursing intervention to provide for patient safety and comfort. This care plan is applicable to all patients receiving this therapy. Although a detailed discussion of the various neuromuscular blockers exceeds the scope of this plan, general information is provided.

Neuromuscular blocking agents act by preventing neural impulse transmission at the skeletal-neuromuscular junction. Both types (depolarizing and nondepolarizing) are most effective when administered intravenously. Most act within 1 to 3 minutes. All, with the exception of succinylcholine, are excreted unchanged in the urine and feces. Succinylcholine is degraded by pseudocholinesterase and eliminated in the urine.

These agents prevent spontaneous respiration by paralyzing the skeletal muscles, including the diaphragm and intercostal muscles. Depending on the specific agent used, neuromuscular blockers also may cause cardiovascular and electrolyte disturbances, such as hypo- or hypertension, elevated serum potassium levels, cardiac dysrhythmias, and asystole. *Potentially lethal drugs, these agents must be given only by persons knowledgeable in their use and side effects. These patients require an artificial airway, mechanical ventilation, and careful hemodynamic monitoring.*

Nursing diagnosis

Potential for fear related to total paralysis secondary to the use of neuromuscular blocking agents.

Note: *Under most circumstances, signs of fear would be recognizable, whether expressed by the patient or inferred through assessment criteria (such as increases in pulse, respiratory rate, and/or blood pressure). However, the effects of these agents preclude expression by the patient, and medications and the patient's physical condition may alter physiologic responses. Therefore, assume that the potential for fear exists and implement interventions to reduce this fear.*

> **GOAL:** Explain the therapy to the patient before it begins and provide continuing support throughout its duration.

Interventions

1. Unless contraindicated because of the situation's critical nature, explain the following to the patient in terms he can understand:
- he will be unable to breathe or move independently
- he will be placed on a ventilator
- someone will always be physically close to him
- other treatments and procedures will be explained to him before they begin.

Also explain the reason for using this drug.

Rationale

This therapy results in complete paralysis and makes the patient entirely dependent on the caregiver for his life, safety, and comfort. An understanding of the reasons for this therapy and its implications may help alleviate his fear. The knowledge that someone will be physically near in the event of any untoward occurrence will help him accept dependency, thereby reducing fear. If the patient's condition precludes giving him this information before drug administration, be sure to explain it when he has stabilized. Also, reexplain the therapy periodically. An ideal time to do this is at the beginning of the shift when the nurse introduces herself to the patient. **Note:** *Give this information to the patient's family and other visitors to lessen their fear. Exercise caution when using the word "paralyzed" to describe the patient's condition; it could easily be misunderstood as indicating that the patient's paralysis is physical as opposed to medically induced.*

2. Be alert for and limit any inappropriate conversations at the bedside.

Patients being treated with neuromuscular blocking agents are capable of recalling events during their paralysis. Also, the patient may not comprehend conversations taking place at his bedside—whether or not they concern him—and this may create additional fear.

3. Administer sedatives, hypnotics, and analgesics as prescribed.

Neuromuscular blocking agents produce paralysis but do not sedate the patient. Medications help lessen fear by decreasing the patient's awareness or recall of this experience. Also, neuromuscular blockers have no analgesic effects; therefore, the patient will experience pain secondary to his injuries. It is imperative to remember this and provide appropriate pain relief.

Nursing diagnosis

Alteration in respiratory function related to the use of neuromuscular blocking agents.

> **GOAL:** Support the respiratory system during the paralysis period.

Interventions

1. Assess the patient's respiratory status and blood gases; inspect ventilator and alarm systems every hour for appropriate settings and proper functioning.

2. Secure an artificial airway with tape or tracheal ribbon. Change the tape when it becomes loose, tight (because of edema), or heavily soiled.

3. Perform chest physiotherapy at prescribed frequency (usually, at a minimum, every 4 hours). Suction the patient's mouth at least every hour and as needed.

4. Remain physically close to the patient and use the alarm systems provided with the ventilator.

Rationale

Neuromuscular blockers eliminate the patient's ability to breathe spontaneously and to clear and protect his own airway. Frequent assessment of respiratory parameters is needed to provide for patient safety and effective ventilation.

Prevent accidental dislodging of the artificial airway and tension on the airway, which may damage vocal cords or irritate the patient. Secretions accumulating on the tape provide a medium for bacterial growth and increase the risk of infection.

These interventions help remove pulmonary secretions normally expelled by the patient. Also, the presence of endotracheal and/or gastric tubes may cause excessive oral secretions, which could result in aspiration if the airway cuff suddenly deflated.

These measures enhance patient safety during the period of complete dependence.

Nursing diagnosis

Impaired mobility related to the use of neuromuscular blocking agents.

> **GOAL:** Maintain joint mobility; prevent contractures.

Interventions

1. Assess the patient, in conjunction with his physicians and physical therapists, for appropriate range-of-motion (ROM) exercises and limitations.

Rationale

Usually, patient complaints of pain or discomfort help determine ROM exercise limits. However, this patient's condition requires assessment to elicit exercise limitations.

*Supplemental nursing diagnosis

2. Perform passive ROM exercises at least every 8 hours, unless contraindicated.

Joint mobility begins to decrease within 24 hours of the onset of decreased activity. Passive ROM exercises assist in maintaining mobility while the patient is immobilized.

3. Frequently assess the patient's position for correct body alignment and make adjustments, as needed. Support the patient's neck while turning or moving him.

Improper body alignment can readily cause injury to the brachial plexus or the peroneal, femoral, or saphenous nerves. Also, the cervical ligaments can readily be injured because of loss of muscular support of the neck.

Nursing diagnosis

Potential for impaired skin integrity related to the use of neuromuscular blocking agents.

GOAL: Maintain skin integrity throughout the immobility period.

Interventions

1. Assess skin condition at the start of each shift and every time the patient is turned.

2. Turn the patient at least every 2 hours.

3. Pad bony prominences.

4. Change soiled linen immediately.

5. Place as few layers of linen as possible between the patient and the "egg crate" mattress, if used.

6. Consult the physician about ordering a specialized bed (such as a Clinitron or Roto-Rest) if the patient is expected to remain immobilized for an extended period.

7. Bathe the patient at least daily and as needed.

8. Provide adequate nutritional support. (See "Malnutrition in the Trauma Patient" in Section IV.)

Rationale

Skin breakdown occurs in immobilized patients because of decreased peripheral circulation (from prolonged pressure on a single area); the presence of a warm, moist environment (which promotes bacterial growth); friction against bed linens; and changes in nutritional status. These efforts are designed to counteract the causes of skin breakdown in these patients.

Nursing diagnosis

Alteration in elimination patterns related to the use of neuromuscular blocking agents.

GOAL: Provide an effective waste elimination method.

Interventions

1. Insert an indwelling urinary catheter using strict aseptic technique.

2. Assess the patient at least once a day for fecal impaction. If necessary, manually disimpact the patient.

Rationale

The patient treated with neuromuscular blocking agents is unable to control elimination of bodily waste. These measures are designed to provide for the patient's elimination needs. Neuromuscular blocking agents do not paralyze smooth muscle; fecal impaction results instead from the patient's immobility and changes in his diet.

3. Assess the patient's need for stool softeners or antidiarrheics, as warranted, and consult his physician.

Nursing diagnosis

Potential for alteration in comfort related to various environmental and physical factors secondary to the use of neuromuscular blocking agents.

> **GOAL:** Anticipate potential sources of discomfort and intervene to maintain the patient's comfort level.

Interventions

1. Maintain the environmental temperature within a comfortable range, or provide sheets or blankets as appropriate.

2. Assess the patient's position frequently (between scheduled turnings) for awkward or potentially uncomfortable positions, and realign as needed.

3. Maintain awareness of the patient's ability to experience pain; remember, he may need a local anesthetic during a painful procedure.

4. Assess all dressings between dressing changes for constriction from edema and, unless contraindicated, change them as needed.

5. Keep bed linens clean and dry.

Rationale

All these interventions are designed to alleviate potential sources of discomfort. The patient being treated with neuromuscular blocking agents will be unable to signal his sense of discomfort. He will depend on you to anticipate these and other factors that may cause discomfort and to intervene on his behalf. Autonomic signs of pain may include hypertension, tachycardia, tearing, and dilated pupils. The patient must be assessed carefully, however, before attributing these signs to pain as they may also be caused by other problems.

Associated care plan

Malnutrition in the Trauma Patient

MALNUTRITION IN THE TRAUMA PATIENT

Note: *Without aggressive nutritional management, the trauma patient is at risk of developing malnutrition. While nutritional assessments or interventions are not generally carried out in the acute resuscitation area, some baseline measurements (by examination or history) should be made early in the patient's hospital stay. For example, the patient must be weighed within the first 24 hours of admission regardless of where he is. His nutritional status and management have a direct bearing on his prognosis. While nutritional support is not usually a priority in initial resuscitation and surgical intervention, it must become a prime consideration thereafter if the patient is to recover.*

Assessment

Mechanism of injury/ etiology:
A hypermetabolic, hypercatabolic state results from increased metabolic demands related to traumatic injury. The patient's protein, fat, and carbohydrate metabolisms are altered in an attempt to meet his energy needs. The result is proteolysis with weight loss, delayed wound healing, and increased infection susceptibility.

This problem may be complicated by the patient's inability to ingest food, necessitating alternative feeding methods.

Physical findings:
• decreased fat stores— reflected by testing triceps skin-fold thickness
• decreased lean muscle mass—reflected by testing midarm muscle circumference
• weight loss

Diagnostic studies

• laboratory data
  □ albumin—levels more reliably indicate long-term than short-term protein deficiency. This protein has a long half-life, increasing the interval between the beginning of its loss and albumin level decreases. Also, infusion of I.V. fluids influences albumin levels. Colloid or blood infusion may raise this level, while large crystalloid infusions or overhydration from any cause can reflect a false low value.
  □ transferrin—with a shorter half-life than albumin, it should reflect alterations in protein metabolism sooner
  □ total lymphocyte count and skin testing—these studies test the patient's cell-mediated immunocompetency, which may reflect his nutritional status. Total lymphocyte count decreases in protein-calorie malnutrition. The patient may exhibit delayed responses to intradermal skin testing during decreased protein synthesis because antibody production also decreases. Other causes of delayed reactions to skin tests may also develop, such as the trauma- or sepsis-related immunosuppressive responses.
• nitrogen balance—its calculation (from the patient's protein intake and urinary urea nitrogen) reflects the relationship between protein synthesis and catabolism. The ideal is a positive nitrogen balance, showing that protein synthesis is greater than breakdown. A patient in a post-traumatic hypermetabolic state usually has a negative balance.
• indirect calorimetry—calculations from the measurement of respiratory gases reflect the patient's resting energy expenditure. This information helps in planning the patient's caloric and other nutritional needs.
• triceps skin-fold thickness and midarm muscle circumference—serial measurements of these areas are compared to standard charts; together with height, weight, and body frame size, the values reflect percentage loss or gain of fat and lean muscle mass

Nursing diagnosis

Potential for alterations in nutrition, less than body requirements, related to hypermetabolic, hypercatabolic responses to traumatic injury.

GOAL #1: Determine the patient's baseline nutritional status within 24 hours of admission.

Interventions

1. Assess the patient's nutritional status by history and examination, including:
- height and weight
- triceps skin-fold thickness
- midarm muscle circumference
- dietary history
- eating patterns
- food allergies
- food preferences
- religious dietary customs
- medical conditions affecting nutrition
- current medications
- chewing or swallowing difficulties
- alcohol use
- recent weight loss or gain.

Rationale

Baseline assessment of the patient's nutritional status is essential to discover any preexisting nutritional deficits. More aggressive nutritional support will compensate for these deficiencies. Baseline measurements must be made within the first 24 hours to obtain an accurate picture of the patient's nutritional status before it begins to change. The patient's dietary history may be obtained from either him or his family and friends. Ideally, the patient should be weighed daily with steps taken to minimize variables, such as time of weighing, the clothes the patient wears, or scale calibration. Serial measurements should also be made of triceps skin-fold thickness and midarm muscle circumference to analyze trends in fat and protein loss or gain. Nutritional assessment is ongoing and aimed at meeting the trauma patient's changing nutritional needs.

Note: *Soon after traumatic injury, the patient experiences a hypermetabolic, hypercatabolic response, which usually ends after 4 to 5 days. In the first 24 hours after injury, the appropriate priority is treating him promptly for injuries and maintaining his perfusion and oxygen needs. Rapid attention to these priorities will minimize infection, sepsis, and multiple organ failure, all of which only increase nutritional demands. Nutritional support has a low priority during this time, but it should not be totally ignored. Nutritional assessment is begun and gastrostomy or jejunostomy tubes may be inserted in the patient requiring abdominal surgery in anticipation of future enteral feeding. After this initial period, the patient remains in a hypercatabolic state, continuing to lose protein and fat stores. At this point, the goal of nutritional therapy is to preserve as much peripheral muscle mass as possible. When the hypermetabolic stage has ended, nutritional support becomes a high priority. The goals are to replace lost stores and to provide sufficient calories and protein to promote wound healing and enable the patient to resist infection.*

GOAL #2: Provide nutritional support appropriate to the patient's needs.

Interventions

1. Consult the physician on appropriate type, amount, and route of dietary supplements.

Rationale

Among the factors of nutritional support for the trauma patient are his injuries and physical condition, his specific caloric and protein needs, effectiveness of the various available supplements, and safety of the various systems. An awake, alert patient usually is managed with a high-calorie, high-protein diet. A patient with functional intestines but who is unable to eat (because of head injury or mandibular fixation) needs enteral feedings through a gastric tube, either passed through the upper GI tract or surgically inserted into the stomach or small intestine. A patient with a nonfunctional bowel, such as one with ileus or abdominal trauma, needs total parenteral nutrition (TPN), containing high concentrations of glucose, protein, electrolytes, vitamins, and minerals. Generally, the patient is also given infusions of fat emulsions as an extra source of calories. A TPN solution can be administered through either peripheral or central veins, but a solution with glucose concentrations greater than 10% is given centrally. When possible, enteral nutrition is preferable because evidence suggests that enteral supplements are more effectively utilized than are parenteral ones.

2. Promote the patient's compliance with his diet:
- teach him to plan his diet and assist as needed
- have his family or friends bring in foods he likes as long as they meet dietary requirements.

The patient recovering from multiple trauma typically requires a high-calorie, high-protein diet to resist infection and replace lost muscle mass. These steps promote the patient's cooperation in meeting his nutritional needs.

GOAL #3: Prevent or minimize nutritional therapy complications.

Interventions

1. Elevate the head of the bed before, during, and after tube feedings, unless contraindicated.

2. Check the feeding tube for proper placement. Aspirate tubing for residual solution and recheck placement of the tube before each feeding.

3. Withhold feeding and contact the physician if you are uncertain of tube placement or if residual solution is greater than the physician's order; document actions. (The physician's order for tube feeding should include maximum residual solution permitted.)

4. Administer tube feedings as prescribed. If the solution is diluted on the unit, precisely measure diluent and feeding.

5. Observe the patient for diarrhea. Notify the physician if it develops.

6. Assist with chest radiography after insertion of a central line for TPN.

7. Use the TPN line only to administer I.V. nutritional supplements.

8. Change TPN line dressings with strict aseptic technique in accordance with hospital policy.

9. Maintain absolute sterility of the TPN system when changing tubing or adding bottles.

Rationale

Pulmonary aspiration is a primary complication of tube feedings. These interventions minimize the patient's vomiting from gastric distention or his physical position.

Diarrhea can develop if the tube-feeding concentration is too high or increases too fast. Diarrhea causes fluid and electrolyte loss. Accurate mixing and administration of feedings and slow increases in concentration should prevent this complication. If diarrhea develops it may be necessary to alter the feedings' progression.

Radiographs establish the correct placement of the central catheter before infusing TPN. Correct placement guarantees infusion into the central circulation. They also evaluate the patient for a pneumothorax.

These steps prevent breaks in the system or sterile technique, which can lead to infection. Under no circumstances should TPN lines be used to draw blood samples or infuse blood products.

10. Change I.V. tubing while the patient holds his breath or performs a Valsalva maneuver. Change tubing of a ventilated patient at the end of inspiration.

The patient is at greatest risk for an air embolism when the I.V. tubing is disconnected. These interventions prevent air embolism by increasing intrathoracic pressure while the tubing is disconnected.

11. Observe the line insertion site for signs of inflammation (redness, edema, pain, or drainage) during dressing changes. Notify the physician of any findings; document all observations.

Promptly recognizing possible infection permits changing the line to eliminate the source of inflammation and minimize infection.

12. Monitor laboratory results of a patient receiving TPN, including:
- blood glucose level
- serum creatinine level
- blood urea nitrogen level
- electrolyte concentration
- liver enzyme concentration
- partial thromboplastin time
- CBC
- serum magnesium level
- serum phosphate level
- chemistry profile
- serum triglyceride levels.

A TPN infusion can lead to metabolic complications, such as hyper- or hypoglycemia, fluid and electrolyte disturbances, carbon dioxide retention, and fatty liver syndrome. These steps aid early detection and rapid correction of such potential problems.

13. Observe the patient for signs of hypo- or hyperglycemia.

14. Gradually wean the patient from the TPN solution to prevent insulin reactions.

PERITONITIS

Assessment

Mechanism of injury/etiology:
- symptoms may appear in an acute or crescendo manner after or in conjunction with:
  - ☐ blunt or penetrating abdominal trauma
  - ☐ recent abdominal surgery
  - ☐ rupture of any hollow organs (such as the gallbladder, appendix, or stomach, as with peptic ulcer disease)
  - ☐ chronic urinary or female genital tract infections

Physical findings:
Respiratory
- rapid, shallow respirations

Cardiovascular
- fever—usually low grade initially
- chills
- tachycardia
- shock state

Gastrointestinal
- abdominal pain/tenderness—constant; increased by movement, breathing, coughing, palpation; generalized or localized; also, complaints of a burning sensation
- pain referred to shoulder, back, chest

- abdominal guarding because of the pain
- abdominal distention, rigidity, ascites
- hypoactive or absent bowel sounds
- anorexia
- nausea/vomiting
- altered bowel habits/constipation

Genitourinary
- decreased urinary output

Diagnostic studies

Note: *In many cases the patient's history, symptoms, and physical examination provide enough information to identify the cause of peritoneal inflammation signs.*
- cultures of specimens from suspicious sites (for example, the urinary tract or an abdominal wound)—may reveal such organisms as *E. coli*, streptococci, or pneumococci
- laboratory data
  - ☐ WBC count—elevated in response to inflammatory process
  - ☐ hemoglobin/hematocrit levels—may be abnormally low if the patient has a concurrent hemorrhagic process
  - ☐ electrolyte levels—may reveal imbalance with profound peritonitis
- abdominal radiography—free air indicates bowel perforation; may visualize bowel obstruction
- abdominal computerized tomography (CT) scan, liver/spleen scans, and ultrasound—may reveal the causative factor, such as intraabdominal fluid, hematoma accumulation, or ruptured viscera
- diagnostic peritoneal lavage (DPL—indicated with a history of blunt abdominal trauma)—returned fluid analysis may reveal WBC count greater than 500 mm³, indicating possible injury to the bowel or other hollow organs (which may produce signs suggesting peritonitis)

Note: *An exploratory laparotomy may be indicated if the patient has penetrating abdominal trauma; positive DPL, CT, liver/spleen scan, or ultrasound results; or if the patient presents and persists in an unexplained shock state after blunt or penetrating abdominal or thoracic trauma.*

Nursing diagnosis

Potential fluid volume deficit related to hemorrhage and fluid volume shift into extravascular space.

GOAL: Restore and maintain a normovolemic state.

Interventions

1. Monitor the patient for signs of hypovolemic shock; monitor/document vital signs every 5 to 15 minutes during initial shock state, then every hour after the patient stabilizes, or as his condition warrants.

Rationale

Profound shock may result from hemorrhage secondary to intraabdominal injury and from fluid shifts (which occur when peritoneal fluid accumulates in large quantities and decreases the circulating blood volume). Analysis of vital sign trends helps determine the effectiveness of resuscitative measures on hemodynamics.

2. Ensure adequate I.V. access with large-bore peripheral catheters; administer fluids, as ordered.

Rapid and substantial fluid replacement facilitates the return to a normovolemic state.

3. Monitor laboratory data (CBC; ABG, electrolyte, amylase, and bilirubin levels; liver function tests; and coagulation studies) frequently.

Evaluating laboratory data helps identify causative factors, diagnose fluid/electrolyte imbalances, and evaluate resuscitative efforts to improve tissue perfusion.

4. Insert an indwelling urinary catheter; monitor intake/output balance closely.

Monitoring urine output helps evaluate hemodynamic status. Decreased urinary output may reflect inadequate fluid replacement, poor tissue perfusion, or toxic effects.

Nursing diagnosis

Potential for impaired gas exchange related to decreased respiratory reserve.

GOAL: Promote and maintain optimal respiratory status.

Interventions

1. Monitor the patient for signs of respiratory distress or failing respiratory effort (such as shallow, rapid respirations with decreased air exchange).

2. Evaluate/document breath sounds, ABG results, chest radiographs.

3. Anticipate the use of supplemental oxygen and possible intubation.

4. Provide optimal pulmonary hygiene, including:
- breathing exercises
- frequent suctioning
- turning and placement in semi-Fowler's position unless contraindicated.

Rationale

Abdominal pain and distention make it difficult for the patient to breathe deeply and cough effectively. This patient may fatigue easily.

Decreased respiratory effort and resultant poor tissue perfusion predispose this patient to pulmonary complications, such as atelectasis and pneumonia. You may note diminished breath sounds and auscultate adventitious sounds, such as rales. ABG results may reveal respiratory acidosis with a decreased $PaCO_2$ resulting from hyperventilation.

The patient in shock, with a circulating volume deficit and decreased respiratory effort, requires oxygen administration to optimize tissue perfusion. In severe cases, the patient may require mechanical ventilation.

These measures facilitate drainage of respiratory secretions, promote adequate gas exchange and expansion, and prevent pooling of secretions in the lower lobes.

Nursing diagnosis

Potential for infection related to pathogens introduced into the peritoneum by free blood, feces, bile, or urine.

GOAL: Recognize early signs of infection; prevent or minimize further infection.

Interventions

1. Monitor/document vital signs (including temperature); note trends in laboratory data, especially WBC count.

2. Anticipate cultures of suspicious areas (for example, an abdominal wound, incision, or blood).

3. Administer antibiotics as ordered.

4. Use aseptic technique when caring for wounds, dressings, drains.

5. Prepare the patient for surgical intervention. (See "Preparation for Surgery" in Section VII.)

Rationale

Trend analysis of vital signs and laboratory data aids early recognition of a septic process. Leukocytosis usually occurs as the infectious process advances. Toxins entering the circulation may result in profound septic episodes.

These studies help identify the cause of the infection and provide baseline information.

Antibiotic therapy may be prophylactic (as with a penetrating abdominal injury) or directed toward halting the growth of specific identified organisms. The current trend in infectious disease treatment is to determine the causative factor before antibiotic administration.

This prevents further contamination and isolates the contaminant.

Surgical procedures may be required to diagnose or treat peritonitis.

Nursing diagnosis

Alteration in bowel elimination related to paralytic ileus secondary to peritoneal inflammation.

GOAL: Prevent or minimize paralytic ileus.

Interventions

1. Ensure insertion and proper placement of a gastric decompression tube and maintain NPO status.

2. Maintain gastric decompression with 80 to 120 mm Hg (intermittent) or 30 to 40 mm Hg (continuous) suction.

3. Irrigate and aspirate both ports of the gastric tube at least every 2 hours (more frequently with continuous suction).

Rationale

Decompression lessens the risk of aspiration of acidic gastric contents should the patient vomit and prevents aggravating the ileus by relieving stomach pressure on the bowel.

Controlled and carefully monitored suction limits lessen the risk of gastric mucosal injury. Continuous suction, although not the optimal method, can be used initially (until the stomach has been emptied) if you stay within recommended suction limits and irrigate the lumen frequently.

Frequent irrigation maximizes patency and proper functioning of the air vent and drainage port. The risk of mucosal damage increases with air vent obstruction.

4. Assess/document the amount and characteristics of gastric secretions; document drainage pH every 2 to 4 hours; include gastric drainage in output totals.

This provides baseline and diagnostic information that aids ileus evaluation. A gastric pH of less than 5 to 7 usually requires antacid therapy. Increased gastric drainage usually occurs with an ileus and, if excessive, may require fluid replacement to prevent dehydration.

5. Monitor/document the quality and quantity of bowel sounds; note trends.

This provides a baseline assessment of GI function. Paralytic ileus produces hypoactive or absent bowel sounds.

Associated care plans

Intraabdominal Trauma: Blunt and
    Penetrating
Vasogenic Shock
Paralytic Ileus

Associated procedures and study

Diagnostic Peritoneal Lavage
Nuclear Medicine Imaging
Preparation for Surgery

ACUTE PANCREATITIS

Note: *The three major concerns for a patient with acute pancreatitis are respiratory compromise, hypovolemia, and pain control. The patient arriving in the emergency department may be in profound hypovolemic shock and need resuscitation in the ABC format, with pain control having a very low priority. Intervention priority for a patient with mild-to-moderate pancreatitis generally includes gastric decompression, relief of pain, and fluid replacement. Reducing gastric secretions and easing pain may prevent the occurrence of more serious respiratory and cardiovascular complications.*

Assessment

Mechanism of injury/etiology:
- edema, hemorrhage, vascular changes, and necrosis caused by lipolytic, proteolytic, and other enzymatic autodigestion of the pancreas
- chronic alcoholism, biliary tract disease—especially cholelithiasis—and trauma
- other precipitating factors may include peptic ulcer disease; infectious diseases, such as infectious hepatitis, viral mumps, and hemolytic streptococcus; drug therapy; hyperparathyroidism; metabolic disorders; cancer; pregnancy; and hereditary and idiopathic causes

Physical findings:
Gastrointestinal
- pain (attack initially may be painless):
  - ☐ mild-to-highly debilitating
  - ☐ slow-to-acute onset, gradually intensifying
  - ☐ located in the left upper quadrant, midepigastrium, subcostal area
  - ☐ radiates or bores through to the back
  - ☐ becomes generalized in the abdomen
  - ☐ no relief from antacids; pain may increase after narcotics administration
  - ☐ some relief when the patient is upright and motionless
- decreased or absent bowel sounds
- nausea/vomiting—fecal vomitus from an ileus may be present
- anorexia—possible history of recent weight loss
- abdominal distention with rigidity and guarding
- Grey Turner's sign—dissection of blood into flanks and retroperitoneal space
- palpable upper abdominal mass
- ascites—not always present

Cardiovascular
- mild fever—from tissue injury, inflammation
- tachycardia
- shock state
- color changes—jaundice, cyanosis
- diaphoresis

Respiratory
- pleuritic chest pain
- painful, uneven respirations
- hiccoughs

Neurologic
- apathy
- confusion

Genitourinary
- mild hematuria
- pyuria

Diagnostic studies

The patient's history and physical examination often provide sufficient data for diagnosis.
- laboratory studies
  - ☐ amylase, lipase levels—elevations indicate need for further diagnostic studies; rising or constantly elevated amylase levels indicate probable pancreatic injury
  - ☐ hemoglobin/hematocrit levels—may be lowered due to hemorrhagic process
  - ☐ WBC count, sedimentation rate—elevated from infection
  - ☐ serum glucose level—transient elevation
  - ☐ calcium, magnesium levels—may be low
  - ☐ fibrinogen and Factor VIII levels—may be elevated
- radiography
  - ☐ chest film—may reveal effusion, atelectasis, elevated diaphragm
  - ☐ abdominal film—may show an ileus, pancreatic calcification
- contrast studies
  - ☐ oral or I.V. cholecystography—reflects biliary tract obstruction or gallbladder disease
  - ☐ upper GI series—reflects pancreatic enlargement, stomach and duodenal involvement
  - ☐ excretory urography or intravenous pyelography—reflects renal involvement
- computed tomography—may locate hematoma, organ enlargement, or blood/fluid accumulation

Nursing diagnosis

Potential for ineffective breathing patterns and decreased gas exchange related to pain, pulmonary effusions, and a paralytic ileus secondary to pancreatic edema and inflammation.

GOAL #1: Reduce respiratory effort; optimize gas exchange.

Interventions

1. Monitor the patient's respiratory status for signs of fatigue or distress, including:
- tachypnea
- dyspnea
- an uneven breathing pattern
- hiccoughs
- deteriorating ABG results.

2. Assist with intubation and initiation of mechanical ventilation as needed. (See "Endotracheal Intubation" in Section VII.)

3. Assist with chest radiography.

Rationale

Pain caused by pancreatic inflammation and edema and abdominal distention from an ileus impair or minimize respiratory effectiveness. Pleural effusions from pancreatic fluid leakage and diaphragmatic irritation exacerbate respiratory embarrassment. Hiccoughs and uneven, painful respirations signal diaphragmatic irritation. The patient with acute pancreatitis usually needs intubation and ventilatory support to optimize gas exchange.

GOAL #2: Minimize the risk or severity of a paralytic ileus.

Interventions

1. Insert a gastric decompression tube. Maintain proper tube position, patency, and appropriate suction levels. Keep the patient NPO.

Rationale

A paralytic ileus occurs in response to pancreatic inflammation. It especially affects the transverse colon because that segment of colon lies in proximity to the pancreas. Abdominal distention causes diaphragm elevation and pain, both of which aggravate respiratory compromise. Gastric decompression and eliminating oral intake prevent additional air and fluid from entering and accumulating in the nonfunctioning intestine. Decompression also prevents or severely limits acid flow from the stomach to the small intestines, decreasing pancreatic stimulation and allowing the gland to rest.

GOAL #3: Optimize the patient's physical comfort.

Interventions

1. Assess the patient's pain level and administer analgesics as ordered.

2. Maintain the patency and proper functioning of the gastric decompression tube.

3. Administer anticholinergics as ordered.

Rationale

Analgesia is usually required during acute pancreatitis. Selective and limited use of narcotics is necessary, since they may heighten pain by increasing ductal and sphincter pressure or tone. Alternative analgesics may be indicated.

Decompression and gastric secretions removal promote comfort.

These drugs reduce gastric acid secretion and may also reduce pancreatic metabolic activity.

Nursing diagnosis

Potential for decreased tissue perfusion related to fluid volume deficit caused by hemorrhage, plasma extravasation into the bowel and retroperitoneal space, and kinin release secondary to pancreatic inflammation and autodigestion by proteolytic, lipolytic, and other pancreatic enzymes.

GOAL: Restore and maintain normovolemia; optimize tissue perfusion.

Interventions

1. Monitor the patient for signs of hemorrhagic shock as listed in Table 2.1 in "Hemorrhagic Shock" in Section II. Monitor vital signs every 5 to 15 minutes while the patient's condition is unstable and every hour after stabilization, or as his condition warrants.

2. Ensure placement of large-bore peripheral I.V. catheters. Assist with placing a peripheral artery or pulmonary artery (PA) catheter. Administer fluid replacement as ordered.

3. Administer blood and clotting factors as ordered.

4. Monitor electrolyte and glucose levels. Administer supplements as ordered.

5. Insert an indwelling urinary catheter and closely monitor urine output, sugar, and acetone.

6. Administer vasopressors as ordered.

Rationale

Early recognition and prompt treatment of shock can minimize subsequent complications.

Acute pancreatitis can trigger profound shock, necessitating resuscitation with excessive volumes of crystalloid or colloid solutions. Monitoring PA and arterial pressures helps accurately evaluate vital signs and resuscitation effectiveness and dictates what other stabilization efforts are needed.

Replacing blood and components helps in resuscitation.

Altered endocrine function related to pancreatitis, together with shock and preexisting diseases, often causes an electrolyte imbalance. Calcium and magnesium supplements may be necessary. Abnormal insulin secretion may cause transient hyperglycemia and require insulin coverage.

Close monitoring of urine output has several purposes. Pancreatic pseudocysts may compress or displace the left kidney, causing hematuria or pyuria. Glucose spillage may reflect endocrine dysfunction. Output is a valuable indicator of adequate perfusion.

Shock unresponsive to fluid resuscitation may require vasopressors to optimize perfusion.

Nursing diagnosis

Potential for infection related to spillage of proteolytic pancreatic enzymes into the peritoneal and retroperitoneal spaces, increased bowel permeability, and autodigestion of the pancreas.

GOAL: Early recognition of, and prompt therapy for, infection.

Interventions	Rationale
1. Monitor the patient closely for signs of infection. Obtain or assist with obtaining cultures as requested.	Increased bowel permeability and leakage of proteolytic pancreatic enzymes can cause significant peritonitis. A pancreatic abscess should be suspected in a patient in a prolonged febrile state. Cultures of blood, effusions, and abscesses aid direction of therapy.
2. Administer antibiotics as ordered.	Administering antibiotics before culture identification of specific microorganisms may precipitate superinfections, which are very difficult to control. Multiple antibiotics may increase therapeutic effectiveness.
3. Prepare the patient for surgical intervention. (See "Preparation for Surgery" in Section VII.)	Pancreatitis unresponsive to the previously mentioned therapy and characterized by persistent fevers and elevated amylase levels often requires surgical intervention.

Associated care plans	Associated procedures and study
Hemorrhagic Shock	Intrahospital Transport of the Shock Trauma Patient
Vasogenic Shock	Positive Contrast Study
Malnutrition in the Trauma Patient	Pulmonary Artery Catheterization
Peritonitis	Preparation for Surgery
Paralytic Ileus	Endotracheal Intubation

Medical diagnosis

PARALYTIC ILEUS

Assessment

Mechanism of injury/ etiology:
Paralytic ileus may develop after, or in conjunction with, any of the following:
- electrolyte/acid-base disturbances
- general anesthesia
- hypoxia
- myocardial infarction
- narcotic administration
- pelvic or vertebral

fractures
- peritonitis
- premature oral intake following surgery or trauma
- premature gastric tube removal
- respiratory failure
- retroperitoneal hematoma
- sepsis
- shock
- spinal cord injury

- surgery
- trauma

Physical findings:
Cardiovascular
- may mimic a septic episode: elevated WBC count, fever, shock

Gastrointestinal
- hypoactive or absent bowel sounds

- increased gastric drainage/vomiting
- abdominal pain/discomfort described as generalized, dull, cramplike
- abdominal distention or tightening
- hiccoughs (from increased pressure on the diaphragm)
- constipation

Diagnostic study

- abdominal radiography—reveals distention of small bowel, colon, or stomach with fluid and air

Nursing diagnosis

Alteration in bowel elimination related to decreased or absent peristalsis secondary to above-listed mechanisms and etiologies.

GOAL #1: Prevent or minimize the risk of paralytic ileus.

Interventions

1. Ensure gastric decompression tube insertion and proper placement; maintain NPO status.

2. Perform frequent abdominal assessments:
- Auscultate the quality and quantity of bowel sounds.

- Measure abdominal girth.

Rationale

The bowel cannot transport gas and fluid effectively in this adynamic or immobile state. Thus any fluid or gas currently in the stomach or bowel becomes trapped and acts as an intestinal obstruction. Early intervention can prevent complications. For example, inserting a gastric decompression tube and restricting additional oral intake reduce gastric contents and relieve pressure on the already distended small bowel. These measures usually prevent the normal transient post-trauma or postoperative sluggish bowel state from progressing to an acute paralytic ileus.

Acute changes or downward trends in bowel sounds (for example, hypoactive or absent sounds) indicate ineffective or absent peristalsis.

Increased abdominal girth measurements confirm abdominal distention, which occurs with gas and fluid accumulation in the paralyzed bowel.

• Assess the amount and characteristics of gastric secretions; document pH every 2 to 4 hours; include gastric drainage in output totals.

This baseline and diagnostic information aids ileus evaluation. A gastric pH less than 5 to 7 usually requires I.V. and tube-instilled alkalinizing agents. Gastric drainage usually increases with an ileus and, if excessive, may necessitate fluid replacement to prevent dehydration.

• Note characteristics of abdominal pain/discomfort.

Pain accompanying a paralytic ileus may be generalized, cramplike, dull, and unrelenting. When administering analgesics (such as narcotics), remember that narcotics may precipitate or aggravate an ileus and, therefore, necessitate alternative analgesia.

GOAL #2: Maintain patency, position, and proper functioning of the decompression tube.

Interventions

1. Maintain gastric decompression with 80 to 120 mm Hg (intermittent) or 30 to 40 mm Hg (continuous) suction via a tube with an air vent system.

Rationale

Controlled and carefully monitored suction levels lessen the risk of injury to gastric mucosa. Continuous suction, although not the optimal method, can be used initially (until the stomach has been emptied) if you stay within the recommended suction levels and irrigate the lumen frequently. For ongoing gastric decompression, only those tubes with built-in air vent systems are recommended.

2. Check gastric tube placement at the beginning of every shift, before instilling any air or liquid, and as needed. Instill 30 cc of air into the drainage port while auscultating at the lower border of the left ribs.

Proper tube function depends on maintaining correct placement. Do not instill liquid without checking placement first. This rule decreases the risk of iatrogenic aspiration.

3. Irrigate the air vent with 30 cc of air and the suction port with 30 cc of normal saline solution (NSS) every 2 hours (more frequently if using continuous suction). Manually aspirate the suction port to ensure the return of NSS and air.

Frequent irrigation maximizes patency and proper functioning of both the air vent and the drainage port. Air vent obstruction increases the risk of mucosal damage.

GOAL #3: Promote patient comfort.

Interventions

1. Assess the patient's pain level and institute relief measures.

Rationale

The pain associated with a paralytic ileus can be intense, constant, and difficult to alleviate. Encourage the ambulatory patient to walk around. The movement may disrupt the gas accumulation and provide some relief. Similarly, the patient confined to bed rest may find relief by turning frequently and moving about in bed. Rectal tubes may hasten gas and fluid elimination as the ileus begins to improve. When administering analgesics (such as narcotics), remember that narcotics may precipitate or aggravate an ileus and, therefore, necessitate alternative analgesia.

Nursing diagnosis

Potential fluid volume deficit related to decreased fluid absorption in the bowel and excessive vomiting/gastric drainage secondary to hypoactive or inactive intestinal tract.

GOAL: Restore and maintain a normovolemic state and electrolyte balance.

Interventions

1. Monitor the patient for signs of dehydration and hypovolemia: take vital signs every hour (or as the patient's condition warrants), maintain ongoing intake/output balance.

2. Ensure adequate I.V. access for hydration.

3. Monitor trends in laboratory studies, such as CBC and electrolyte levels and ABG studies.

Rationale

Decreased or ineffective peristalsis resulting in an intestinal obstruction permits gas and fluid accumulation in the GI tract. The bowel loses its ability to absorb fluids, which places the patient at risk for dehydration. The dehydrated state may progress to hypovolemia unless recognized and corrected promptly with adequate volume replacement.

Electrolyte absorption is interrupted as the bowel remains immobile and nonfunctioning. Supplemental electrolytes and alkalinizing agents may be necessary to restore normal electrolyte and acid-base balances.

Nursing diagnosis

Potential for impaired respiratory function related to diaphragmatic elevation or aspiration of vomitus secondary to abdominal distention.

GOAL #1: Promote and maintain optimal respiratory efforts.

Interventions

1. Monitor the patient for signs of respiratory distress or failing respiratory effort, such as shallow, rapid respirations with decreased air exchange.

2. Evaluate and document breath sounds, ABG results, chest radiographs.

3. Provide optimal pulmonary hygiene:
• encourage coughing and deep breathing
• have the patient use incentive spirometry
• turn him frequently
• place the patient in semi-Fowler's position, unless contraindicated
• suction, as indicated.

4. Anticipate the need for supplemental oxygen and possible intubation.

Rationale

The abdominal distention that occurs with a paralytic ileus causes diaphragm elevation and increases the patient's respiratory efforts. Distention and associated abdominal pain or discomfort make it difficult for the patient to take deep breaths and cough effectively. He may also fatigue easily.

Decreased respiratory effort and resultant poor tissue perfusion predispose the patient to pulmonary complications (such as atelectasis and pneumonia). You may note diminished breath sounds and adventitious sounds (such as rales). ABGs may reveal respiratory acidosis with decreased $PaCO_2$ from hyperventilation.

These measures facilitate respiratory secretion drainage, promote adequate gas exchange and lung expansion, and prevent pooling of secretions in the lower lobes.

Supplemental oxygen enhances tissue perfusion by increasing oxygen availability at the alveolar/capillary membrane. Patients with deteriorating respiratory efforts may require endotracheal intubation and mechanical ventilation until their overall status improves.

*Supplemental nursing diagnosis

GOAL #2: Prevent or minimize the risk of aspiration.

Interventions

Rationale

1. Maintain the patency, position, and proper functioning of the decompression tube.

As discussed, this patient requires vigilant care to maintain a properly working gastric tube. This includes aggressively maintaining tube patency, even during patient transport. Clamping or obstructing the drainage port predisposes the patient to aspiration should vomiting occur.

2. Ensure the availability of suction apparatus.

Immediate oropharyngeal suctioning may reduce the risk of aspiration should vomiting occur.

Additional considerations

Paralytic ileus can occur as a complication of almost any surgical procedure and many medical conditions. It can also lead to other complications, such as aspiration, further increasing the length of hospitalization. So be aggressive about preventing paralytic ileus in all at-risk patients. The two major aggravating factors are easily avoided: premature postoperative oral intake and premature gastric tube removal (before the bowel is ready to function). Keep this patient NPO for an extra day or two; it is a minor inconvenience, given the risk.

Associated care plan
Lower Airway Obstruction

MECHANICAL BOWEL OBSTRUCTION (M.B.O.)

Assessment

Mechanism of injury/etiology:
MBO may be complete or partial, transient or persistent, strangulating or nonstrangulating; most common in the small bowel; caused by intrinsic, extrinsic, or intraluminal problems, including:
• abscess
• adhesions—most common in small bowel (proximal)
• carcinoma—most common in large bowel (distal)

• foreign body
• gallstones—usually large
• hematoma
• hernia
• barium or fecal impaction
• intussusception—telescoping of bowel
• ischemia
• strictures

Physical findings:
Gastrointestinal

• profuse vomiting (proximal MBO)
• feculent vomiting (dis-

tal MBO)
• abdominal distention (distal MBO)
• hyperactive, high-pitched bowel sounds (may be intermittently absent)
• middle to lower abdominal pain: sharp, cramping; intervals coinciding with peristaltic movement
• diffuse abdominal tenderness
• absent bowel movements if MBO is complete; diarrhea if MBO is

partial
• signs and symptoms of peritonitis or gas gangrene if strangulation occurs (refer to respective care plans)

Cardiovascular
• dehydration
• shock state
• sepsis

Genitourinary
• oliguria
• azotemia

Diagnostic studies

• abdominal radiographs
  ☐ plain film—reveals large amount of localized air in obstructed area
  ☐ upright or lateral decubitus—may show air/fluid levels

• barium enema—aids in differentiating small-bowel from colonic obstructions
• sigmoidoscopic examination—aids in diagnosing colonic obstruction

Alteration in bowel elimination related to physical obstruction of the bowel lumen secondary to internal, external, or intraluminal blockage.

GOAL #1: Recognize patients at risk for MBO and minimize the risk.

Interventions

1. Alert the oncoming nurse or receiving unit when the patient has undergone a barium study. Initiate cathartics as ordered. Monitor trends in the patient's bowel elimination closely after a barium study.

Rationale

If the proper cathartics, stool softeners, and enemas are not administered appropriately after a barium study, the risk of barium impaction leading to an MBO increases, especially in the immobilized patient.

GOAL #2: Minimize gastric and intestinal distention and pressure.

Interventions

1. Maintain the patient NPO. Insert a gastric decompression tube and maintain suction. Assist with insertion of an intestinal decompression tube as needed. Follow established hospital protocol and manufacturer's instructions for safe insertion and proper maintenance of intestinal tubes.

Rationale

The obstructed, and now nonfunctional, bowel causes fluid and gas to accumulate proximal to the obstruction. The bowel rapidly becomes distended, exerting retrograde pressure on the stomach. Restricting all oral intake lessens fluid accumulation in the nonfunctional bowel segment. Gastric decompression prevents added pressure on the bowel and lowers the risk of aspiration if vomiting occurs. Increased intraluminal pressure caused by fluid and gas buildup can impair circulation to the obstructed site. Long intestinal tubes, such as the Cantor or the Miller-Abbott, promote proximal decompression, reducing intraluminal pressure. Both tubes have distal mercury-filled balloons, which maintain the tubes' desired position in the distal duodenum or proximal jejunum. Serious complications associated with both tubes mandate strict compliance with manufacturer's package insert instructions.

Nursing diagnosis

Potential for fluid volume deficit related to accumulation of intestinal secretions, extracellular fluid depletion, and profuse vomiting secondary to obstructed and nonfunctional bowel.

GOAL #1: Restore and maintain a normovolemic state.

Interventions

1. Monitor the patient for hypovolemic shock; record vital signs and urine output hourly or more often as the patient's condition warrants.

2. Ensure adequate peripheral I.V. access and replace fluids as ordered. Assemble necessary equipment for inserting a central venous catheter.

Rationale

Every 24 hours, the GI tract secretes about 8 liters of fluid to promote digestion and nutrient absorption. The distention from an MBO causes this secretion to increase. But, due to its immobility, the small bowel can neither reabsorb nor eliminate the fluid. The blocked bowel, distended with air and fluid, can trigger profuse vomiting. Also, protein secreted into the bowel lumen causes a third-space fluid depletion. In all, a patient with MBO may lose 3 or more liters of fluid in 24 hours. Close monitoring and adequate fluid replacement are essential to prevent hypovolemic shock. In severe volume depletion, central venous pressures help to evaluate and direct fluid replacement.

GOAL #2: Restore and maintain electrolyte balance.

Interventions

1. Obtain baseline laboratory data and monitor trends in CBC; serum sodium, chloride, potassium, hydrogen, creatinine, and blood urea nitrogen levels; and ABGs. Collect and send urine samples for analysis as requested.

2. Administer electrolyte replacements as ordered.

Rationale

In an MBO, severe electrolyte imbalances with metabolic alkalosis result from excessive fluid and nutrient loss. Hemoconcentration, resulting from plasma leakage into the bowel, and uremic azotemia and oliguria from severe dehydration are all MBO-related complications.

Nursing diagnosis

Potential for infection related to proliferation of intestinal bacteria, intestinal ischemia, and possible bowel rupture secondary to fluid and gas stasis in the bowel and possible intestinal strangulation.

GOAL: Recognize early signs of localized or systemic infection.

Interventions

1. Monitor the patient closely for signs of peritonitis, gas gangrene, and vasogenic-septic shock, including:
- severe, constant abdominal pain
- specific area of increased pain with strangulation
- fever spikes
- increased abdominal girth
- profound shock state
- deterioration in mental status.

2. Administer antibiotics as ordered.

3. Prepare the patient for surgical intervention. (See "Preparation for Surgery" in Section VII.)

Rationale

The small-bowel bacterial count is normally low. But in a patient with MBO, bacteria proliferate rapidly because of fluid and gas stasis. The colon, however, normally contains large numbers of bacteria, and an MBO there can be devastating. The toxins elaborated by the bacteria can escape through the bowel wall and enter the peritoneal cavity, where they are absorbed into the systemic circulation. Strangulation develops when the MBO impairs both circulation and tissue perfusion to the affected segment. A closed-loop obstruction, in which blockage occurs both proximally and distally, severely impedes circulation to the strangulated bowel loop. The combination of (1) bowel distention with toxic products and (2) impaired circulation to the affected segment greatly aggravates the risk of gangrene, bowel rupture, and peritonitis. Unless the complications are promptly recognized and effectively treated, profound septicemia can develop.

Broad-spectrum antibiotics are usually indicated, especially if strangulation is suspected.

An MBO often mandates an emergency exploratory laparotomy, especially if strangulation, rupture, or peritonitis occurs. Intervention may be as simple as lysis of adhesions or as extensive as bowel resection with a colostomy.

Associated care plans

Vasogenic Shock
Peritonitis

Associated procedure

Preparation for Surgery

Medical diagnosis

ACUTE RENAL FAILURE (A.R.F.)

Assessment

Mechanism of injury/etiology:
- oliguria/anuria
- trauma or shock, such as hypovolemic shock from hemorrhage, burns, dehydration, third-space shifting, vasodilating drugs; ARF may be an end-stage complication of any shock state
- diminished cardiac output
- renal artery disorder
- genitourinary trauma, such as obstruction, vasculitis, vascular tumor, fibrosis, calculi, strictures, hematoma, clot formation
- disseminated intravascular coagulation
- aortic surgery
- acute tubular necrosis
- ischemia/hypoperfusion
- drugs, such as salicylates, methyl alcohol, inorganic agents, organic solvents, nephrotoxic agents, anesthetic agents, antimicrobials, organic radiograph contrast media, or heroin overdose
- gram-negative or -positive sepsis
- any disorder or injury (such as a crush injury) precipitating the release of heme or myoglobin
- hemolysis, transfusion reactions, obstetric complications

ARF classifications:
- prerenal—decreased renal perfusion and decreased glomerular filtration rate
- renal/intrarenal/intrinsic—parenchymal damage from disease or nephrotoxins
- postrenal—obstruction caused by alterations in tract integrity (from renal tubules to urinary meatus)

Note: *In impending renal failure secondary to hypovolemia and consequent renal hypoperfusion, therapy should focus on restoration of fluid volume and cardiac output. This may require large volume infusion and inotropic agents, therapy similar for other hypovolemic states discussed in this text.*

ARF phases:
ARF can manifest as anuric, oliguric, nonoliguric, or diuretic phases of failure. Obstruction or acute renal parenchymal damage usually produces anuria. Oliguric and nonoliguric failure generally occur secondary to hypovolemia, sepsis, or drug toxicity. Nonoliguric failure can be difficult to diagnose—urine output may remain normal while inability to concentrate urine may be the only

manifestation. The diuretic phase usually occurs 2 to 6 weeks after the initial insult or injury and may herald the onset of high-output renal failure or the recovery phase of ARF. Differential diagnosis is imperative; however, this care plan will focus solely on the initial management of the later phases of ARF.

Physical findings:
Note: *Physical and diagnostic findings depend on the type, cause, and phase of ARF.*

Respiratory
- Kussmaul's respirations
- rhonchi, moist rales
- dyspnea
- pink, frothy secretions
- pulmonary edema

Cardiovascular
- ECG changes
- dysrhythmias
- tachycardia
- full, bounding pulse
- hypertension
- jugular vein distention (JVD)
- elevated pulmonary artery, central venous, and pulmonary capillary wedge pressures (PAP, CVP, PCWP)
- increased body weight
- congestive heart failure

Neurologic
- headache
- irritability
- drowsiness
- restlessness
- anxiety
- muscle weakness
- flaccid paralysis
- hyporeflexia
- muscle twitches
- seizures
- uremic coma

Gastrointestinal
- nausea/vomiting
- anorexia
- thirst
- dry mucosa
- diarrhea or constipation
- GI bleeding
- stomatitis
- uremic breath

Genitourinary
- oliguria with urine output < 400 cc/24 hours
- enlarged prostate
- dysuria
- pain (type, location, and severity depend on ARF etiology)
- difficulty maintaining a steady, strong stream of urine

Dermatologic
- dry skin
- pruritus
- periorbital edema
- uremic frost (extremely rare)

Diagnostic studies

- laboratory data
  - ☐ blood urea nitrogen (BUN)/creatinine levels—elevated
  - ☐ phosphate, magnesium, potassium levels—elevated
  - ☐ sodium, calcium, hemoglobin/hematocrit, platelet levels—lower than normal
  - ☐ ABGs—reveal metabolic acidosis
  - ☐ urinalysis—reveals presence of protein, casts, RBCs, WBCs, debris
  - ☐ specific gravity—>1.020 indicates oliguria (prerenal)
  - ☐ urine osmolality—elevated in prerenal
  - ☐ urine sodium level—decreased in prerenal; elevated in renal
- radiography (radiographic, media contrast, and sonographic studies assist in confirming genitourinary obstruction, damage, hydronephrosis, and renal calculi)
  - ☐ chest radiograph—may reveal interstitial changes indicative of pulmonary edema

Nursing diagnosis

Potential for fluid volume excess related to inability of the kidneys to eliminate body fluid.

GOAL: Recognize fluid volume excess and restore a normovolemic state.

Interventions

1. Assess the patient for:
- peripheral edema
- JVD
- elevated PAP, CVP, PCWP
- dyspnea
- moist rales
- Kussmaul's respirations
- pink, frothy secretions, if intubated.

2. Weigh the patient at the same time each day and with the same amount of clothing.

3. Measure urine output every hour via an indwelling catheter. Test urine specific gravity every 8 hours.

4. Restrict oral intake as necessary.

5. Assess fluid volume lost through vomiting, diarrhea, fever, and insensible loss. Administer fluid based on calculated losses.

6. Monitor laboratory data for serum and urine studies.

Rationale

Tubular damage/ischemia, increasing angiotensin levels, increased vascular resistance, and reduced renal blood flow cumulatively cause decreased glomerular perfusion, filtration, and tubular flow, and oliguria and fluid retention. JVD and elevated CVP and pulmonary pressures indicate excess intravascular volume. Increased hydrostatic pressure pushes fluid into the interstitial space, causing peripheral and pulmonary edema (PE). PE is usually evidenced by dyspnea, moist rales, rhonchi, and frothy sputum. Kussmaul's respirations are a compensatory response to acidosis caused by retention of metabolic wastes.

The kidneys' inability to excrete body fluids causes a daily increase in body weight. Body weight changes serve as effective indicators of volume status. Minimizing the variables permits more accurate daily weight comparisons.

The goal of volume management is to promote optimal cellular hydration without causing fluid overload. Urine specific gravity, although not accurate in intrinsic renal disease, is a simple, inexpensive test of renal concentrating ability.

Thirst and dry mucosa may prompt patients to drink to excess, if permitted.

A guide to volume administration is based on the following equation:

> urine output in the last 24 hours
> + 600 to 800 cc—insensible loss
> + other losses
> + 100 cc/each degree C. above normal in febrile patients

= volume replacement for the next 24-hour period.

Evaluating laboratory test results aids ongoing assessment of fluid and electrolyte balance.

7. Administer diuretics as ordered.

Diuretic therapy for ARF patients is controversial. For example, in the patient with prerenal failure from hypovolemia, the use of diuretics can further diminish renal blood flow.

8. Assist with dialysis, according to established hospital protocol and procedure.

Dialysis assists management of fluid and electrolyte balance, acidosis, coagulopathy, and uremic encephalopathy. The choice between peritoneal and hemo/ultrafiltration dialysis is based on numerous factors, such as relative safety, equipment availability, presence of or potential for infection, effectiveness, side effects, management of drug therapy, and potential complications. The nursing roles and responsibilities vary according to the method of dialysis chosen.

Nursing diagnosis

Potential for hyperkalemia related to the inability of the kidneys to excrete potassium.

> **GOAL:** Recognize early signs of hyperkalemia and intervene appropriately.

Interventions

1. Monitor serum potassium trends.

2. Monitor and report signs of hyperkalemia, including ECG, neuromuscular, and respiratory changes.

3. Maintain awareness of all sources of K^+ and administer an antihyperkalemic regimen as ordered:
- calcium
- sodium bicarbonate
- dextrose/insulin
- resin agents (observe for possible hypernatremia as a side effect).

Rationale

Increased tissue catabolism, hemolysis, and infection can impair the kidneys' ability to excrete K^+, evidenced by elevated serum potassium K^+ levels. Hyperkalemia alters transmission of nerve impulses at the cellular membrane. Elevated K^+ levels and resultant flaccid paralysis can impair breathing patterns as the respiratory muscles lose function. Hyperkalemia can cause dysrhythmias and ECG changes such as flattened or absent P waves; prolonged PR intervals; widened QRS complexes; ST segment depression; and peaked and elevated T waves, which can progress to asystole. Hyperkalemia potentiates cardiac response to digitalis preparations.

Certain drugs, intravenous fluids, and stored blood all contain K^+. Calcium antagonizes K^+'s action on the myocardium. Sodium bicarbonate, dextrose, and insulin administered simultaneously cause a transient shift of K^+ into the cells. The above measures temporarily lower serum K^+ levels until excess K^+ can be permanently removed through the use of resin agents or dialysis. Exchange resins substitute sodium for K^+ through the bowel wall; then K^+ is bound to the resin and excreted in the stool.

Nursing diagnosis

Potential for fluid volume deficit related to acute GI bleeding secondary to the effects of uremia.

> **GOAL #1:** Minimize the risk for and promptly recognize GI bleeding.

Interventions

1. Test gastric pH every 4 hours and administer non-magnesium-based antacids, as ordered.

Rationale

Antacids reduce acidity, restore normal gastric pH, and minimize the risk of ulcerations. **Note:** *The use of magnesium-based antacids is contraindicated as ARF patients' kidneys are unable to excrete magnesium.*

---

*Supplemental nursing diagnosis

2. Test gastric drainage and stools for occult blood.

Early detection of occult bleeding permits prompt institution of corrective measures.

3. Assess for the presence of:
- bloody stools
- diarrhea
- abdominal pain
- an increase in abdominal girth
- hematemesis.

These findings can signal the presence of ulcers, blood accumulation in the abdomen, and GI bleeding. (See "Acute Upper Gastrointestinal Bleeding" in Section II.)

4. Monitor for trends in hemoglobin/hematocrit levels and platelet count and for signs of hemorrhagic shock.

Renal damage causes diminished erythropoietin production; thus the patient may be anemic prior to GI bleeding. Trend analysis of hemoglobin/hematocrit levels aids detection of acute GI bleed onset. The uremic patient produces excessive amounts of parathyroid hormone, which increases gastric acid secretion. Increased acidity, in combination with the patient's physiologically and psychologically stressed state, can precipitate bleeding ulcers. Platelet dysfunction, common in patients with BUN levels >100 mg/dl, further potentiates bleeding. The ARF patient in a volume excess state can quickly become severely volume depleted, and progress to hypovolemic shock in the presence of massive GI bleeding.

GOAL #2: Restore a normovolemic state.

Interventions

1. Estimate blood loss; administer blood and component therapy as ordered.

2. Prepare the patient for surgery. (See "Preparation for Surgery" in Section VII.)

Rationale

Replacement is based on estimated blood loss, hemoglobin/hematocrit levels, and assessment findings.

Surgical intervention may be necessary for definitive care if other measures are ineffective.

Nursing diagnosis

Potential for injury related to alteration in level of consciousness secondary to uremia.

GOAL: Maximize patient safety.

Interventions

1. Keep side rails up at all times, pad side rails, use therapeutic restraints appropriately, as ordered; institute seizure precautions.

Rationale

Uremia affects the central nervous system, causing confusion, altered perception, dizziness, agitation, and seizures.

Nursing diagnosis

Potential for infection related to uremia and catabolism secondary to ARF.

GOAL: Minimize the risk for, and recognize early signs of, infection.

Interventions

1. Maintain pulmonary hygiene with coughing and deep-breathing exercises, incentive spirometry, suctioning, and chest physiotherapy.

2. Provide good oral hygiene at least four times a day.

3. Prevent skin breakdown by:
• turning the patient every 2 hours
• applying antiembolic stockings as ordered
• providing skin care every 2 to 4 hours
• using special beds and mattresses.

4. Use aseptic technique when:
• changing dressings
• caring for invasive lines, dialysis sites, endotracheal tubes, urinary catheters.
Remove any unnecessary invasive lines.

5. Monitor vital signs, temperature, WBC count, dressings, wound sites, and nature of drainage.

Rationale

Retention of urea, uric acid, and creatinine and increased catabolism impair the healing process and may lead to infection. Immobility, retained secretions, and pulmonary edema predispose the patient to atelectasis, infiltrates, and pneumonia.

Ammonia-producing bacteria increase irritation, which can cause stomatitis and lead to parotitis. Therefore, meticulous oral hygiene must be instituted.

These measures promote venous return, increase circulation, and prevent dryness, itching, and friction. Specialized beds and mattresses spread pressure evenly over a larger area and decrease the opportunity for decubiti formation.

Any interruption in the skin barrier provides direct entry for bacterial contaminates. Aseptic technique and removal of nonessential lines minimize the risk of pathogen introduction. The dialyzed patient usually does not require an indwelling urinary catheter.

Fever, tachycardia, elevated WBC count, nonhealing wound sites, and foul, purulent drainage indicate infection. **Note:** *Pericarditis, another secondary infection, can occur in up to 20% of ARF patients. If not promptly recognized and treated, pericarditis may cause pericardial effusion resulting in tamponade. The nurse should remain alert for early signs and symptoms of tamponade and report them immediately.*

Additional considerations

Drug therapy in the ARF patient can be extremely tenuous. Hyperkalemia may alter the myocardial response to medications. Dosages must be adjusted considering the ARF patient's kidneys' inability to excrete many drugs, the interference with GI absorption, and dialysis treatments. Analgesics require titration in the pre- and postdialysis phases for optimal effectiveness. Nutritional support of the ARF patient requires planned balancing of protein, potassium, sodium, and glucose. This may be accomplished through a restricted diet, gastric feedings, or total parenteral nutrition. Disseminated intravascular coagulation may complicate ARF, so maintain a high index of suspicion to facilitate early detection and intervention.

Associated care plans

Acute Upper Gastrointestinal Bleeding
Psychosocial Support of the Trauma Patient
Acute Pericardial Tamponade
Malnutrition in the Trauma Patient
Vasogenic Shock
Disseminated Intravascular Coagulation

Associated procedure

Preparation for Surgery

FAT EMBOLISM SYNDROME (F.E.S.)

Assessment

Note: *Always suspect FES in at-risk patients to promote early recognition and diagnosis.*

Mechanism of injury/ etiology:
- history of long-bone fractures, multiple fractures, burns, massive soft tissue or arterial injuries, multisystem trauma, recent open reduction–internal fixation

Physical findings:

Respiratory
- sudden onset of respiratory distress
- shortness of breath
- tachypnea (>30 breaths/minute)
- productive cough, hemoptysis
- moist rales

Cardiovascular
- normo- to hypotensive
- tachycardia
- ECG changes
- chest pain
- fever (102.2° to 104° F./39° to 40° C.)
- cyanosis
- hypovolemic shock state

Neurologic
- headache
- sudden deterioration in sensorium after a previously normal state of mentation
- confusion, restlessness, agitation, wild-eyed stare, anxiety, stupor, unresponsiveness
- convulsions (may resemble delirium tremens)
- pupillary changes
- retinal lesions

Genitourinary
- hematuria
- sudden incontinence
- oliguria, anuria

Skin
- flat, nonblanching petechiae (grouped on the chest, axilla, shoulders, flanks, conjunctiva, oral mucosa) that appear on 2nd to 4th day; may appear and disappear in waves

Diagnostic studies

- laboratory data
  - ☐ ABGs—reflect hypoxemia (PaO$_2$< 60 mm Hg), commonly the first or only indication in high-risk patients
  - ☐ hemoglobin/hematocrit levels—may drop precipitously
  - ☐ WBC count and fibrin split products—rise
  - ☐ platelet count—falls
  - ☐ lipase and free fatty acid levels—rise
  - ☐ sputum and urine samples—may reflect the presence of fat
- radiography—chest film reveals snowstorm picture, indicating patchy, fluffy pulmonary infiltrates
- ECG—shows nonspecific changes that reflect right ventricular strain
- cryostat-frozen section of clotted blood—reveals fat globules
- lung, renal, petechiae biopsy—may reveal embolic fat

Potential for decreased tissue perfusion related to mobilization of fat globules and altered fat metabolism secondary to fractures, burns, arterial or soft tissue injuries, multisystem trauma, postoperative open reduction–internal fixation procedure.

GOAL #1: Reduce or minimize the risk of FES.

Interventions

1. Identify and closely monitor high-risk patients for early signs of FES:
- sudden change in mentation
- rapid onset of respiratory distress
- fever.

Rationale

Many multisystem trauma patients have subclinical levels of FES. This syndrome commonly goes unrecognized or is diagnosed as a pure respiratory syndrome. Help reduce the risk of FES by recognizing at-risk patients early and instituting proven therapeutic measures. Clinical findings have been noted as soon as 1 hour and as late as 4 days after injury; on average, findings appear 24 to 48 hours after injury.

2. Immobilize fractures and soft tissue injuries as soon after the injury as possible; use caution and handle the patient gently when movement is necessary.

Immobilization reduces movement of bone ends or fragments, which release fat globules from the marrow into circulation after injury. Align and immobilize the fracture as soon as possible and maintain positioning until definitive care occurs. Unnecessary movement may cause further bone end disruption, increasing fat globule release.

3. Watch for early signs of hypovolemic shock, institute preventive measures, and be prepared to intervene immediately. Monitor vital signs and neurologic status, ensure I.V. access, analyze laboratory data trends, replace fluids.

Some theories equate FES incidence and severity with the duration and class of the postinjury shock state and the duration of hypoxia. For example, a sustained Class III or IV shock state increases the FES risk. Closely evaluating laboratory data trends and assessment parameters helps identify impending shock and determine therapeutic requirements. Fluid replacement and supplemental oxygen administration are essential to minimize or reverse the shock state.

4. Obtain baseline laboratory data specific for FES; analyze further trends in levels of lipase, free fatty acids, platelets, fibrin split products.

Although the value of some laboratory studies is controversial, the following may aid FES diagnosis:
- lipase level—rises in normal response to trauma, especially fractures. Because lipase breaks down neutral fats to free fatty acids, circulating free fatty acids increase after injury. These acids bind with proteins.
- hematocrit level—may drop suddenly as a result of increased RBC aggregation and associated pulmonary hemorrhage.
- platelet count—falls as the platelets adhere to fat globules.
- fibrin split products level—increases result from fibrinolytic system failure. The altered fibrinolysis occurs because of altered fat metabolism.

GOAL #2: Optimize pulmonary perfusion.

Interventions

1. Obtain a baseline respiratory assessment and monitor the patient closely for sudden deterioration; investigate any sudden changes in ABG trends, breath sounds, and ventilatory pattern and function.

2. Administer supplemental oxygen as ordered at the first signs of respiratory deterioration; anticipate the need for intubation and mechanical ventilation.

Rationale

Baseline findings usually include clear breath sounds, ABG results within the accepted normal range, and effective ventilatory rate and rhythm. Sudden onset of respiratory distress with tachypnea, dyspnea, cyanosis, moist rales, and hypoxemia indicates pulmonary vascular obstruction. The lungs filter out the fat globules, which then obstruct the capillary membranes. Capillary damage and serotonin release cause increased capillary permeability, leading to interstitial edema, pneumonitis, and possible pulmonary hemorrhage.

Begin therapy to promote or maintain adequate oxygenation early, to avoid later complications of hypoxia. Most severe cases of FES require intubation, sedation, and mechanical ventilation with high levels of positive end-expiratory pressure. These patients have clinical findings and needs similar to those of patients with adult respiratory distress syndrome. The capillary membrane damage causing interstitial edema progresses to decreased surfactant production, decreased compliance, alveolar collapse, and increased shunting.

3. Monitor trends in ABGs and chest radiographs.

A decreased PaO_2 commonly provides the first sign of FES. A baseline ABG and follow-up studies (as indicated by the patient's condition) aid early hypoxia detection. Although the initial chest radiograph (performed on admission) may not reveal any pathology, subsequent films will begin to exhibit a snowstorm picture as FES progresses.

4. Administer steroids, as ordered.

The effectiveness of steroid therapy to decrease the inflammatory effects of FES remains controversial.

GOAL #3: Recognize and ensure patient safety during periods of neurologic deterioration secondary to decreased cerebral perfusion and hypoxemia.

Interventions

1. Document a baseline neurologic assessment; monitor closely for trends or changes in behavior (such as restlessness, anxiety, agitation) or alterations in level of consciousness, ranging from confusion to unresponsiveness.

2. Restrain the patient, as appropriate (obtain physician order).

Rationale

A classic sign of FES is a rapid change in behavior or level of consciousness after a period of normal mentation. Possible causes of this deterioration include globule occlusion of specific cerebral vessels and generalized hypoxemia. Additional findings may include retinal lesions, convulsions that mimic delirium tremens, and possible abnormal flexion positioning.

The patient in an acute state of agitation and confusion may easily disrupt I.V. lines, airways, and other tubes and drains. Therapeutic restraint usually requires written orders.

GOAL #4: Maximize cardiac function.

Interventions

1. Monitor the patient closely for signs of cardiac strain, such as a change in vital signs, increased cardiac output, complaints of chest pain, ECG changes.

2. Monitor and document hourly intake and output balance.

3. Anticipate the need for pulmonary artery (PA) catheter insertion; ensure availability of necessary equipment; assist as needed.

Rationale

Fat globules obstructing the pulmonary vasculature cause increased resistance to pulmonary blood flow. The heart attempts to compensate by increasing the rate and cardiac output. ECG changes indicative of right ventricular strain may include right bundle branch block, inverted T waves, depressed RST segments, and dysrhythmias.

This patient requires close and careful balancing of intake and output to prevent cardiac failure and to minimize pulmonary edema.

PA monitoring provides valuable information and aids in determining and directing fluid replacement. This patient can rapidly develop pulmonary edema and cardiac failure.

Associated care plan
Adult Respiratory Distress Syndrome

Associated procedure
Pulmonary Artery Catheterization

COMPARTMENT SYNDROME

Assessment

Note: *The clinician must maintain a high index of suspicion when caring for patients with blunt trauma so that signs of compartment syndrome are recognized early and irreversible muscle damage is prevented.*

Mechanism of injury/ etiology:
- open or closed fractures
- arterial or venous injuries
- intraarterial injection
- postischemic swelling
- soft tissue injury
- burns
- crush injury
- joint dislocations
- limb compression during unconscious state
- toxicity syndromes (such as from snakebites)
- external constriction of fascial compartment (such as by a cast, splint, dressing, or pneumatic antishock garment)
- exercise

Physical findings:
Musculoskeletal

- pain (disproportionately intense for injury type; deep, continuous, and localized to involved compartment; increased on stretching of involved muscles)
- firm fascial compartments on palpation
- paresthesia (decreased tactile sensation in area innervated by involved nerve)
- paresis
- muscle weakness
- paralysis (late sign)

Note: *Intracompartment pressures of 30 to 60 mm Hg can cause muscle ischemia. Because the diastolic pressure of the main artery traveling through the compartment is greater than 30 to 60 mm Hg, the quality of pulses and capillary refill times (CRTs) distal to the compartment will not be affected. Therefore, pulse quality and CRTs are not useful as assessment criteria. The exception is in compartment syndrome of the hands and feet, where the normal distal end arterial pressures are lower. In these situations the compartment pressures above can easily impair arterial flow, diminishing pulse and slowing CRT.*

Table 4.1

Indicators of Compartment Involvement

Deltoid compartment
- pain on passive shoulder adduction
- reduced active shoulder abduction
- paresthesia of superior lateral aspect of upper arm
- firmness of compartment

Upper arm—anterior compartment (biceps brachialis)
- pain over anterior upper arm area on passive elbow extension
- weakness on elbow flexion
- paresthesia in area innervated by ulnar, median, radial, and lateral antebrachial cutaneous nerve

Upper arm—posterior compartment (triceps)
- pain over posterior upper arm area on passive elbow flexion
- paresthesia over posterior surface of hand
- paresis of muscles innervated by radial and ulnar nerves

Forearm—volar compartment
- pain in compartment area and on passive finger extension
- fingers in flexed position
- paresis of thumb and finger flexors
- paresthesia of palmar surface of hand
- compartment firmness

Forearm—dorsal compartment
- pain on finger and wrist extension
- paresis of finger extensors
- extension of the hand

Hand—central palmar compartment
- paresthesia of volar surface of the fingers
- compartment firmness

(continued)

Indicators of Compartment Involvement *(continued)*

Hand—thenar compartment

- pain on passive flexion or extension
- paresis of thumb on opposition and flexion
- compartment firmness

Hand—hypothenar compartment

- pain on passive extension or flexion of the little finger
- paresthesia of the little finger
- compartment firmness

Hand—interossei compartment

- pain on flexion of interphalangeal joints
- flexed metacarpophalangeal joints with extended interphalangeal joints

Gluteal compartments

- pain in compartment area and with hip flexion or adduction
- paresthesia of muscles innervated by sciatic nerve
- compartment firmness

Pelvis—iliacus compartment

- pain around inguinal ligament and on passive hip extension after flexion
- paresthesia around medial aspect of lower leg

Thigh—anterior compartment

- pain in compartment area and on active flexion or extension of knee
- paresthesia around the knee and medial aspect of lower leg and foot
- compartment firmness

Thigh—posterior compartment

- pain in compartment area and on passive knee extension
- paresthesia of medial aspect of upper leg
- compartment firmness

Lower leg—anterior compartment

- pain in compartment area and on plantar flexion of foot, toe, or ankle
- paresthesia in first web space area
- compartment firmness

Lower leg—lateral compartment

- pain on passive foot inversion and active foot eversion
- paresthesia on the dorsum of the foot and in the first web space

Lower leg—superficial posterior compartment

- pain on active plantar flexion and passive dorsiflexion
- paresthesia over lateral aspect of the foot

Lower leg—deep posterior compartment

- pain on passive dorsiflexion of foot and toes and on eversion of the foot
- paresis of toes and foot
- paresthesia of plantar aspect of foot

Foot—medial compartment

- pain on passive movement of great toe
- compartment firmness

Foot—lateral compartment

- pain on passive movement of the toes
- compartment firmness

Foot—central compartment

- pain on passive extension of the toes
- compartment firmness

Foot—interosseous compartment

- pain on passive movement of the toes
- paresthesia of the toes
- compartment firmness

Diagnostic studies

- clinical findings alone can establish diagnosis
- intracompartment pressure measurement—confirms diagnosis

Nursing diagnosis

Potential for decreased muscle tissue perfusion and motor and sensory deficit related to increased intracompartment pressure.

> **GOAL #1:** Prevent or minimize the risk of compartment syndrome.

Interventions

1. Elevate affected extremities when possible.

2. Monitor splints, casts, dressings, or other potential constrictors for tightness.

Rationale

Elevation increases venous return, thereby reducing edema formation.

External devices can constrict compartment volume, increasing intracompartment pressures. Removal of external constrictors will be necessary to reduce compartment pressure.

> **GOAL #2:** Identify early signs of compartment syndrome.

Interventions

1. Assess fascial compartments at risk for compartment syndrome every hour. Notify the physician of positive findings immediately.

2. Assist with intracompartment pressure measurement.

3. Communicate with operating room personnel concerning preparation of the patient for surgery if fasciotomy is required.

Rationale

Signs and symptoms of compartment syndrome can occur from 3 hours to 4 days after injury. Increased muscle tissue fluid pressures can occlude intracompartment microcirculation, leading to muscle ischemia and muscle and nerve necrosis within 6 hours. Early recognition facilitates prompt surgical intervention to reduce compartment pressure, thus minimizing damage.

Intracompartment pressure measurement supplements clinical examination and helps confirm diagnosis of compartment syndrome.

Surgical decompression of the compartment may become necessary. This involves incising the fascia enclosing the muscle to allow room for the increase in compartment volume.

Nursing diagnosis

Potential for renal dysfunction related to precipitation of myoglobin and hemoglobin in the renal tubules, secondary to myonecrosis.

> **GOAL:** Minimize the risk of tubular necrosis.

Interventions

1. Monitor urine output and pH levels. Administer bicarbonate and diuretics, as ordered.

Rationale

Myonecrosis releases hemoglobin and myoglobin into the plasma. These can precipitate out in the renal tubules, causing tubular necrosis. Techniques for preventing tubular necrosis include maintaining alkaline urine and diuresis.

Associated care plan	**Associated procedures**
Acute Renal Failure	Intracompartment Pressure Measurement
	Preparation for Surgery

*Supplemental nursing diagnosis

Medical diagnosis

GAS GANGRENE

Assessment

Mechanism of injury/ etiology:
- trauma
- wounds contaminated by soil
- GI tract injuries or surgery
- female genital tract injuries or surgery
- foreign objects
- devitalized tissue

Note: *Gas gangrene may develop rapidly, 4 to 48 hours postinjury or postsurgery.*

Physical findings:
Local response
- local wound pain out of proportion to severity of wound
- sudden local puffiness with discoloration of tissue

- foul-smelling, brownish exudate
- crepitation in tissue (may occur late)

Systemic response
- tachycardia
- tachypnea
- hypotension
- fever
- toxic delirium (early sign—initial euphoric state progressing to incoherence and disorientation; believed to be caused by clostridial endotoxins)
- profound toxemia (late sign)
- circulatory collapse (late sign)

Diagnostic studies

Note: *Early diagnosis—and thus timely intervention—relies on clinical findings. Laboratory verification takes time, and clostridial infection progresses rapidly, with a high mortality rate.*
- Gram stain—for gram-positive bacilli

- cultures—for clostridium
- WBC count—for leukocytosis
- radiographs of involved tissue—for evidence of gas in tissues

Nursing diagnosis

Potential for fluid volume deficit related to increased cellular permeability secondary to exotoxic activity of clostridial invasion.

GOAL: Prevent hypovolemia or restore normovolemia.

Interventions

1. Ensure adequate venous access with two large-bore catheters. Administer fluid replacement, as ordered.

Rationale

Patients with gas gangrene exhibit signs and symptoms of developing septic shock. Systemic exotoxic activity increases cellular permeability, creating a fluid volume deficit by third-space shifting of intravascular fluid.

Nursing diagnosis

*Potential for clostridial infection related to trauma or wound contamination.

GOAL #1: Recognize early signs of infection.

*Supplemental nursing diagnosis

Interventions

1. Monitor all patients with abdominal or extremity wounds, especially if contaminated by soil, and those recovering from GI or female genitourinary (GU) tract surgery for indications of clostridial invasion, particularly:
• sudden local edema
• foul-smelling, brownish exudate
• pain out of proportion to severity of wound
• tissue crepitus.

2. Observe for signs of toxic delirium:
• incoherence
• disorientation.

3. Check for elevated temperature.

4. If you note any combination of the above symptoms, notify the physician immediately.

5. Prepare for radiographs and the following laboratory studies:
• CBC
• cultures
• Gram stain.

Rationale

Clostridial organisms normally inhabit the GI and female GU tracts and are also prevalent in soil. These organisms most commonly invade an extremity or abdominal wound or the uterus during trauma or surgery.

Toxic delirium is one of the most unique and characteristic findings in true gas gangrene. It appears very early in the disease.

Early recognition of gas gangrene is the key to early, aggressive management, vital for this rapidly developing and often fatal infection.

Differential diagnostic tests are indicated, because other organisms (such as *E. coli* and *Klebsiella*) may produce gas in the tissues. These gram-negative organisms may produce necrotizing fasciitis. Although treatment is similar, the mortality rate is less than that of gas gangrene.

GOAL #2: Initiate prompt therapy.

Interventions

1. Obtain the patient's allergy history. Administer antibiotic therapy as ordered and observe for adverse reactions.

2. Prepare the patient for surgery. (See "Preparation for Surgery" in Section VII.)

3. Anticipate the need for hyperbaric oxygen therapy.

4. Place the patient in isolation, according to institutional policy. (See "The Critically Ill or Injured Patient Requiring Special Care" in Section VII.)

Rationale

In vitro antimicrobial sensitivity tests demonstrate penicillin G to be the most effective in killing the clostridium organism. For patients allergic to penicillin, tetracycline or chloramphenicol may be used.

Rapid tissue necrosis and systemic toxicity are caused by clostridial toxins and the breakdown of muscle and soft tissue. Clostridium spreads rapidly, following fascial lines. Extensive surgical debridement is necessary to prevent this spread. Amputation of the involved extremity may be needed to prevent death.

While not used extensively, hyperbaric oxygenation—supersaturation of oxygen, generally under 3 atmospheres of pressure—may benefit some patients.

Isolation measures are taken to prevent cross contamination.

Associated care plan	Associated procedures
Vasogenic Shock	Preparation for Surgery The Critically Ill or Injured Patient Requiring Special Care

TRANSFUSION REACTIONS

Assessment

Mechanism of injury/ etiology:
• recent homologous blood or blood products transfusion (reactions may occur within minutes of, or as long as several weeks after,

transfusion)
• hemolytic reaction:
  ☐ ABO/Rh antigen-antibody incompatibility—donor's blood is incompatible with recipient's blood
• nonhemolytic reaction:

☐ febrile—leukocyte and platelet antigen incompatibility
☐ allergic or anaphylactic—IgA plasma protein sensitivity
☐ infectious or sep-

tic—bacterial or viral contamination

Physical findings:
See Table 4.2.

Diagnostic studies

• laboratory data
  ☐ hemolytic reactions
    • hemoglobinemia/uria
    • positive Coombs' (antiglobulin) test
    • blood urea nitrogen (BUN)/creatinine levels—elevated due to azotemia or renal failure
    • bilirubin level—elevation 5 to 7 hours postreaction reflects RBC hemolysis
    • coagulation profile—demonstrates shortened clotting times
    • urine—positive for casts, RBCs, heme particles
    • return donor and recipient blood samples to blood bank for further analysis
  ☐ nonhemolytic reactions
    • febrile—return donor and recipient blood samples to blood bank for further analysis

• allergic—return donor and recipient blood samples to blood bank for further analysis
• infectious—positive cultures of blood, tubing, bag; increased WBC count, BUN and creatinine levels; return donor and recipient blood samples to blood bank for further analysis
☐ radiography
  • chest radiograph may reveal bacterial infiltrates

Note: *Although prevention is the best treatment for transfusion reactions, an early differential diagnosis is imperative for prompt, appropriate therapy. Follow established institutional policy and protocol. Laboratory analysis varies after transfusion reaction; however, most blood banks will repeat the ABO, Rh, and antibody typing and will run a serum haptoglobin, bilirubin, and blood culture. Urine analysis for free hemoglobin may be required as well.*

Hemolytic reactions

Note: *Judicious protocols to ensure proper identification when patient samples are drawn, during laboratory testing, and before starting a transfusion prevent most hemolytic reactions.*

Potential for decreased tissue perfusion related to hemolysis, vasoconstriction, and clot formation secondary to antigen-antibody reaction.

GOAL: Recognize early signs of circulatory impairment; prevent or minimize further circulatory compromise.

Interventions

1. Assess the patient's cardiovascular status before, during, and after transfusion, including:
- pulse, blood pressure, ECG
- temperature (skin and core)
- skin color
- central venous pressure (CVP), pulmonary arterial pressure (PAP), cardiac output (CO)—if available
- evidence of bleeding disorders (oozing at suture or I.V. insertion sites, ecchymosis, petechiae)

- level of consciousness (LOC)
- urine output/urinalysis.

2. Stop the transfusion, change the tubing, change the fluid to normal saline solution (NSS), and notify the physician.

3. Return the unused blood component container to the blood bank and obtain blood and urine samples for laboratory testing.

4. Anticipate the need to treat shock and hypotension by administering the following:
- large volume infusion
- vasopressors
- inotropic agents
- anticoagulants
- antipyretics.

Rationale

These parameters provide a baseline for trend analysis, reflect cardiovascular function, and aid differential diagnosis and treatment.

Decreasing LOC and urine output reflect impaired cerebral and renal perfusion.

These actions prevent further infusion of the component causing the reaction, clear the I.V. tubing, and ensure that I.V. access remains available. The physician will order appropriate treatment.

Sample results can be diagnostically informative (see laboratory data in the "Diagnostic studies" section of this care plan).

Small blood clot formation and vasoconstriction can occlude the intravascular compartment. Large volume infusion promotes system flushing and diuresis. Vasopressors improve intractable histamine- and serotonin-induced hypotension. Inotropic agents improve cardiac output and perfusion; increased renal perfusion and diuretics may prevent renal failure. Systemic anticoagulants may prevent or minimize disseminated intravascular coagulation (DIC). Antipyretics reduce the febrile response by inhibiting prostaglandin release.

Nursing diagnosis

Impaired gas exchange related to decreased pulmonary tissue perfusion secondary to sluggish circulation.

GOAL: Optimize pulmonary tissue perfusion.

Interventions

1. Assess the patient's respiratory status, including:
- respiration rate and quality
- chest pain
- anxiety and restlessness
- ABG levels
- chest radiographic findings.

2. Anticipate the need for supplemental oxygen, an artificial airway, and mechanical ventilation.

Rationale

Pulmonary vessel vasoconstriction and circulatory system sluggishness limit available alveolar end space for gas exchange, impairing respiratory function, which requires adjunctive therapy. Assessing the patient's respiratory status assists in defining respiratory function alterations.

Nonhemolytic reactions: Febrile

Nursing diagnosis

Hyperthermia related to hypothalamic stimulation by serotonin released secondary to leukocyte and platelet antigen incompatibility.

GOAL: Recognize and promptly treat early signs and symptoms of febrile transfusion reaction.

Interventions

1. Assess the patient for signs and symptoms of febrile reactions (see Table 4.2).

2. Stop the transfusion, change the tubing, change the solution to NSS, and notify the physician.

3. Draw a blood sample for culture and sensitivity; return the unused blood component container to the blood bank.

4. Administer antipyretics as ordered.

Rationale

Febrile reaction and symptoms develop secondary to the antigen-antibody response or to the reaction of the recipient's antibodies to the donor's components. Recognizing the signs and symptoms helps make a differential diagnosis.

These actions prevent further infusion of components that caused the reaction, clear the I.V. tubing, and ensure that I.V. access remains available. The physician will order appropriate treatment.

An initial febrile response can develop in both septic and nonhemolytic febrile transfusion reactions. Septic reactions may result in positive blood cultures, whereas febrile reactions do not. This information assists the differential diagnosis.

Antipyretics reduce fever by inhibiting prostaglandin release.

Nonhemolytic reactions: Allergic

Nursing diagnosis

Potential for decreased tissue perfusion related to vascular permeability and smooth muscle contraction secondary to IgA plasma protein sensitivity.

GOAL: Recognize an allergic transfusion reaction promptly and minimize its progression.

Interventions

1. Assess the patient for signs and symptoms of allergic reaction (see Table 4.2).
Note: *Allergic reactions as manifested by urticaria can develop in as many as 3% of recipients.*

2. Stop the transfusion, change the tubing, change the solution to NSS, and notify the physician. Return the unused blood component container to the blood bank.

3. Monitor the patient's vital signs every 5 to 15 minutes, including heart rate and rhythm and blood pressure.

Rationale

Immediate identification of an allergic reaction facilitates rapid treatment, which is imperative because death can occur precipitously.

These actions prevent further infusion of components that caused the reaction, clear the I.V. tubing, and ensure that I.V. access remains available. The physician will order appropriate treatment.

Vascular collapse and shock can develop within minutes.

4. Infuse I.V. fluids as ordered.

Rapid volume resuscitation with crystalloid solution maintains the vascular space's integrity, improving cardiac output and blood pressure.

5. Administer as ordered:
- vasopressors and inotropic agents
- steroids.

Vasopressors and inotropic agents increase cardiac output and perfusion to vital organs. Giving steroids, although controversial, is thought to inhibit the anaphylactic response.

Nursing diagnosis

Ineffective airway clearance related to bronchospasm and glottal edema secondary to IgA plasma protein sensitivity.

GOAL: Restore and maintain effective airway clearance.

Interventions

1. Monitor the patient's respiratory status, including respiratory rate and quality, breath sounds, and ABG levels.

2. Administer supplemental oxygen as ordered.

3. Administer bronchodilators as ordered.

4. Anticipate the need for emergency intubation, cricothyroidotomy or tracheostomy, and mechanical ventilation. (See "Endotracheal Intubation," "Needle Cricothyroidotomy," and "Surgical Cricothyroidotomy" in Section VII.)

Rationale

Upper airway obstruction is a life-threatening situation requiring early recognition and immediate therapy.

The use of supplemental oxygen increases the oxygen available for gas exchange.

Pulmonary vasoconstriction impedes gas exchange. Bronchodilators minimize bronchospasms and increase alveolar end space available for gas exchange.

Delaying intubation can lead to airway swelling, which may require surgical intervention for airway management. Mechanical ventilation ensures optimal oxygenation.

Nonhemolytic reactions: Septic

Nursing diagnosis

Potential for infection related to introduction of pathogens through homologous transfusion.

GOAL: Recognize early signs of infection and prevent or minimize a septic episode.

Interventions

1. Monitor the patient for signs and symptoms of infection or sepsis (see Table 4.2).

2. Stop the transfusion, change the tubing, change the solution to NSS, and notify the physician.

Rationale

Promptly recognizing the signs of an infection or septic episode promotes rapid, aggressive treatment, minimizing septic consequences.

These actions prevent further infusion of components that caused the reaction, clear the I.V. tubing, and ensure that I.V. access remains available. The physician will order appropriate treatment.

3. Monitor the patient's vital signs every 5 to 15 minutes, including:
- heart rate and rhythm
- blood pressure
- CVP, PAP, and CO (if available).

A septic episode may deteriorate rapidly to septic shock. Frequent assessment of vital signs will detect impending shock and permit rapid intervention.

4. Return the unused blood component container to the blood bank and draw a blood sample for culture and sensitivity.

Samples from the patient, blood container, and filter should be cultured for bacterial identification.

5. Administer the following, as ordered:
- I.V. fluids

Septic-process endotoxins stimulate serotonin and histamine release, which may cause circulatory collapse and subsequent shift of fluid into the interstitial space. I.V. therapy maintains fluid and electrolyte balance.

- antibiotics

Broad-spectrum antibiotics may be given immediately. Antibiotics specific for the causative organism should be ordered after the blood culture results become available.

- vasopressors or inotropic agents

Vasopressors and inotropic agents support the cardiovascular system, increasing cardiac output and promoting kidney and other vital organ perfusion.

- steroids

Although still controversial, steroid administration is sometimes beneficial. (See "Vasogenic Shock" in Section II.)

- antipyretics.

Antipyretics reduce fever and, indirectly, metabolic demand by inhibiting prostaglandin release.

Note: *In any transfusion reaction, make sure that all relevant documentation describing the reaction and nursing and medical interventions is in the nurses' notes and that specific institutional standard forms for transfusion reactions are completed.*

Associated care plans	**Associated procedures**
Vasogenic Shock	Endotracheal Intubation
Psychosocial Support of the Trauma Patient	Needle Cricothyroidotomy
	Surgical Cricothyroidotomy

Table 4.2

Signs and Symptoms of Hemolytic and Nonhemolytic Transfusion Reactions

Hemolytic

Acute or delayed—within first few minutes or as long as 2 weeks post-transfusion[1]:
- fever, chills, flushing
- chest heaviness or constriction
- bleeding abnormalities (mild to DIC)
- jaundice
- hemoglobinemia
- azotemia
- purpura
- shock
- dyspnea deteriorating to adult respiratory distress syndrome (ARDS)
- pleuritic chest or back pain
- anxiety or apprehension
- restlessness
- headache
- nausea and/or vomiting
- hemoglobinuria
- oliguria deteriorating to anuria and renal failure
- abnormal bleeding
- tachycardia
- hypotension

Nonhemolytic

Febrile:
- reaction within 1 to 2 hours post-transfusion
- tachycardia
- flushing, fever, chills
- headache
- back and generalized muscle pain
- tachypnea

Allergic or anaphylactic:
- reaction within minutes of transfusion
- hypotension, tachycardia
- flushing—*no fever*
- urticaria, hives, itching
- dyspnea—wheezing, rales, bronchospasms, glottal edema deteriorating to cardiopulmonary arrest
- vomiting, abdominal cramps, diarrhea

Septic:
- reaction ranging from immediate to 2 hours post-transfusion
- shock
- chills, fever, flushing
- nausea, vomiting, abdominal cramps
- oliguria deteriorating to anuria and renal failure
- ARDS, DIC (end-stage complications)

[1]Hepatitis can develop as late as 6 months after a hemolytic transfusion reaction.

DISSEMINATED INTRAVASCULAR COAGULATION (D.I.C.)

Assessment

Mechanism of injury/ etiology:
- any condition that activates procoagulant activity, causes endothelial or reticuloendothelial injury, or promotes venous stasis
- severe acidosis, hypoxia, hemolysis, anticoagulant therapy, hemolytic transfusion reaction, massive transfusions, obstetric complications, heatstroke, toxic shock syndrome, metastatic malignancies, pulmonary and fat emboli, polycythemia, liver or spleen disease or trauma, near drowning, snakebites, vitamin K deficiency, and complications of all shock states (particularly vasogenic)

Note: *DIC occurs as a sequela of a preceding disorder, injury, or disease. It may be acute or chronic, and the treatment is primarily aimed at correcting the underlying cause.*

Physical findings:
Chronic
- deep vein thrombosis (DVT)
- recurrent ecchymosis

Acute
Respiratory
- tachypnea
- hemoptysis
- pulmonary embolus

Cardiovascular (bleeding)
- tachycardia
- hypotension
- cyanosis
- shock state

- petechiae
- ecchymosis
- abnormal or prolonged bleeding from puncture sites, wounds, tubes, and orifices
- mucous membrane oozing
- painful joint swelling
- decreased central venous, pulmonary artery, and pulmonary capillary wedge pressures

Cardiovascular (clotting)
- cool, mottled skin
- cyanosis affecting the extremities
- weak or absent peripheral pulses
- DVT signs and symptoms

Neurologic
- restlessness

- lethargy
- decreased level of consciousness
- vision changes
- retinal hemorrhages
- intracerebral bleeding
- headache
- aphasia
- epistaxis

Gastrointestinal
- hematemesis
- occult blood in stool
- increased abdominal girth
- bloody diarrhea

Genitourinary
- hematuria
- oliguria
- flank or back pain (from dissection of blood)
- renal failure
- increased menstrual bleeding

Diagnostic study

- laboratory data—specific DIC profiles vary institutionally as do normal laboratory values. No single test confirms DIC; however, Table 4.3 summarizes those studies recommended as essential.

Table 4.3

Hemoglobin	female, <14 g/100 cc; male, <17 g/100 cc
Hematocrit	female, <42%; male, <52%
Platelets	<150,000
Fibrinogen	<170 mg/100 cc
Fibrin split products	>10mcg/cc
Prothrombin time	>15 to 17 seconds
Activated partial thromboplastin time	>35 seconds
Lee-White clotting time	>15 minutes
Plasma thrombin time	>15 seconds
Blood urea nitrogen/creatinine levels	elevated with renal failure

Nursing diagnosis

Potential for decreased tissue perfusion related to accelerated capillary clotting and uncontrolled hemorrhage.

GOAL #1: Recognize early signs of coagulopathy.

Interventions

1. Monitor laboratory studies often in patients with conditions that may trigger DIC. **Note:** *If possible, do not draw blood samples for coagulation studies from a heparinized line.*

2. Inspect all bodily secretions and test them for occult blood.

3. Monitor the patient for signs of bleeding, clotting, and hemorrhagic shock. (See "Hemorrhagic Shock" in Section II.)

Rationale

DIC is most effectively managed when treatment is initiated early. Therefore, maintain a high index of suspicion when assessing patients with underlying disorders. Trend analysis of laboratory data reflects early coagulation profile changes. Blood samples drawn from a heparinized line may reflect false prolongation in clotting times.

Occult bleeding may occur before obvious bleeding is apparent.

Increased bleeding and clotting times reflect a clotting-process abnormality. Several factors in the shock state are believed to trigger DIC.

GOAL #2: Prevent or minimize further bleeding.

Interventions

1. Assist in determination of the estimated blood loss:
- weigh the patient daily, if possible
- evaluate the volume of blood lost in dressings, linen, and blood specimens
- monitor hemoglobin and hematocrit levels
- closely monitor intake and output.

2. Administer blood and component therapy as ordered.

3. Apply pressure, cool packs, and topical clotting agents to bleeding areas as ordered.

4. Administer anticoagulant or antifibrinolytic agents as ordered.

Rationale

Measure blood loss as accurately as possible since it determines the plan for adequate replacement. Hemoglobin/hematocrit values aid blood loss calculation; however, the current values may lag behind actual bleeding. Poor renal perfusion, as evidenced by decreased urine output, may reflect impending renal failure or hypovolemia.

This treatment is controversial in some institutions since it is sometimes thought to potentiate the clotting/bleeding cycle. Blood and component therapy, however, can compensate for blood loss and correct the coagulation deficit and hypovolemia.

These measures all help control bleeding. Local hemostasis may occur, since cool packs cause vasoconstriction and slow blood flow through the vessels. By decreasing vessel diameter, vasoconstriction allows a smaller clot to occlude the lumen. Thrombin, present in most topical clotting agents, promotes a stable, localized clot that enhances hemostasis.

This mode of therapy is also highly controversial and often contraindicated because anticoagulants can promote bleeding and antifibrinolytics cause indiscriminate clot formation. Anticoagulants are contraindicated in intracerebral hemorrhage, necrotizing lesions, metastatic disease, and hepatic failure.

5. Protect the patient from further blood loss by:
- administering all medications by P.O. or I.V. routes if possible (minimize I.M. or S.Q. injections, use the smallest-gauge needle possible and apply direct pressure to the site after injection)
- gently turning and positioning the patient
- using a flotation pad, sheepskin, and padded side rails
- administering passive range-of-motion exercises
- avoiding brisk rubbing, scrubbing, and vigorous physiotherapy
- suctioning gently
- ensuring humidification of inhaled supplemental oxygen
- providing gentle oral hygiene
- using tape sparingly (use paper tape if possible)
- using an electric razor to shave the patient
- withdrawing laboratory specimens through an I.V. or arterial line.

The patient with DIC is particularly vulnerable to anything producing friction, irritation, or local trauma. All such factors can promote hemorrhage. Since the patient with DIC cannot form a stable clot, even slight trauma can cause hemorrhage. Inadvertent removal of existing clots can also precipitate bleeding.

GOAL #3: Maximize oxygen availability, utilization, and tissue perfusion.

Interventions

1. Administer supplemental oxygen as ordered.

2. Ensure the availability and proper functioning of equipment needed for endotracheal intubation and mechanical ventilation.

3. Initiate measures to reduce temperature, if the patient is febrile.

4. Provide patient care in blocks of time.

5. Administer vasoactive drugs as ordered.

6. Closely monitor the patient for hypoxemia, hypotension, acidosis, and electrolyte imbalance.

Rationale

These measures all lower the oxygen deficit. Blood loss and the resultant anemia decrease the amount of oxygen-carrying RBCs. Controlled oxygen delivery promotes acid-base balance. Pulmonary capillaries may become clogged with microthrombi, inpeding or preventing optimal oxygen/carbon dioxide exchange.

Decreased body temperatures lower metabolic demands and oxygen consumption.

This affords the patient the rest periods necessary to minimize oxygen demands and to regain strength.

These drugs enhance cardiac output and perfusion.

These conditions may potentiate the DIC cycle, since they all are generally present in shock, a precursor of DIC.

Nursing diagnosis

Alteration in comfort related to tissue necrosis secondary to inadequate tissue perfusion.

GOAL: Promote comfort.

Interventions

1. Assess the patient for area and intensity of pain.

2. Avoid administering aspirin- or other anti-coagulant-containing analgesics.

3. Administer analgesia via P.O. or I.V. routes as ordered.

4. Assess the patient for both analgesic effectiveness and cardiovascular and respiratory changes.

Rationale

Pain in DIC is usually caused by tissue ischemia.

These agents promote bleeding.

S.Q. and I.M. injections can increase bleeding sites. P.O. and I.V. routes minimize further bleeding.

Analgesics can induce hypotension and respiratory depression and may have to be changed according to the above findings and their degree of effectiveness.

Additional considerations

Nutritional support is imperative because protein, vitamin K, and calcium are needed to manufacture clotting factors. Tube feedings or hyperalimentation should be initiated early. Remember that patients with DIC may require peritoneal dialysis or hemodialysis to remove metabolites and to correct acid-base imbalances in acute renal failure.

Associated care plans

Psychosocial Support of the Trauma Patient
Deep Vein Thrombosis
Pulmonary Thromboembolus
Hemorrhagic Shock
Malnutrition in the Trauma Patient
Acute Renal Failure

REFERENCES

COMPLICATIONS

Diabetes Insipidus

Carpenito, L.J. *Handbook of Nursing Diagnosis.* Philadelphia: J.B. Lippincott Co., 1984.

Diseases, 2nd ed. Nurse's Reference Library. Springhouse, Pa.: Springhouse Corp., 1987.

Fairchild, R.S. "Diabetes Insipidus: A Review," *Critical Care Quarterly* 3(2):111-18, September 1980.

Smith, J. "Nursing Management of Diabetes Insipidus," *Journal of Neurosurgical Nursing* 13(6):313-17, December 1981.

Pulmonary Thromboembolus

DeWeese, J.A. "Venous and Lymphatic Disease," in *Principles of Surgery,* 4th ed. Edited by Schwartz, S.I. New York: McGraw-Hill Book Co., 1984.

Diseases, 2nd ed. Nurse's Reference Library. Springhouse, Pa.: Springhouse Corp., 1987.

Roberts, W. "Thromboembolic Complications in Patients with Cardiac Disease," in *Cardiac Nursing.* Edited by Underhill, S.L., et al. Philadelphia: J.B. Lippincott Co., 1982.

Sivarajan, E.S., and Christopherson, D.J. "Anticoagulant, Antithrombotic, and Platelet-Modifying Drugs," in *Cardiac Nursing.* Edited by Underhill, S.L., et al. Philadelphia: J.B. Lippincott Co., 1982.

Woodruff, M.L. "Pulmonary Thromboembolism: Risk Factors, Pathophysiology, and Management," *Critical Care Nurse* 52-63, July/August 1984.

Pulmonary Edema

Diseases, 2nd ed. Nurse's Reference Library. Springhouse, Pa.: Springhouse Corp., 1987.

Niarchos, A.P., and Laragh, J.H. "Cardiovascular Problems in the Trauma Patient," in *Care of the Trauma Patient.* Edited by Shires, G.T. New York: McGraw-Hill Book Co., 1979.

Niles, N.A., and Wills, R.E. "Heart Failure," in *Cardiac Nursing.* Edited by Underhill, S.L., et al. Philadelphia: J.B. Lippincott Co., 1982.

Adult Respiratory Distress Syndrome

Carpenito, L.J. *Handbook of Nursing Diagnosis.* Philadelphia: J.B. Lippincott Co., 1984.

Carrico, C.J., and Horovitz, J.H. "Postinjury Acute Pulmonary Failure," in *Care of the Trauma Patient,* 2nd ed. Edited by Schires, G.T. New York: McGraw-Hill Book Co., 1979.

Daily, E.K., and Schroder, J.S. *Techniques in Bedside Hemodynamic Monitoring,* 2nd ed. St. Louis: C.V. Mosby Co., 1981.

Glennon, S.A., et al. "Respiratory Disorders," in *AACN Clinical Reference for Critical-Care Nursing.* Edited by Kinney, M.R. New York: McGraw-Hill Book Co., 1981.

Hudson, L.D. "Ventilatory Management," in *Care of the Trauma Patient,* 2nd ed. Edited by Shires, G.T. New York: McGraw-Hill Book Co., 1979.

Deep Vein Thrombosis

DeWeese, J.A. "Venous and Lymphatic Disease," in *Surgery,* 4th ed. Edited by Schwartz, S.I. New York: McGraw-Hill Book Co., 1984.

Perry, M.O. "Deep Vein Thrombosis," in *Care of the Trauma Patient,* 2nd ed. Edited by Shires, G.T. New York: McGraw-Hill Book Co., 1979.

Roberts, W. "Thromboembolic Complication in Patients with Cardiac Disease," in *Cardiac Nursing.* Edited by Underhill, S.L., et al. Philadelphia: J.B. Lippincott Co., 1982.

Sivarajan, E.S., and Christopherson, D.J. "Anticoagulant, Antithrombotic, and Platelet-Modifying Drugs," in *Cardiac Nursing.* Edited by Underhill, S.L., et al. Philadelphia: J.B. Lippincott Co., 1982.

Wessler, S. "The Role of Antithrombotic Prophylaxis Among Patients Subjected to Trauma," in *Principles and Practice of Trauma Care.* Edited by Worth, M.H. Baltimore: Williams & Wilkins Co., 1982.

Woods, S.L., and Laurent-Bopp, D. "Laboratory Tests Using Blood and Urine," in *Cardiac Nursing.* Edited by Underhill, S.L., et al. Philadelphia: J.B. Lippincott Co., 1982.

Use of Neuromuscular Blocking Agents

Carpenito, L.J. *Handbook of Nursing Diagnosis.* Philadelphia: J.B. Lippincott Co., 1984.

Drugs, 2nd ed. Nurse's Reference Library. Springhouse, Pa.: Springhouse Corp., 1984.

Procedures. Nurse's Reference Library. Springhouse, Pa.: Springhouse Corp., 1983.

Vitello-Cicciu, J.M. "Recalled Perceptions of Patients Administered Pancuronium Bromide," *Focus on Critical Care* 2(1):28-35, February 1984.

Malnutrition in the Trauma Patient

Assessment. Nurse's Reference Library. Springhouse, Pa.: Springhouse Corp., 1983.

Guenter, P. "Nutritional Care of the Trauma Patient," in *Trauma Nursing.* Edited by Cardona, V.D. Oradell, N.J.: Medical Economics Books, 1985.

Hoppe, M.C. "Nutritional Management of the Trauma Patient," *Critical Care Quarterly* 6(1):1-16, June 1983.

Neel, C.J., and Wallerstein, M.B. *A Pocket Guide for Medical-Surgical Nursing.* Bowie, Md.: Robert J. Brady Co., 1985.

Procedures. Nurse's Reference Library. Springhouse, Pa.: Springhouse Corp., 1983.

Shires, G.T., et al. "Fluid, Electrolyte, and Nutritional Management of the Surgical Patient," in *Surgery,* 4th ed. Edited by Schwartz, S.I. New York: McGraw-Hill Book Co., 1984.

Wiles, C.E., and Cerra, F.B. "The Exogenous Substrate Support of the Trauma Patient," in *Principles and Practice of Trauma Care.* Edited by Worth, M.H. Baltimore: Williams & Wilkins Co., 1982.

GI Complications

Broadwell, D.C., and McGarity, W.C. "Gastrointestinal Disorders," in *AACN Clinical Reference for Critical Care Nursing.* Edited by Kinney, M.R., et al. New York: McGraw-Hill Book Co., 1981.

Jones, R.S. "An Approach to the Acute Abdomen and Intestinal Obstruction," in *Gastrointestinal Disease.* Edited by Sleisenger, M.H., and Fordtran, J.S. Philadelphia: W.B. Saunders Co., 1973.

Roberts, S.L. *Physiological Concepts and the Critically Ill Patient.* Englewood Cliffs, N.J.: Prentice-Hall, 1985.

Shahinpour, N. "Disorders of the Hepatic System and Pancreas," in *Little-Brown Manual of Medical-Surgical Nursing.* Edited by Hincker, E.A., and Malasanos, L. Boston: Little, Brown & Co., 1983.

Strange, J.M. "An Expert's Guide to Tubes and Drains," *RN* 46:34, April 1983.

Strange, J.M. "Gastrointestinal Bleeding," in *Gastrointestinal Problems.* Oradell, N.J.: Medical Economics Books, 1985.

Strange, J.M. "The Riddle of Abdominal Trauma...How Much Damage and Where?" *RN* 46:42, March 1983.

Waitkoff, B. "Disorders of the GI System," in *Little-Brown Manual of Medical-Surgical Nursing.* Edited by Hincker, E.A., and Malasanos, L. Boston: Little, Brown & Co., 1983.

Acute Renal Failure

Cowley, R.A., and Dunham, C.M. *Shock Trauma/Critical Care Manual.* Baltimore: University Park Press, 1982.

Emergencies. Nurse's Reference Library. Springhouse, Pa.: Springhouse Corp., 1985.

McGeown, M.G. "Renal Failure after Trauma," in *Trauma Care.* Edited by Odling-Smee, W., and Crockard, A. New York: Grune & Stratton, 1981.

O'Boyle, C.M., et al., eds. *Emergency Care—The First 24 Hours.* East Norwalk, Conn.: Appleton-Century-Crofts, 1985.

Perry, A.G., and Potter, P.A., eds. *Shock—Comprehensive Nursing Management.* St. Louis: C.V. Mosby Co., 1983.

Schrier, R.W. "Acute Renal Failure: Pathogenesis, Diagnosis and Management," *Hospital Practice* 16(3):93-112, 1981.

Thomson, G.E. "Acute Renal Failure," *Medical Clinics of North America* 57:6, 1973.

Fat Embolism Syndrome

Arlington, R.G. "Internal Fixation of the Lower Extremity: Care Considerations," in *Assessment and Fracture Management of the Lower Extremities.* Monograph Library of the National Association of Orthopedic Nurses, A.J. Jannetti, Inc., October 1984.

Brunner, L.S., and Suddarth, D.S., eds. *Lippincott Manual of Nursing Practice,* 3rd ed. Philadelphia: J.B. Lippincott Co., 1982.

Burgess, A., and Mandelbaum, B.R. *Management of Acute Orthopedic Injuries in the Critically Injured Patient,* in press.

Cardea, J.A. "Complications of Fractures," in *Complications in Surgery and Trauma.* Edited by Greenfield, L.J. Philadelphia: J.B. Lippincott Co., 1984.

Evarts, C., and Mayer, P.J. "Complications," in *Fractures in Adults,* vol. 1, 2nd ed. Edited by Rockwood, C.A., and Green, D.P. Philadelphia: J.B. Lippincott Co., 1984.

Guenter, C.A., and Braun, T.E. "Fat Embolism Syndrome: Changing Prognosis," in *Chest* 79(2):143-45, February 1981.

Lanros, N.E. "Major Trauma," in *Assessment and Intervention in Emergency Nursing,* 2nd ed. Bowie, Md.: Robert J. Brady Co., 1983.

Talucci, R.C., et al. "Early Intramedullary Nailing of Femoral Shaft Fractures: A Cause of Fat Embolism Syndrome," *American Journal of Surgery* 146:107-11, July 1983.

Wilson, R.F., and Norton, M.L. "Respiratory Failure in Trauma," in *Management of Trauma: Pitfalls & Practice.* Edited by Walt, A.J., and Wilson, R.F. Philadelphia: Lea & Febiger, 1975.

Compartment Syndrome

Garfin, S.R. "Anatomy of the Extremity Compartments," in *Compartment Syndromes and Volkmann's Contracture.* Edited by Mubarak, S.J., and Hargens, A.R. Philadelphia: W.B. Saunders Co., 1981.

Hargens, A.R., and Mubarak, S.J., eds. "Definition and Terminology," in *Compartment Syndromes and Volkmann's Contracture.* Philadelphia: W.B. Saunders Co., 1981.

Mubarak, S.J. "Etiologies of Compartment Syndromes," in *Compartment Syndromes and Volkmann's Contracture.* Edited by Mubarak, S.J., and Hargens, A.R. Philadelphia: W.B. Saunders Co., 1981.

Owen, C.A. "Clinical Diagnosis of Acute Compartment Syndromes," in *Compartment Syndromes and Volkmann's Contracture.* Edited by Mubarak, S.J., and Hargens, A.R. Philadelphia: W.B. Saunders Co., 1981.

Rorabek, C.H. "The Treatment of Compartment Syndromes of the Leg," *Journal of Bone and Joint Surgery* 66-B(1):93-97, 1984.

Thorpe, D.M. "Neurovascular Assessment of the Lower Extremity," in *Assessment and Fracture Management of the Lower Extremities.* Monograph Library of the National Association of Orthopedic Nurses, A.J. Jannetti, Inc., October 1984.

Trunkey, D.D. "Trauma Principles and Penetrating Neck Trauma," in *Current Therapy of Trauma.* Edited by Trunkey, D.D., and Lewis, F.R. Philadelphia: B.C. Decker, 1984.

Gas Gangrene

Ballinger, W.F., II. *The Management of Trauma,* 2nd ed. Philadelphia: W.B. Saunders Co., 1973.

Burke, J.F., and Bondoc, C.C. "Wound Sepsis: Prevention and Control," in *The Management of Trauma,* 4th ed. Edited by Zuidema, G.D., et al. Philadelphia: W.B. Saunders Co., 1985.

Dineen, P. "Surgical Infections in Trauma Patients: Management and Prevention," in *Care of the Trauma Patient,* 2nd ed. Edited by Shires, G.T. New York: McGraw-Hill Book Co., 1979.

Fine, D.P., and Postier, R.G. "Infections," in *Manual of Medical Care of the Surgical Patient,* 3rd ed. Edited by Papper, S., et al. Boston: Little, Brown & Co., 1985.

Papper, S., and Williams, G.R. *Manual of Medical Care of the Surgical Patient,* 2nd ed. Boston: Little, Brown & Co., 1981.

Shires, G. T. *Care of the Trauma Patient,* 2nd ed. New York: McGraw-Hill Book Co., 1979.

Transfusion Reactions

Guthrie, M.M. *Shock.* New York: Churchill Livingstone, 1982.

Perry, A.G., and Potter, P.A., eds. *Shock—Comprehensive Nursing Management.* St. Louis: C.V. Mosby Co., 1983.

Smith, L. "Reactions to Transfusion," *American Journal of Nursing* 84(9):1096-1101, 1984.

Disseminated Intravascular Coagulation

Coleman, R. "DIC: A Problem in Critical Care Medicine," *Heart & Lung* 3:787-96, 1979.

Emergencies. Nurse's Reference Library. Springhouse, Pa.: Springhouse Corp., 1985.

Franco, R. "Acute DIC," *Critical Care Update* 8:17-20, 1981.

Guthrie, M.M. *Shock.* New York: Churchill Livingstone, 1982.

Guyton, A. A. *Textbook of Medical Physiology.* Philadelphia: W.B. Saunders Co., 1981.

Perry, A.G., and Potter, P.A., eds. *Shock—Comprehensive Nursing Management.* St. Louis: C.V. Mosby Co., 1983.

SECTION V

PSYCHOSOCIAL
SUPPORT OF THE TRAUMA
PATIENT

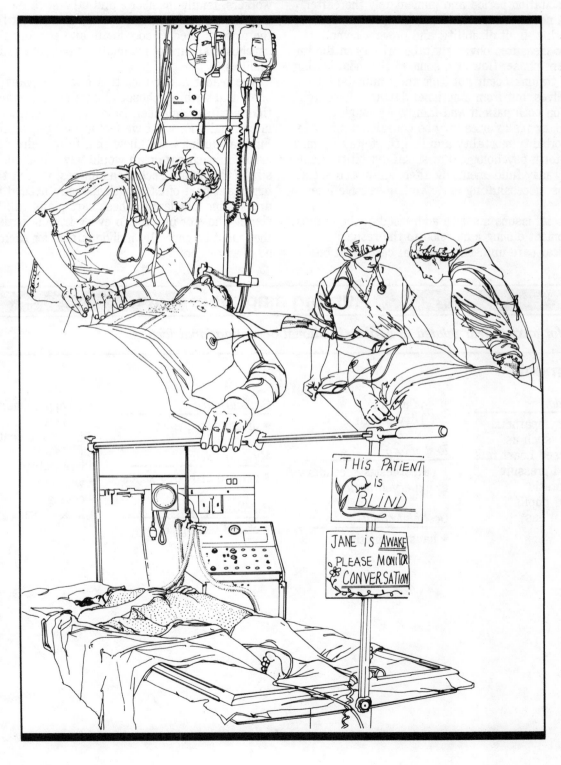

PSYCHOSOCIAL SUPPORT OF THE TRAUMA PATIENT

Introduction

The critically injured trauma patient requires rapid treatment and diagnosis if he is to survive. During the initial resuscitation period and immediately thereafter, this patient needs many technically oriented procedures to preserve life, limit disability, and prevent complications. These measures obviously take priority in the initial treatment phase. However, some of the most lasting sequelae of trauma occur not from the traumatic injuries themselves, but from emotional damage these injuries inflict on both patient and family. Although a particular patient's injuries may be considered minor in terms of morbidity/mortality and length of stay, he may suffer long-term psychological or social disability. Traumatic injury may fundamentally alter family and social relationships, necessitating early and aggressive intervention.

Psychosocial issues must be addressed at the earliest possible moment during admission to the resuscitation area or critical care unit. Psychosocial care must be planned, coordinated, and consistent to be effective. This care will be provided by nurses, physicians, social workers, family members, and others. Nurses, as the health care professionals spending the most time with the patient, need to coordinate and support planned psychosocial care of traumatized patients and their families.

The reader may notice that few care plans in this book deal with psychosocial care of the patient in more than a cursory manner. Be assured that this was done intentionally for what we feel are very good reasons. First, as authors, we knew that fully addressing these issues in each care plan would have easily doubled the size of this book. Second, as nurses, we felt that this important part of each patient's care needed to be addressed independently. These care plans will be applicable, in whole or in part, to every trauma patient; but they must be carefully individualized for each patient to be of any value.

Nursing diagnosis

Potential for anxiety/fear related to varied situational or maturational factors.

Assessment

Cardiovascular
- signs of sympathetic stimulation, such as:
  - ☐ increased heart rate and blood pressure
  - ☐ diaphoresis
  - ☐ dilated pupils
  - ☐ palpitations
- ☐ flushing
- ☐ dry mouth

Respiratory
- paresthesias secondary to hyperventilation

Gastrointestinal
- nausea/vomiting

Genitourinary
- urinary frequency

Musculoskeletal
- generalized body aches

Psychosocial
- stated feelings of:
  - ☐ nervousness
- ☐ apprehension
- ☐ fear
- ☐ loss of control
- ☐ tension
- irritability
- withdrawal
- crying
- lack of concentration

GOAL: Lessen anxiety and support coping mechanisms.

Interventions

1. Assess the patient for current level of anxiety/fear.

2. Acknowledge and accept the presence of anxiety/fear in the patient.

3. Support healthy use of defense mechanisms.

4. Assist the patient in identifying the factor(s) creating anxiety.

Rationale

Anxiety occurs on a continuum from mild anxiety to panic. Mild anxiety may actually benefit the individual as it characteristically heightens his sense of awareness, which helps him deal effectively with actual physical or emotional threats. However, as anxiety approaches panic, the patient becomes progressively less able to interrupt this process without assistance. When the patient reaches a panic state, he becomes completely unable to deal with the precipitating factor or his anxiety without outside intervention. Fear elicits many of the same emotional and physical reactions from the patient and progresses along much the same continuum. The primary difference between the two is the patient's ability to identify the threat causing feelings of fear.

Discussing anxious feelings provides the patient an opportunity to consider these emotions and their possible causes. Anxiety is caused by either real or perceived threats. Regardless of how realistic the threat is—or what the nurse's perception of the threat is—the patient's perception of his being threatened is only too real to him. Accepting the patient's feelings as valid will permit discussion without fear of ridicule.

Defense mechanisms distance the individual from a real or perceived threat. These protections are only pathologic if they interfere with the patient's ability to function. Healthy defense mechanisms are used until the patient is able to confront the threat openly, or, in some situational threats, until the problem resolves itself. As an example, the patient anxious about insertion of a central line may use a regressive defense, becoming more dependent. Even if the patient does not identify the cause of his anxiety, this source is self-limiting. Once the line has been inserted, the source of anxiety has been eliminated, and the patient's behavior should revert to his pre-stressor level. Intervention would be needed if the patient's behavior did not revert from its regressive stance after the line was inserted.

Anxiety is characterized by a set of emotions and physical alterations experienced in response to a threat that the patient cannot clearly identify. This threat may be related to basic needs for air, food, and comfort, such as the patient being in pain, on a ventilator, or having difficulty breathing. It may be related to biological threats, such as anticipated invasive procedures or surgery. Patient concerns with self-concept may also create anxiety. (See the nursing diagnoses on disturbances in self-concept in this section.) Alternatively, the anxiety may be unrelated to the traumatic episode but stem instead from family, job, maturational, or social concerns prior to admission. The traumatic injury may simply exacerbate or heighten these feelings and concerns. The patient's willingness to discuss the subject openly indicates his readiness to cope with anxiety. Through discussion, he may identify the source of his anxiety, which may lead to the discovery of potential resolutions.

Nursing diagnosis

Impaired verbal communication.

Note: *Impaired verbal communication is usually a physical problem related to interference with speech by injuries to the face, throat, or chest; treatment modalities; or neurologic injury. However, this diagnosis is presented as a psychosocial care plan because the ability to communicate is essential for an individual to meet his basic and higher-level needs. The inability to communicate also creates additional emotional problems for the patient such as anxiety/fear, frustration, and increased feelings of powerlessness.*

Assessment

Neurologic
- aphasia
- closed head injury
- cerebral vascular acci-

dent
- motor deficits

Maxillofacial
- mandibular fracture

- mandibular fixation

Respiratory
- endotracheal intubation

- tracheostomy
- respiratory distress

GOAL: Provide the patient with alternative means of communication.

Interventions

1. Assess the patient's ability to verbally communicate. In consultation with his physician, arrange for appropriate referrals/consultations, as needed.

2. In collaboration with the patient's physician, refer the patient to speech/communication specialists, as appropriate.

3. Assess the patient's ability to communicate nonverbally. Provide for an alternative to verbal communication appropriate to the patient's abilities, such as
- note writing
- picture/word boards
- sign language.

Rationale

If verbal impairment is noted, first investigate the patient's ability to communicate prior to the trauma. If a communication deficit existed before injury, find out which alternative means of communication the patient had been using.

In the patient with no previous verbal disability, impairment can occur either through direct injury to the speech apparatus (including the mouth, throat, and mandible) or through neurologic impairment. Direct injury or certain treatments (such as intubation, tracheostomy, or mandibular fixation) can interfere with or prevent verbal expression without interfering with the ability to interpret thoughts. Therefore, adopting an alternative mode of communication probably will not be difficult with this patient.

However, verbal communication is a complicated task requiring many intricate steps. The ability to translate mental images into words is essential. Then adequate muscular control over the diaphragm, vocal cords, tongue, and mouth must exist. Finally the patient must be able to breathe adequately and with sufficient control to produce sound. Additionally, two-way communication requires that the patient be able to hear or have some other means of receiving data and to interpret and process this information. Neurologic injuries may produce a deficit in any of these areas.

Patients with deficits of this nature will require assessment and intervention by speech therapists, audiologists, and other communication specialists.

Patients who are unable to communicate verbally because of temporary problems interfering with speech (intubation, tracheostomy) need to have some alternative means of communication provided. These patients will need assessment of their abilities to write, gesture, silently mouth words, and draw or point to pictures indicating their needs. This assessment should include the patient's physical and intellectual abilities to complete these tasks. Providing an alternative method allows the patient to communicate his needs and desires and helps reduce his anxiety or fear, level of frustration, and feelings of powerlessness.

Nursing diagnosis

Ineffective individual coping related to varied internal and environmental factors.

Assessment

Causative factors:
• factors that precipitate inability to cope or alter the patient's physical, emotional, or intellectual ability to cope; especially likely with treatment/injury causing immobility or altered body image

Physical
• amputation
• scars
• change in appearance secondary to treatment/injury
• closed head injury resulting in aphasia, amnesia, confusion, or ataxia
• spinal cord injury
• orthopedic injuries

Environmental
• sensory overload secondary to admission to resuscitation area or intensive care environment

Developmental
• preexisting unresolved conflict related to patient's developmental stage

Observed behaviors:
• unhealthy use of defense mechanisms
• stated inability to cope
• inability to problem-solve, given alternatives
• violent or destructive behavior

GOAL: #1: Assess appropriate coping with preexisting or trauma-related stressors.

Interventions

1. Identify and assess the patient's ineffective coping through observation and discussion concerning items under observed behavior.

2. Assess the patient's coping abilities including:
• stressors the patient currently faces
• ability to cope with these stressors
• patient's existing support system
• physical limitations of coping ability resulting from injury
• patient's ability to accept assistance with coping.

Rationale

Effective coping is the ability to successfully encounter, identify, and manage internal and environmental stressors. Effective coping requires the physical, intellectual, and emotional abilities to problem-solve and adapt to change. The trauma patient's ability to cope may be overwhelmed because of either limited coping resources or the sudden, unexpected increase in stressors associated with traumatic injury. Identification of the patient's inability to cope indicates the need for further interventions either to increase his coping abilities or to decrease stressors.

Each individual has varying abilities to cope with problems. Although a person may be able to cope with day-to-day problems without assistance, he may be overwhelmed by the added stresses of traumatic injury and hospitalization. Understanding the number and types of stressors the patient faces aids adequate assessment of his ability to cope with these stressors.

Most trauma-related stressors can be readily seen. However, the challenge is to elicit the stressors with which the patient was struggling prior to injury and those unseen stressors created by the injury. These may include problems associated with money, family or other relationships, or work. Also, the patient's personality or value system may attach a great deal of significance to independence; therefore, hospitalization may greatly increase this patient's stress level. The patient may be unwilling to accept assistance because doing so would indicate an intolerable level of weakness or dependency.

The patient's pre-injury support system needs to be assessed. The members of the support system (family/friends) and their strengths and weaknesses need to be determined. Also, this system may no longer be capable of supporting the patient because of its members' inability to cope with the patient's injuries and their effect on the system. In this circumstance, an interim support system may be substituted while interventions seek to enable family/friends to resume support of the patient.

The patient whose injury alters his body image or renders him immobile faces additional stressors, burdens, or limitations that may exceed his coping boundaries. The common sequelae of head injuries—confusion, headache, decreased attention span, decreased frustration tolerance, ataxia, amnesia, and aphasia—critically interfere with the skills needed for effective problem solving. The patient may no longer have the emotional and intellectual abilities needed to cope with even the smallest levels of stress or frustration.

GOAL #2: Support the patient during periods of inability to cope. Balance the patient's coping abilities and level of stress.

Interventions

Rationale

1. Identify and eliminate unnecessary stressors, such as:
- environmental noise
- excess light
- pain/discomfort
- unnecessary sleep interruptions
- inappropriate bedside conversations.

Some sources of stress can be eliminated or drastically reduced. Such controls decrease the energy the patient must waste dealing with unnecessary burdens. This permits him to devote more energy to solving more demanding concerns.

2. Offer the patient opportunities to discuss his concerns through techniques of open-ended questioning and active listening.

These techniques provide the opportunity and time for the patient to discuss his concerns and alternative solutions. Verbal problem solving with another person may enable the patient to reach a solution.

3. Present the patient with alternatives. Clarify problems and alternative solutions.

The patient may have difficulty problem solving because of a lack of information concerning problems or potential solutions. The patient may be unaware of resources available to assist him with injury-related problems. He may be unable to cope with a problem because he thinks he must cope with it by himself. Informing the patient of available resources and options may help him cope.

4. Promote patient access to his preexisting support system.

If intact, the patient's preexisting support system may provide the most effective initial assistance. He is accustomed to relating to and interacting with this system, in which he has an established level of trust. Before health care providers can effectively assist the patient, they need to establish a level of trust, but even then, the patient's original support system retains primary importance. The bonds between members of his original system are usually stronger than those with health personnel, primarily because of their longevity. Because of its importance, this support system requires assessment of its continuing coping abilities just as the patient does. Any alteration to the norm, such as the patient's traumatic incident, can produce a variety of effects on the entire system. The system may strengthen as its members draw together for mutual support, or it may deteriorate along a continuum from diminished effectiveness to negative, destructive behaviors.

Nursing diagnosis

Potential for powerlessness related to traumatic injuries and hospitalization.

Assessment

Observed behaviors:
- patient expresses feelings of lack of control
- over events
- patient refuses to or reluctantly participates
- in decision making
- patient may express
- emotions ranging from apathy to violence

GOAL: Minimize the patient's feelings of powerlessness.

Interventions	Rationale
1. Maintain awareness of probable feelings of powerlessness in the patient.	Feelings of powerlessness are almost inherent in hospitalization for any cause, but may be more pronounced in trauma victims or other critically ill persons. Usually the state designates which centers will treat trauma or other critical or emergent problems. This designation process, while effective from medical and financial viewpoints, removes the patient's power to decide where he will be taken for health care. This removal of the decision-making power from the patient continues when he arrives at the hospital. He is asked many personal questions (perhaps several times), his personal space is violated continually, and his personal possessions (clothing and valuables) are taken from him. Also, during initial resuscitation, the trauma patient generally does not participate in choices concerning who will care for him or what care he will receive, and everything is being done to or for him instead of by him. Remaining aware that these feelings are likely is the first step in helping the patient cope with this loss of power and in returning power to him.
2. Assess the patient and situation to determine his ability to make decisions.	In light of the patient's probable feelings of powerlessness, critically assess which decisions are appropriate for the patient to make and which must be made by the health care team. The type of injuries and the number and rapidity of necessary procedures dictate the appropriate degree of the patient's control over his care. During admission of an acutely ill patient, it may only be possible to recognize the existence of the patient's feelings.
3. Provide the patient with explanations of all treatments and procedures.	Knowledge gives the patient some sense of control. Keeping him informed about what is happening and why helps him understand his condition, upcoming procedures, and the need for his compliance. Although he may not be able to influence the progression of his care, he does need to make the decision to comply with the health care team's requests.

4. Give the patient the opportunity to make all decisions appropriate to his condition and knowledge level.

Almost all patients are able to exercise some decision-making ability. Patients unable to engage in this process include those who are anesthetized or unconscious. Patients who are confused, mentally disabled, or lacking in sufficient knowledge have an altered ability to make decisions. The decisions made by the patient may seem relatively small—such as choosing which arm to inject or on which side to turn—but these decisions give him some control over his environment.

5. Make sure that the patient is offered only appropriate choices. For example, do not ask him to which side he wants to turn if he can only turn to the right.

Giving the patient a choice that does not really exist sets the patient up for failure and compounds his feelings of powerlessness. Giving the patient a number of choices, any of which would be acceptable, helps ensure successful decision making.

6. Gradually increase the number and complexity of decisions made by the patient as his condition improves.

This process slowly increases the patient's independence and decision-making capacity. Inherent in this intervention is patient education, to provide the patient with the knowledge necessary to make rational, intelligent decisions.

7. Support and encourage appropriate expressions of powerfulness by the patient.

Having been temporarily stripped of his decision-making power, the patient usually requires support to resume decision making. This intervention may require the nurse's critical evaluation of her feelings concerning the patient's expressions of power so she can foster this behavior in the patient.

Nursing diagnosis

Disturbance in self-concept
A. Related to change in body image

Assessment

Causative factors:
- loss of body part
- loss of function
- disfigurement (as from traumatic or surgical scars)

Stages of body image change adaptation
- impact—depersonalization, anxiety
- retreat—denial, un-

realistic plans for the future, avoidance of any mention of injuries or traumatic incident
- acknowledgment—iso-

lation, withdrawal, feelings of worthlessness
- reconstruction—self-acceptance, increased motivation

> **GOAL:** Recognize the patient's stage in dealing with body image change; support normal emotional processes.

Interventions

1. Assess the patient for current stage of adaptation through observation of behaviors and analysis of patient-nurse and patient-visitor interactions.

2. Maintain an awareness of invasive admission procedures as additional psychological stressors.

3. Provide orientation information concerning hospitalization and the nature and extent of injuries. Keep answers short and concise.

4. Assess the patient's perception of his injuries.

5. Recognize denial as a normal adaptive response during the retreat phase. Denial may be indicated by the patient's refusal to participate in his care or by the use of symbolism (the patient assigns his feelings to some other person or object).

6. Promote patient participation in his care by:
- discussing the reason for his refusal to participate
- focusing on his healthy aspects or the positive side of his altered image.

Rationale

All trauma patients undergo some degree of alteration in body image if there is loss of a body part, loss of function, or disfigurement. Four stages of dealing with body image changes have been defined: impact, retreat, acknowledgement, and reconstruction. Behavioral observations and analysis of interactions provide clues to the patient's current stage.

During the impact stage, the patient experiences a psychological shock state that began at the time of injury. Each procedure and the rapid pace of activity during a trauma admission reinforce his conversion from a healthy person to an injured and hospitalized person.

The patient at this stage is primarily focused on the present. This information helps him develop realistic perceptions of events as well as serving the very practical purposes of obtaining consent and cooperation. Information is kept concise because the patient's anxiety level will probably impair his ability to retain extensive, detailed information.

The patient's view of the traumatic incident may provide clues to future behavioral changes. Where the patient places the locus of control for his trauma (his fault or the fault of others) may determine future feelings of guilt, despair, or anger.

Denial gives the patient time to mourn his loss and gather the emotional resources needed to adapt to his altered self-image.

Discussing the reason for the patient's refusal to participate in his care may disclose ways of gaining the patient's participation without forcing him or allowing him to avoid self-care. Focusing on positive aspects helps the patient accept his new body image.

7. Support the patient during the acknowledgment stage by:
- providing requested information concerning his trauma and care
- reassuring the patient regarding prospects for the future (be realistic)
- including him in support groups.

During this stage, the patient works to recognize that his body has changed and begins the process of understanding that change. This is a deeply difficult time as a host of new feelings and sensations are experienced. Support groups may be helpful at this stage as a source of encouragement and mutual aid.

8. Assess the patient's strengths and weaknesses. Utilize his strengths to support him during the reconstruction stage:
- preexisting self-concept, body image, and self-esteem
- external support systems.

In the final stage, the patient works to redefine his body image and incorporate this into his relationships with others.

Nursing diagnosis

Disturbance in self-concept
B. Related to change in role performance
Note: *Whether an injury creates temporary or permanent role changes will depend on the patient's roles prior to injury and thus requires individual assessment. The factors listed serve as general guidelines for consideration.*

Assessment

Causative factors:
Temporary role changes
- hospitalization
- pain

- injuries not creating permanent disability

Permanent role changes
- spinal cord injuries
- amputations

- orthopedic injuries
- chronic pain

GOAL: Support and assist the patient in redefining his self-concept.

Interventions

1. Determine the patient's roles and role performance prior to his injury.

2. Assess the nature and extent of role performance changes.

Rationale

Each individual performs many different roles at any given point in his life. He may simultaneously be a spouse, parent, child, subordinate, supervisor, church member, friend, and many others. The patient may have different levels of vested interest in each and perform them at varying levels of competence. He may enjoy some roles more than others and perform some out of sheer necessity. This assessment gives the nurse a greater understanding of the patient as an individual and is the beginning step in defining role changes related to traumatic injury.

On admission to a hospital essentially all roles but that of patient are interrupted. As the patient continues toward recovery, concern turns to reestablishing roles. The nature of the patient's injuries may negate the performance of certain roles, necessitate changes in the manner in which some roles are performed, and have no effect on other roles. Furthermore, these changes in role performance may be of either a temporary or permanent nature. If a bricklayer lacerates his spleen, he will be temporarily unable to perform that role, but will probably, in time, be able to return to work in the same capacity. If that same patient suffers a complete lesion of the cervical spinal cord, the role of bricklayer will be permanently lost.

3. Assist the patient in reorganizing his self-concept, including:
- grieving for lost or changed roles
- defining new or potential roles
- defining new ways of performing existing roles
- reeducating and retraining for new or altered roles.

Self-concept, simply put, is the totality of what we think and feel about ourselves. This complex concept is composed of our body image (how we think we look), roles (how we define our relationship with the external world), and self-esteem (how we feel about ourselves). Part of our self-concept is externally derived, based on other people's reactions to us, and we use our roles, primarily, to define ourselves to others. Therefore, changes in role performance represent significant alterations in our self-concept, especially permanent changes. Although simple to state, this intervention presents a difficult interdisciplinary challenge.

Additional considerations

Although this plan treats changes in body image and role performance separately, it must be emphasized that they occur simultaneously and act together to alter the patient's self-concept. All potential causes of self-concept disturbance must be considered and treated simultaneously.

Nursing diagnosis

Potential for spiritual distress of patient or family members related to traumatic injury and hospitalization.

Assessment

Family or patient:
- requests spiritual guidance
- requests performance of religious ceremony/ritual
- expresses doubts about religious/spiritual beliefs
- expresses fears of death, spiritual pain

GOAL: Help the patient and his family meet their spiritual needs.

Interventions

1. Identify patient/family need for spiritual counsel via:
- patient/family requests for pastoral counsel (by priest, minister, rabbi)
- patient/family discussions of religious/spiritual needs.

2. Contact or assist in contacting either a personal or a hospital-affiliated spiritual/pastoral counselor for the patient/family. Offer to assist in this area.

3. Provide, whenever possible, for the opportunity to complete requested religious/spiritual ceremonies. Provide the family with access to the chapel if desired.

4. Maintain an open, nonjudgmental attitude concerning the patient's or family's spiritual beliefs.

Rationale

The patient or family may express their spiritual needs either directly or indirectly. A sudden traumatic injury may cause the patient or family to question their religious or spiritual beliefs and request spiritual counseling to resolve these questions.

These interventions provide the patient/family with access to spiritual guidance and counsel. Offering to help locate spiritual counsel indicates acceptance of beliefs and may help the patient or family feel more comfortable in making these requests.

Certain religious ceremonies may hold significance for the patient or family, such as the Sacrament of the Sick for Catholic patients. Completion of these ceremonies provides the patient/family with a great deal of spiritual comfort and impacts significantly on their anxiety level. Every attempt should be made to allow these ceremonies to occur. It is possible, for instance, to have a priest go into the operating room to anoint the patient.

Maintaining a nonjudgmental attitude about the family's and patient's beliefs indicates acceptance and caring.

Nursing diagnosis

Potential for alterations in family processes related to:
A. changes in family members' role responsibilities
B. loss (temporary or permanent) of family wage earner
C. loss of emotional support of family member secondary to traumatic injury of a family member.
Note: *It must be emphasized that the patient's primary support system, especially in our highly mobile society, may or may not be the traditionally defined "family." The patient may be geographically far removed from his family, have no living relatives, or have family relationships that have completely broken down. Additionally, even patients with strong family support systems probably belong to secondary groups of friends, co-workers, and significant others. For convenience, however, in this care plan "family" refers to the patient's support system as a whole, regardless of its component members. The patient's entire support system will be affected by his traumatic injury and may require assistance to optimize its function. Nurses must assess from whom the patient gains support and to whom he gives support and intervene to help maintain that system.*

Assessment

Observed behaviors:
Inability of the family to:
● meet needs of its members it was previously

able to meet
● obtain necessary outside assistance

● overcome the crisis situation
● communicate constructively

● express emotions and needs

GOAL #1: Assist family members in resolving the crisis of traumatic injury and hospitalization.

Interventions

1. Expedite rejoining of family members with the patient:
● maintain flexible visitation policies
● enable the patient and family to speak by phone if visiting is not possible
● take stable patients to the family if they cannot come into the resuscitation area.

2. Provide family members with realistic information concerning the patient's injuries.

3. Keep explanations as brief (but complete) as possible and give information in terms family members can understand. Plan the order in which to give information, and remain sensitive to the family's ability to receive more information.

Rationale

A family member's hospitalization for traumatic injury, almost without exception, precipitates a crisis state for the remaining family members. This crisis is largely based on the family's lack of knowledge about the patient's condition, even whether or not he is alive. Traumatic injury occurs without warning. The family's last contact with the patient may have been over the breakfast table. Suddenly they are informed, usually over the phone or by a police officer arriving at their door, that their family member has been injured and taken to the hospital. Initial information given to the family may be limited, and their first need is to assure themselves that the patient is alive and ascertain his condition. The family's anxiety usually increases as time passes. Rejoining the family with the patient as quickly as possible gives them the knowledge they need to confront the next crisis—dealing with the patient's injuries.

Providing the facts facilitates a realistic perception of events. This helps resolve the crisis by minimizing anxiety-producing speculation.

The family's anxiety level will limit the amount and complexity of information they can assimilate at one time. Therefore, the interview with the family should be planned to provide the most essential information first. The interview should stop before the family reaches the saturation point.

GOAL #2: Determine areas in which the family is unable to function adequately.

Interventions

1. Assess family function through observation of group interactions (internal and external) and initiation of open discussion of potential problems the family may face.

Rationale

The effect of a patient's injury and hospitalization on his family will vary significantly based on many factors. Adverse or beneficial effects may be influenced by preexisting family stability, previous experience with crises, guilt associated with the traumatic incident, and the patient's relative importance to family function. In our experience, the family rarely is completely unable to function in all areas. Observing family interactions—among themselves (internally) and with outsiders (externally)—provides clues to the group's stability and areas in which they may need assistance. Open discussion may reveal problem areas directly or indirectly, signaling problems that require further investigation.

GOAL #3: Support the functional capacity of the family.

Interventions

1. Provide family members with information concerning potential problem areas.

Rationale

Anticipatory guidance based on the nurse's past experience with other families assists the family in two ways. First, the family gains information that may aid problem solving when these problems do occur. Second, the family realizes that others have surmounted the problems they are about to face.

2. Recognize the family's inability to reach decisions and provide them with instructions or assist problem-solving efforts as appropriate.

In most cases, the trauma patient's family is in a new situation. They may feel uncomfortable making decisions or not realize alternatives available. They may forget even the most obvious needs, such as eating, and may neglect themselves out of concern for the traumatized member. They may benefit from simple instructions or help in problem solving, such as being provided with alternatives from which to choose.

3. Provide the family with appropriate referrals for assistance.

The family may need referrals for additional counseling from social workers, family counselors, financial counselors, or support groups. The need for outside help increases as the patient approaches the rehabilitative stages of treatment, particularly in cases of permanent disability.

REFERENCES

PSYCHOSOCIAL SUPPORT OF THE TRAUMA PATIENT

"Assessing Psychological Status," in *Assessment.* Nurse's Reference Library. Springhouse, Pa.: Springhouse Corp., 1983.

Braulin, J.L.D., et al. "Families in Crisis," *Critical Care Quarterly* 5(3):38-46, December 1982.

Groves, M.J. "Initial Communication with Trauma Patients," in *Trauma Nursing.* Edited by Cardona, V.D. Oradell, N.J.: Medical Economics Books, 1985.

Lee, J.M. "Emotional Reactions to Trauma," *Nursing Clinics of North America* 5(4):577-87, December 1970.

"Relating with Patients and Their Families," in *Practices.* Nurse's Reference Library. Springhouse, Pa.: Springhouse Corp., 1984.

Roberts, S.L. *Behavioral Concepts and the Critically Ill Patient.* Englewood Cliffs, N.J.: Prentice-Hall, 1976.

Solomon-Hast, A. "Anxiety in the Coronary Care Unit," *Critical Care Quarterly* 4(3):75-82, December 1981.

PEDIATRIC
TRAUMA

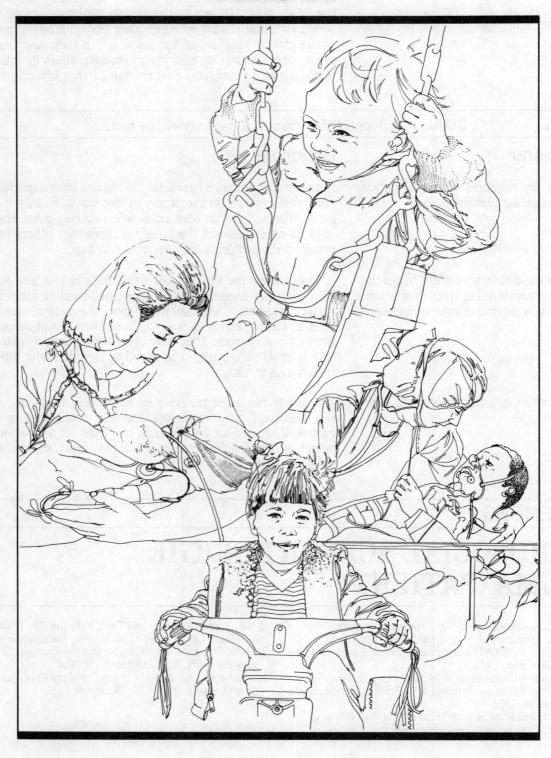

PEDIATRIC TRAUMA

Introduction

The leading cause of child death in the United States is accidental or inflicted trauma. About 10% of all accident-related fatalities are children under age 14. Every year, more than 20 million children sustain injuries serious enough to require medical care; many are major, multisystem injuries.

Prompt, confident, and appropriate nursing care during the initial resuscitation phase can reduce the mortality and morbidity associated with pediatric trauma. Unfortunately, many children in emergency situations are evaluated by physicians and nurses who have limited pediatric experience. Making the correct decisions and applying the proper treatment modalities require preparation—an understanding of the basic differences and difficulties inherent in pediatric emergencies and systematic planning. Therefore, the initial nursing management care plans that follow focus on the unique aspects of emergency pediatric care. A carefully considered, predetermined care plan minimizes the potential for error, reduces the anxiety that a child creates in the trauma resuscitation bay, and maximizes recovery potential.

Dealing with pediatric trauma competently requires recognition of special stabilization and treatment techniques. For example, the primary survey of the injured child presents several unique aspects:

• *Airway*—Although airway management takes precedence, as always, the child's small anatomical proportions complicate the anterior and cephalad position of the larynx. Simply knowing how to adapt airway management with mask-bag ventilation and oral-tracheal intubation for pediatric use can save lives.
• *Breathing*—A child's breathing mechanics differ from an adult's, limiting effective resuscitation techniques and presenting a high risk for tension pneumothorax.
• *Circulation*—Complex pediatric compensatory mechanisms make circulatory assessment difficult; they can mask early signs of shock, potentially delaying recognition until the shock state is full-blown. At the same time, overcautious—potentially insufficient—volume resuscitation compounds the risk of avoidable death in children.

Other typical pediatric emergency problems include the likelihood of central nervous system trauma (occurring in more than 50% of these cases), which complicates management options. In addition, immature, possibly inefficient, thermoregulation can result in hypothermia, which mimics shock and worsens metabolic acidosis.

Even these few examples demonstrate that a commitment by emergency nursing personnel to improve pediatric emergency care methods will benefit many families throughout the country. The ability to provide the essentials of care begins with the proper nursing assessment sequence, which recognizes the special needs of children.

With good teamwork and communication, we can reverse the untoward incidence—reaching epidemic proportions—of trauma that is currently affecting our most precious national resource, our children.

Martin R. Eichelberger, MD
Director, Emergency Trauma Services
Children's Hospital National Medical Center
Washington, D.C.

PEDIATRIC AIRWAY OBSTRUCTION

Assessment

Note: *It is imperative to suspect all trauma patients—including infants and children—of having cervical spine injuries until proven otherwise. Ensure proper alignment of the cervical spine to prevent injury to the spinal cord during airway management. Utilize one person to apply manual in-line traction on the head and cervical spine. Apply a hard collar as soon as possible to immobilize the head and cervical spine in proper alignment.*

Mechanism of injury/ etiology:
- near drowning
- smoke inhalation, chemical/thermal burns
- blunt or penetrating trauma to the face/neck, such as clothesline injury
- tongue occluding airway or blood, vomitus, or other foreign materials in the airway

Physical findings:
Respiratory
- cyanosis

- nasal flaring
- retractions (supraclavicular, intercostal, subxyphoid, sternal)
- change in respiratory rate/depth (dyspnea/ tachypnea)
- decreased or absent breath sounds
- wheezes
- inspiratory stridor (obstruction at/above thoracic inlet)
- expiratory stridor (obstruction below thoracic

inlet)
- snoring (obstruction at laryngeal inlet)
- expiratory grunting (appears early, later decreases as condition deteriorates)
- subcutaneous air in face, neck, upper chest
- rapid progression to respiratory arrest
- signs of pneumothorax, hemothorax

Cardiovascular
- cyanosis

- rapid deterioration to cardiac arrest

Neurologic
- agitation to unresponsiveness and flaccidity

Associated injuries:
- burns
- maxillofacial injury
- tracheal/laryngeal injury
- head/cervical spine injury

Diagnostic studies

- bronchoscopy—provides direct visualization of lower airway
- radiographs of neck and chest—may confirm position

of aspirated foreign objects; may reveal fractures or dissection of air
- ABG results—reflect severity of hypoxic episode

Ineffective airway clearance related to complete or partial obstruction by the tongue, foreign matter, edema.

GOAL #1: Restore a patent airway; avoid stimulation of the gag reflex.

Interventions

1. Assess the patient rapidly for:
- air flow from the nose and mouth
- chest movement
- bilateral breath sounds.

Rationale

Findings from this rapid assessment determine whether the obstruction is complete or partial.

2. Remove any obvious obstructing matter from the nose or mouth, either manually or with suction. Avoid blind manual sweeping of the oropharynx.

Rapid airway management is crucial in the pediatric patient because hypoxia rapidly progresses to complete cardiac arrest. An accumulation of blood or mucus or other foreign matter may easily obstruct the airway. Simple suctioning of the oropharynx or manual removal of debris may clear the airway. All attempts should be made to accomplish this gently and carefully to avoid pushing debris farther into the airway.

3. Perform the jaw-thrust or chin-lift maneuvers.

These maneuvers physically open the airway by elevating the mandible, which in turn lifts the tongue away from the posterior pharyngeal wall. Simultaneously, they allow maintenance of cervical spine alignment. *Do not turn the child's head to either side or hyperextend the head/neck.*

4. Insert an artificial oral airway after measuring for proper size/length; measure from the corner of the mouth to the earlobe.

The large tongue of the infant or young child commonly causes obstruction when neurological injury is also present. Soft tissues relax and permit the tongue to rest against the posterior pharyngeal wall, causing obstruction of the small airway. An oral airway repositions the tongue and may provide temporary relief of the obstruction.

5. Ensure availability of all sizes of uncuffed and cuffed endotracheal tubes, laryngoscopes and appropriate blades, and the suction catheters necessary for each size endotracheal tube. (See "Endotracheal Intubation" in Section VII.)

The unresponsive or maxillofacially injured child usually requires emergency intubation because of his inability to protect and maintain a patent airway. The loss of airway patency may result from loss of the gag reflex, excessive edema or bleeding, or inability to swallow. Uncuffed tubes minimize subglottic edema and later ulceration. Once the required tube size has been determined, have one size smaller and one size larger readily available at the bedside in case of unexpected deviation from the approximated size. Table 6.1 lists the approximate sizes of endotracheal tubes and suction catheters for children from birth to 8 years of age and a general formula for determining appropriate sizes. Between the ages of 8 and 12 years, the child's weight and body build help decide whether he needs adult- or pediatric-size tubes. A stylet, or guidewire, may be needed. Having copies of this or a similar chart affixed to the pediatric resuscitation cart saves time and reduces potential personnel anxiety prior to pediatric intubation.

Note: *Esophageal obturator airways are contraindicated for the pediatric patient under the age of 12.*

6. Secure the endotracheal tube with twill or adhesive tape.

Uncuffed endotracheal tubes can easily become dislodged, causing further airway obstruction or respiratory arrest.

7. Auscultate bilateral breath sounds after intubation and assist with chest radiograph.

The trachea of an infant or small child is short as well as small in diameter. Intubation of the bronchus occurs if the tube is inserted too far below the vocal cords. These measures confirm proper tube positioning.

8. Ensure the availability of appropriately sized manual or mechanical ventilatory devices.

The intubated pediatric patient usually requires assistance with ventilation. Manual bag resuscitators should be kept on the pediatric specialty cart for quick access. The mechanism for rapid acquisition of a volume, time-cycled ventilator should be documented on the pediatric resuscitation cart.

9. Measure and strictly observe appropriate volume limits with manual or mechanical ventilation by watching chest expansion.

Although pediatric patients have smaller lungs and vital capacities, they also have greater resistance to air flow. Aggressive ventilation without regard to lung expansion can easily cause pulmonary rupture. Underinflation of the lungs in an effort to prevent rupture may be equally detrimental as the child does not receive optimal ventilation. Careful monitoring of the rise and fall of the chest aids evaluation of inspiratory forces.

10. Ensure availability of emergency pediatric cricothyroidotomy equipment; assist as necessary. (See "Needle Cricothyroidotomy" in Section VII and "Emergency Airway Tray" in Appendix 3.)

Extensive maxillofacial injury, obvious or suspected laryngeal or tracheobronchial tree injury, or the small size of the anatomical structures may make it physically impossible for even skilled personnel to successfully intubate a child. Advance preparation for this procedure includes having an emergency airway tray available with pediatric surgical instruments and various sizes of tracheostomy tubes. Although this procedure is rarely required in the pediatric patient, it is preferred over a tracheostomy because of reduced blood loss and fewer associated complications.

GOAL #2: Maintain a patent airway.

Interventions

1. Monitor the patient continuously for signs of respiratory distress; ensure the availability of intubation equipment.

2. Monitor the intubated infant or child continuously for endotracheal tube placement.

3. Monitor the intubated infant or child continuously for endotracheal tube patency. Ensure the availability and functioning of appropriate suction apparatus; suction the patient as needed; document characteristics of tracheal secretions.

Rationale

Children who initially are able to protect their own airways may experience subsequent respiratory difficulties from neurologic deterioration, progressive soft tissue swelling, or laryngeal spasms, as with inhalation injury. *Continuous airway assessment is a primary nursing function and an essential fundamental of pediatric trauma care.*

Vigilant monitoring of the endotracheal tube is mandatory in the pediatric patient. Tube placement above the cords increases the risk of tube dislodgement, and placement too far below the cords intubates the right mainstem bronchus only. Any number of events can cause dislodgement or extubation of the uncuffed tube. Simple head movements from side to side, flailing arms, suctioning, and turning may alter tube placement. Pediatric patients are highly intolerant of hypoxia and without aggressive intervention rapidly deteriorate into respiratory arrest followed by cardiac arrest.

Accumulations from continued bleeding and mucus formation may easily obstruct the narrow diameter of the pediatric tube. Retained secretions may cause lower airway obstruction or complications, such as pneumonia or atelectasis, and they provide excellent media for bacterial growth. Documentation of quantity and characteristics of tracheal secretions aids detection of additional respiratory insult, for example, pulmonary contusion.

Nursing diagnosis

Potential for impaired gas exchange related to aspiration of foreign objects into the lungs.

GOAL: Restore and maintain adequate gas exchange.

Interventions

1. Ensure the availability and anticipate the use of supplemental, humidified oxygen or mechanical ventilation.

Rationale

The pediatric patient in any degree of respiratory distress requires early administration of 100% oxygen before, during, and after airway establishment to optimize gas exchange. Upper airway obstruction may lead to obstruction of the small lower airways as aspirated foreign objects decrease alveolar function and impair adequate gas exchange.

2. Monitor the patient closely for indications of respiratory deterioration or distress; obtain a baseline chest radiograph and ABG sample.

The pediatric patient is extremely sensitive to altered oxygen–carbon dioxide exchange. Baseline studies, trend analysis, and continuous physical assessment aid early detection of lower airway complications.

3. Auscultate breath sounds frequently; provide optimal pulmonary hygiene including:
• frequent suctioning
• patient repositioning
• chest physiotherapy
• incentive spirometry (as appropriate for age and airway type).

Wheezes indicate probable lower airway obstruction. Pulmonary hygiene must be initiated early during resuscitation to optimize aeration and prevent complications from aspirated and retained secretions. These measures mobilize secretions, prevent pooling, and promote full lung expansion.

4. Ensure the availability of equipment for a bronchoscopy. (See "Bronchoscopy" in Section VII.)

Bronchoscopy aids diagnosis of aspiration and affords deep pulmonary suctioning.

Nursing diagnosis

Potential for infection related to bacterial growth in lungs or crycothyroidotomy site secondary to aspiration of foreign objects or wound contamination.

GOAL #1: Minimize the risk for bacterial growth in the lungs.

Interventions

1. Provide optimal pulmonary hygiene. (See "Lower Airway Obstruction" in Section II.)

Rationale

Prompt and consistent removal of pulmonary secretions reduces the risk for pneumonia and other pulmonary complications.

GOAL #2: Reduce the risk for bacterial growth in the cricothyroidotomy site.

Interventions

1. Maintain sterile technique, as possible, including the use of:
• masks and gloves
• masks for bedside staff
• sterile tray/instruments.

Rationale

Sterile technique decreases the risk of contaminants entering the wound and ultimately the respiratory tract.

2. Perform aseptic wound care every 8 hours or as often as required if wound drainage is excessive.

Aseptic wound care reduces the risk of bacterial growth. Close attention to the wound site, surrounding tissue, and drainage promotes early detection of infection.

Associated care plans	Associated procedures and study
Lower Airway Obstruction	Bronchoscopy
Pediatric Gastric Distention	Needle Cricothyroidotomy
General Pediatric Care Considerations	Endotracheal Intubation

Table 6.1

Selecting the Perfect Size

Age	Endotracheal tube[1]	Suction catheter
Newborn	3.0	6F
6 months	3.5	8F
18 months	4.0	8F
3 years	4.5	8F
5 years	5.0	10F
6 years	5.5	10F
8 years	6.0	10F

[1]Uncuffed endotracheal tubes are usually used for children under 8 years of age.

Formulas for determining the appropriate size tube

1.
$$\frac{\text{Patient's age in years} + 16}{4} = \text{internal diameter of tube (mm)}$$

2. Width of the child's little finger = diameter of the trachea

PEDIATRIC HYPOVOLEMIC SHOCK

Assessment

**Mechanism of injury/
etiology:**
Blunt

- automobile, motorcycle accidents
- pedestrian/motor vehicle collisions
- bicycle, sledding accidents
- gymnastic, athletic accidents
- falls
- assault, abuse

Penetrating

- knife or bullet wounds
- explosion or blast injuries
- iatrogenic causes, such as insertion of chest, gastric, and endotracheal tubes

Physical findings:
Respiratory

- rapid, shallow respirations

- irregular respiratory pattern

Cardiovascular

- pallor or cyanosis
- clammy skin
- cool, mottled extremities
- tachycardia
- thready pulse

- sluggish capillary refill time
- hypotension (late sign)

Neurologic

- decreased level of consciousness, or agitation

Genitourinary

- oliguria

Diagnostic studies

- ABG results
  - ☐ respiratory alkalosis—$PCO_2 < 34$ (early sign)
  - ☐ metabolic acidosis—$PCO_2 > 45$, pH < 7.3 (late sign)
- hemoglobin/hematocrit levels—decreased because of blood loss
- WBC, platelet counts—increased in response to trauma

Potential for decreased tissue perfusion related to fluid volume deficit secondary to hemorrhage.

GOAL #1: Recognize early signs of shock.

Interventions

1. Monitor vital signs every 5 to 15 minutes or as the child's condition warrants. Provide continuous ECG monitoring. Ensure availability of a chart or reference that defines normal heart rate and blood pressure based on age.

Rationale

Children have a great compensatory ability to vasoconstrict; therefore, obvious signs of shock, such as hypotension, generally do not become evident until after a significant blood volume loss (15% to 20%). Constant vital sign evaluation promotes early detection of change. Auscultating blood pressure with a Doppler device maximizes accurate evaluation, especially during hypotensive episodes. Machines that automatically measure the blood pressure at predetermined time intervals enable more precise evaluation, especially in neonates and infants. Reference charts permit comparison with expected norms by age, promoting accurate data evaluation.

2. Assess closely for signs of hemorrhagic shock:
- tachycardia
- cold, mottled extremities
- prolonged capillary refill time
- hypotension
- tachypnea
- decreased level of consciousness
- decreased urine output.

The margin for error is quite small in children; their condition may rapidly change and deteriorate. Blood volume totals between 7% and 9% (70 to 90 cc) of their total body weight. For example, a child weighing 10 kg (22 lb) has a total blood volume of approximately 800 cc. Thus a blood loss that would seem harmless in an adult may rapidly precipitate a shock state in an infant or child. Vigilant physical assessment helps direct further therapeutic interventions.

GOAL #2: Maximize oxygenation.

Interventions

Rationale

1. Assess the child's respiratory status constantly for signs of distress:
- tachypnea, dyspnea
- retractions, nasal flaring
- stridor, snoring, grunting
- cyanosis
- decreased or absent breath sounds.

Children are highly intolerant of any respiratory compromise. Respiratory distress may occur suddenly and require emergency airway support. Use of a pulse oximeter during resuscitation, surgery, and critical care enables early detection of respiratory compromise.

2. Administer supplemental oxygen at 100% fraction of inspired oxygen, as ordered, to all pediatric trauma patients.

Small airway passages and tidal volumes in infants and young children increase their sensitivity to any disturbances in the gas exchange process. Early oxygen therapy maximizes the amount of oxygen available for transport and utilization and reduces the risk of hypoxia-induced systemic complications. Supplemental oxygen therapy should continue until ABG results reflect adequate ventilation.

3. Ensure availability of equipment for intubation and mechanical ventilation. Assist as necessary. Refer to Table 6.1 in "Pediatric Airway Obstruction" for age and approximate tube sizes. (See "Pediatric Airway Obstruction" in Section VI and "Endotracheal Intubation" and "Needle Cricothyroidotomy" in Section VII.)

In infants and young children, increased lung compliance, increased airway resistance, and overall metabolic rate lead to significant calorie expenditure during respiration. The infant has little respiratory reserve function; therefore, any problems that increase airway resistance further stress the infant. The child's small airway and delicate tissues predispose him to obstruction even after minimal trauma or edema. Early tracheal intubation and ventilatory support promote optimal pulmonary function.

4. Guard against airway obstruction and dislodging or extubation of an uncuffed tube.

Sudden respiratory distress may follow any compromise in airway patency or any change in the endotracheal tube's position. Maintenance of the proper position (2 to 3 cm below the vocal cords) and airway patency must be a constant priority because of the child's intolerance to hypoxia. The child's airway is shorter than the adult's, and tube positioning slightly above the cords may dislodge it; positioning too far below the cords results in right mainstem intubation.

5. Monitor and report trends in ABG results.

Because of the child's narrow tolerance range, even subtle changes may indicate gas exchange problems. Trend analysis of blood gas data promotes early detection of subtle changes.

6. Provide optimal pulmonary hygiene as appropriate for age and airway type. Suction the endotracheal tube gently.

Pulmonary measures, such as turning, suctioning, incentive spirometry, and chest physiotherapy, optimize full lung expansion and alveolar aeration, prevent secretion accumulation or pooling, mobilize secretions, and minimize the risk of pulmonary complications. Vigorous tracheal suctioning or advancing the suction catheter too far may injure the tracheobronchial tree or cause a pneumothorax.

7. Insert the gastric decompression tube gently and carefully, or assist as needed. Maintain position, patency, and proper tube function. Use a syringe for manual aspiration of air and gastric contents. (See "Pediatric Gastric Distention" in Section VI.)

Gastric distention, a common problem in infants and young children, causes diaphragmatic elevation, which impairs lung expansion and reduces tidal volume. The distended stomach also predisposes the patient to vomiting. Remember that uncuffed endotracheal tubes, used in infants and young children, increase the risk of aspiration if vomiting occurs. Careful, gentle gastric tube insertion minimizes the risk of esophageal injury.

GOAL #3: Restore normovolemia. Minimize further blood loss.

Interventions

1. Assist with insertion of appropriate-size intravenous catheters. Assemble equipment needed for cutdown procedures (see "Cardiovascular considerations," page 314). Secure all I.V.s with adequate padding, tape, and arm or foot boards.

2. Assist with weighing the patient or estimating his weight.

3. Administer fluid volume replacement via syringe bolus or volume-limited drip, as ordered, based on body weight (usually 10 to 20 cc/kg), volume loss, and signs of shock. Maintain a continuous intake record. Repeat the initial bolus as ordered if the patient does not respond.

4. Assemble equipment and assist with insertion of peripheral artery, central venous, and pulmonary artery catheters.

5. Administer blood and component therapy, as ordered, based on volume loss, signs of shock, and body weight as follows:
- 10 cc/kg—packed RBCs
- 20 cc/kg—fresh-frozen plasma.

Rationale

Early, rapid volume replacement may restore hemodynamic stability and prevent deterioration to a shock state. Shock may increase the difficulty of intravenous catheterization in the infant or small child. Cutdowns may offer optimal access; the distal saphenous vein is the preferred site. Keep in mind that intravenous access above and below the diaphragm is essential when intraabdominal injury is suspected. Protective padded dressings minimize the risk for I.V. dislodgement and infiltration.

Calculations for fluid replacement and drug dosage are based on the child's weight. Determination of urine output adequacy and blood loss severity also require weight estimation.

Carefully estimated fluid replacement amounts, administered by methods that offer close control, promote accurate fluid replacement. Precise measurements and recording of fluid intake aid in determining fluid balance. Patient assessment must continue during fluid resuscitation as calculated fluid replacement amounts may prove inadequate for excessive or persistent blood loss or fluid shifts into interstitial spaces. **Note:** *Fluid resuscitation must be accomplished prior to certain procedures, such as closed-tube thoracostomy for a hemothorax, or the child may exsanguinate.*

These monitoring devices provide valuable data that aid precise hemodynamic evaluation and guide further volume replacement therapy. Radial artery catheters promote accurate blood pressure monitoring and offer easy access for blood sampling. Generally, pulmonary artery and central venous catheters are not indicated during early resuscitation and may not be necessary if the patient responds appropriately and stabilizes after the initial intravenous fluid bolus.

The small blood volume–body weight ratio in the child predisposes him to a shock state after trauma. Excessive crystalloid resuscitation dilutes the remaining circulating volume and impairs oxygen transport. Persistent hemodynamic instability after the initial crystalloid boluses usually indicates the need for blood replacement.

6. Avoid excessive, repeated blood sampling. Draw the minimum amount of blood necessary for the laboratory study requested.

Any unnecessary blood loss may cause further deterioration of the shock state.

7. Apply direct pressure or a pressure dressing over bleeding sites. Apply a pediatric pneumatic antishock garment (PASG) as indicated. Use caution when inflating the abdominal compartment. (See "The Pneumatic Antishock Garment" in Section VII.)

Direct pressure and pressure dressings promote hemostasis without causing further tissue damage. A PASG provides tamponade to external and internal bleeding sites by compressing underlying structures. This garment can also enhance circulation to vital organs as it may translocate blood from the extremities. Abdominal compartment inflation may increase intraabdominal pressures and impede diaphragmatic movement. This can cause respiratory embarrassment or arrest and precipitate pulmonary edema. Ventilatory adjustments and even intubation may become necessary to compensate for impaired ventilation.

8. Administer inotropic agents, as ordered.

Inotropic agents, although not usually indicated in hypovolemic shock, may aid hemodynamic stabilization when fluid resuscitation is ineffective.

9. Prepare the child for surgery. (See "Preparation for Surgery" in Section VII.)

Persistent hemodynamic instability after blood transfusions of more than 30 cc/kg generally indicates the need for surgical intervention.

GOAL #4: Maintain an adequate fluid balance.

Interventions

1. Include the following fluids in the intake record:
- intravenous boluses and infusions
- flush solutions
- fluid used to mix medication
- retained peritoneal lavage fluid.

Include the following in the output record:
- weight or cc measurement of saturated dressings
- gastric drainage
- chest tube drainage
- blood drawn for laboratory analysis
- urine output.

2. Infuse all fluid replacements through a volume-limiting chamber or infusion pump.

3. Ensure accurate measurements of urine output by weighing diapers or measuring output via an attachable urine collection bag or indwelling catheter. Test urine samples for occult blood and specific gravity.

4. Monitor all available hemodynamic parameters and the child's respiratory status continuously.

Rationale

Inclusion of administered and drawn fluids, drainage, and outputs in ongoing intake and output records promotes accurate fluid balance determination.

Fluid replacement requires controlled administration routes to minimize the risk of fluid overload.

Urine output indicates adequacy of volume replacement and tissue perfusion. An hourly output of less than 1 cc/kg is considered oliguria in the pediatric patient. Accurate output records necessitate precise measurement of every obtainable cc of urine. The child's age and stability determine the appropriateness of various collection devices. Renal injury may easily occur, because a child's kidneys lack sufficient fascial protection. Microscopic hematuria, therefore, requires further diagnostic investigation. Urine specific gravity indicates adequacy of volume replacement and renal function.

The condition of an infant or young child can change rapidly and thus requires continuous reassessment to detect early changes and to direct further therapy.

Additional considerations

The pediatric trauma patient requires the services of a variety of specialists, including a pediatrician, a pediatric surgeon, a pediatric neurosurgeon, a radiologist, a pediatric orthopedist, a neonatologist (when appropriate), pediatric trauma nurses, and the general trauma team. These specialists and the therapy they may request are not always available in the local hospital. Rapid, safe transfer to a regional pediatric trauma center may be a lifesaving measure if instituted immediately after patient stabilization. The initial resuscitative phase, however, requires the availability of emergency equipment in appropriate sizes and quantities for this special patient population. A mobile cart dedicated to pediatric equipment aids effective patient management. Rapid access to appropriate personnel, such as nurses from the neonatal or pediatric intensive care units, and to resource manuals that include pediatric drug dosages, tube and drain sizes, and normal vital sign ranges also promotes quality care.

Associated care plans

Pediatric Airway Obstruction
Pediatric Gastric Distention
General Pediatric Care Considerations
Hemorrhagic Shock

Associated procedures

Preparation for Surgery
Pulmonary Artery Catheterization
Diagnostic Peritoneal Lavage
The Pneumatic Antishock Garment
Endotracheal Intubation
Needle Cricothyroidotomy

PEDIATRIC HYPOTHERMIA

Assessment

Mechanism of injury/ etiology:
- environmental exposure (cold outdoor temperature; lack of clothing or covering in ambulance, helicopter, and resuscitation area)
- infusion of I.V. fluids at or below room temperature
- burns or shock state

Physical findings:
Cardiovascular
- cyanosis
- skin cool or cold to touch

- shock state

Respiratory
- mild to severe distress

Diagnostic studies

- core temperature—less than 36° to 37° C.
- ABGs—reveal metabolic acidosis

Nursing diagnosis

Potential for hypothermia related to increased body surface area to body mass ratio, a limited amount of subcutaneous tissue, thin skin, inability to shiver in an unconscious state, and environmental exposure.

GOAL #1: Recognize and closely monitor patients at risk for hypothermia.

Interventions

1. Obtain the baseline temperature of all pediatric trauma patients on admission. Monitor core temperatures every 2 hours, or more frequently as the patient's condition warrants.

Rationale

Children, especially infants under the age of 6 months, have a large body surface area covered with relatively thin skin and limited subcutaneous tissue, which permit greater convectional heat loss. These anatomic features and immature homeostatic compensatory mechanisms predispose this patient to hypothermia. The risks increase dramatically when the infant or young child experiences environmental or physical changes that alter body temperature. Baseline and ongoing core temperature evaluation can aid early detection of hypothermia.

GOAL #2: Minimize further body heat loss. Maintain normothermia.

Interventions

1. Institute measures to prevent further heat loss including:
- removing wet diapers or clothing
- covering the child with warm, dry linen
- wrapping the infant's head in stockinette
- wrapping the child's head in a towel or sheet.

Rationale

The infant's or young child's thin skin and limited subcutaneous fat promote rapid body heat loss through evaporation. Admission priorities must include body heat preservation measures.

2. Institute passive rewarming measures, including:
- heated bed linen
- warming lights (with caution)
- hyperthermia blankets (with caution)
- warmed I.V. bags placed at the groin, axilla, neck
- isolette with warming unit, as available and appropriate for age and size.

Early institution of these passive rewarming techniques may suffice to restore and maintain a normal core temperature.

GOAL #3: Restore a core temperature of 36° to 37° C.

Interventions

1. Institute measures to rewarm core temperature, such as:
- warming all I.V.s either prior to infusion (in a warming machine) or during infusion (through a heated coil device)
- using heated nebulizers for supplemental oxygen administration or warming cascades for patients on mechanical ventilators
- warming blood prior to infusion either by mixing with warm normal saline solution (NSS) or by infusing through a heated coil device
- using warmed NSS or Ringer's lactate solution for diagnostic peritoneal lavage
- lavaging the stomach via a gastric decompression tube with warmed NSS.

2. Monitor the child's cardiovascular and respiratory status closely during rewarming, including:
- heart rate
- blood pressure
- ECG rhythm
- respiratory rate
- ABG results.

Rationale

Core rewarming measures are essential to prevent shock. This can occur when external rewarming is performed too rapidly or without regard to the core temperature. The heart, which is still cool, cannot adequately handle the sudden rush of blood from the periphery. In addition, external rewarming causes a rapid entry of acidotic blood into the central circulation, potentiating severe acidosis.

Calories and energy are expended as the child's body attempts to produce heat and restore a normal temperature. Catecholamine release during hypothermia affects the pulmonary vasculature, causing pulmonary hypertension and increased oxygen consumption through nonshivering thermogenesis. The results include energy depletion, hypoxia, and metabolic acidosis. Impaired tissue perfusion, life-threatening dysrhythmias, and severe acidosis are common sequelae of hypothermia.

Associated care plans

Hypothermia
General Pediatric Care Considerations

Associated procedure

Diagnostic Peritoneal Lavage

Medical diagnosis

PEDIATRIC GASTRIC DISTENTION

Assessment

Note: *Pediatric patients, especially infants, swallow a large amount of air as they cry. This accumulation of air in the stomach can lead to major ventilatory problems as the enlarged stomach pushes up on the diaphragm. Increased intrathoracic pressure impairs lung expansion, decreasing vital capacity.*

Mechanism of injury/ etiology:
- swallowed air (aerophagia) resulting from fear, crying
- incorrect placement of endotracheal tube
- paralytic ileus

Physical findings:
Gastrointestinal
- abdominal distention (crescendo or sudden onset)
- decreased or absent bowel sounds
- abdominal pain and discomfort (especially in left upper quadrant)

Respiratory
- shallow respirations
- tachypnea
- dyspnea
- respiratory distress or arrest (onset may be acute)

Diagnostic studies

- abdominal radiograph—may reveal distended stomach, bowel
- chest radiograph—may reveal elevated diaphragm
- gastric tube aspiration—detects large quantities of air

Nursing diagnosis

Ineffective breathing patterns related to diaphragmatic elevation secondary to gastric distention.

> **GOAL:** Prevent or minimize gastric distention.

Interventions

1. Avoid maneuvers that externally compress the stomach.

2. Ensure proper placement of a gastric decompression tube; maintain position, patency, and proper tube functioning.

3. Monitor the infant or child with an endotracheal tube continuously for proper tube placement, especially after suctioning and turning; auscultate breath sounds at least every hour and with any change in respiratory status; observe chest expansion.

Rationale

Any external pressure on the abdomen can further compress the stomach, causing the patient to vomit. *Aspiration is a major risk should this occur.*

Any severely injured pediatric trauma patient should receive a nasal or oral gastric decompression tube. A nasal tube is tolerated better but is contraindicated by head or facial injuries. An oral tube, although safer for a child with head or facial trauma, may become a problem if the child has teeth. Maintenance principles are the same as for the adult decompression tube.

The uncuffed pediatric endotracheal tube can easily become dislodged and slip into the esophagus, causing rapid gastric distention and respiratory distress. The child swiftly deteriorates to respiratory arrest without immediate intervention.

Associated care plans

Paralytic Ileus
Pediatric Airway Obstruction
General Pediatric Care Considerations

GENERAL PEDIATRIC CARE CONSIDERATIONS

To maximize the quality of care provided for the pediatric trauma patient, adult-oriented emergency care personnel must *be prepared prior to admission*. Waiting until this patient arrives in the resuscitation area to develop a plan and procure specially sized equipment is too late! Many aspects of traumatic injuries and principles of trauma care of the infant and child are similar to those of the adult trauma patient. Clearly, however, both prehospital and in-hospital personnel must recognize the problems inherent to this particular patient population and adapt their trauma knowledge base to meet these special needs. This section devotes primary attention to those areas in which care must be altered and priorities must be expanded.

Mechanism of injury

The pediatric patient falls victim to the same variety of traumatic mechanisms of injury as the adult; however, the patterns and zones of injury usually differ. A classic example is the pedestrian-automobile collision. The adult generally sustains tibia-fibula injuries, the so-called bumper fractures, whereas the child commonly sustains a femur injury. In adult trauma, specific mechanisms raise the suspicion of specific associated injuries. In pediatric trauma, this focal range of associated suspicions must shift slightly to facilitate accurate detection of underlying injuries.

Age and weight

Essentially all calculations for fluid replacement, drug administration, and tube and drain size and accurate evaluation of vital signs and output depend on the child's weight and age. Obtain the child's approximate age and weight as soon as possible, preferably prior to the child's arrival. This information individualizes preparation for resuscitation.

Equipment

All emergency care facilities should stock lifesaving equipment in pediatric sizes and adequate quantities. Rapid access to a sufficient selection of equipment is paramount to optimizing pediatric trauma care. This equipment should include airways, oxygen masks, a laryngoscope and blades, intravenous catheters, thoracostomy tubes, cervical collars, gastric tubes, urinary collection bags or indwelling catheters, internal and external defibrillator paddles, and surgical instruments. The pediatric inventory can be easily stored in a designated mobile cart or, if available, in the dedicated pediatric resuscitation room. Appendix 3, "Sample Trays and Specialty Carts Lists," lists the contents of a sample pediatric admission cart. This equipment should undergo routine checks for availability and proper functioning.

Drug dosages

Drug administration in the pediatric trauma patient commonly stresses even the most experienced emergency care personnel. Drug cards, with a variety of commonly used emergency drugs and precalculated dosages according to weight, offer one solution to ensure accuracy and allay personnel anxiety. After determining the child's weight, simply select the appropriate drug card from the file. See Table 6.2 for a basic sample that can be used as a guide.

Table 6.2

Weight—5 kg (11 lb)

Drug and concentration	Usual dose	Amount required
Sodium bicarbonate 1 mEq/cc	1 to 2 mEq/kg	5 to 10 mEq (5 to 10 cc)
Epinephrine 1:10,000 (0.1 mg/cc)	0.01 mg/kg (0.1 cc/kg)	0.5 cc
Atropine 0.1 mg/cc	0.02 mg/kg (0.02 cc/kg)	1 cc
Lidocaine 2% (20 mg/cc)	1 mg/kg (0.05 cc/kg)	0.25 cc

Respiratory considerations

Airway management is always the first priority in the pediatric trauma patient. Anatomic differences influence the incidence of potentially life-threatening pediatric injuries. The child's flexible thorax increases the risk of pulmonary contusions and traumatic asphyxia, yet it simultaneously decreases the incidence of sternal and rib fractures. Additionally, therapeutic measures (such as endotracheal intubation and suctioning, tube thoracostomy, and mechanical ventilation) carry greater risks in the infant and child because of their fragility and smaller anatomical size. Immediate and continuous evaluation of the child's airway and overall respiratory status promotes early detection of subtle changes and deteriorating trends. Rapid correction of airway and breathing problems minimizes the occurrence of further morbidity. The following formulas and guides facilitate appropriate management of pediatric respiratory problems.

- Endotracheal tube (ETT) size approximation

$$\frac{16 + \text{age in years}}{4}$$

For example, a 4-year-old would probably require a size 5 ETT.

☐ Premature infants generally require a 2.5-mm tube; newborns, a 3.5-mm tube.

☐ Other quick correlative estimators are the diameter of the child's fifth finger and external nares measurement.

Note: *These methods only provide a general guide. Tubes one size larger and one size smaller should be readily available at the bedside.*

- Tidal volume—6 cc/kg = appropriate tidal volume
- Chest tube sizes and suction amounts

☐ small children—#12 French tube/10 cm water suction

☐ larger children/adolescents—#20 to #24 French tube/20 cm water suction

- Chest tube drainage

☐ >1 to 2 cc/kg/hour without slowing requires further investigation

Cardiovascular considerations

The emphasis in this area is on constant observation and monitoring and accurate data evaluation. Early detection of a shock state in the infant or child is more difficult because of the delayed appearance of obvious signs and symptoms of shock. The following formulas aid accurate evaluation of hemodynamic data and may be used as guides for resuscitation:

- Normal vital signs

☐ systolic pressure—80 + twice the child's age (ages 1 to 20 yrs)

☐ diastolic pressure—⅔ the systolic pressure

- Blood volume per body weight

☐ 8% to 9% of total body weight (80 to 90 cc/kg)—all ages

- I.V. access—listed in order of preference with appropriate catheter sizes (sizes vary, however, with age/weight of the child)

☐ distal saphenous vein cutdown (ankle)—at least 20G

☐ upper extremity vein—20G to 25G

☐ femoral vein percutaneous—22G for small infants, 20G for older children

☐ proximal saphenous or femoral vein cutdown—18G to 20G

☐ external or internal jugular percutaneous or cutdown—difficult during resuscitation

☐ subclavian vein percutaneous—LAST RESORT

- Fluid resuscitation guidelines

☐ initial bolus—10 to 20 cc/kg of Ringer's lactate solution given as an I.V. push

☐ repeat I.V. bolus—if no significant hemodynamic change

☐ blood transfusion—started if patient remains unstable after two I.V. boluses of crystalloid solution

  - packed RBCs—10 cc/kg
  - whole blood—20 cc/kg
  - fresh-frozen plasma—20 cc/kg
  - platelets—10 cc/kg
  - 5% albumin—20 cc/kg
  - 25% albumin—4 cc/kg

- Fluid maintenance guidelines

☐ 0 to 10 kg—100 cc/kg/24 hours

☐ 11 to 20 kg—1,000 cc + 50 cc/kg/24 hours over 10 kg

☐ 21 to 40 kg—1,500 cc + 20 cc/kg/24 hours over 20 kg

☐ 40 kg—2,500 cc/24 hours
- Defibrillation guidelines
  ☐ 2 watt-seconds/kg—external defibrillation of the child
- Urine output

☐ generally 1 to 2 cc/kg/hour of urine output for the younger child represents adequate volume and tissue perfusion; 0.5 to 1 cc/kg/hour is satisfactory in older children.

Neurologic considerations

Head injuries, occurring in approximately 50% of all pediatric trauma victims, and the pediatric concussion syndrome demand early recognition and prompt intervention for optimal outcomes. Close observation of clinical signs and intracranial pressure via subarachnoid bolts and use of computerized tomography (CT) scans facilitate appropriate care. Definitive care for head-injured children is similar to that for adults. Measures to prevent further cerebral edema, lower intracranial pressure, and optimize oxygenation and perfusion must be initiated. Suspected spinal cord injuries in the child require the same precautions and precise care as in the adult. Rigid cervical collars available in various sizes should be readily available on the pediatric cart. Some small adult collars can be cut down to the appropriate size for younger children. Remember—a collar that is too small can impinge on the child's airway; one too large will be ineffective. Manual in-line cervical traction is a priority if such equipment is not immediately available. Additionally, the frightened child will not lie still and generally requires restraints, even with a collar in place, to prevent twisting.

Gastrointestinal considerations

The spleen and liver are the organs most commonly injured by abdominal trauma, in the child as in the adult. Diagnosis of intraabdominal injury may be confirmed by diagnostic peritoneal lavage (DPL) or a CT scan, the preferred tool. The indications and procedures for these diagnostic studies are the same as in the adult. Indwelling urinary catheter and gastric decompression tube insertion prior to DPL are essential to reduce the risk of complications as in the adult. A child's bladder sits higher in the abdomen than an adult's bladder and therefore is at greater risk for injury. Gastric distention is a common complication in the young child and requires treatment prior to DPL. The recommended ratio for infusing fluid for DPL is 15 cc/kg. Surgical intervention generally occurs only when the child remains unstable. Although surgical techniques are similar for the child and the adult, therapy is usually more conservative. Salvage of the spleen and liver are high priorities in the pediatric patient.

Resources and referrals

The involvement of specialty personnel—such as pediatricians, pediatric surgeons, neonatologists, and pediatric or neonatal nurses—on the emergency resuscitation team optimizes recovery potential. To maximize the chances of involving these specialists in the acute resuscitation phase, notify them as soon as possible of an incoming pediatric admission. Keep pertinent information, such as *current* phone numbers, readily accessible on top of the pediatric admission cart. For circumstances in which these specialists and dedicated pediatric or neonatal intensive care units are unavailable, a system for referral and transfer to a regional pediatric trauma center should be established. Rapid, safe transport of the injured child to such a specialty center by personnel proficient in pediatric care is essential.

Summary

Adult-oriented emergency care personnel may have understandable difficulty remembering all the formulas for pediatric calculations. A well-formatted "Resuscitation Reminders" sheet can make pediatric resuscitation guidelines readily accessible. Using Table 6.3, similar sheets can be developed for a wide range of patient weights and kept in a binder or file box on the pediatric admission cart for easy access and quick referral. Table 6.3 has been precalculated for the child weighing 5 kg. If a computer system is available in your facility, this information can be programmed for quick bedside access. Hard copies can be printed and kept at the bedside for continued use after resuscitation.

Table 6.3

Sample Resuscitation Reminders Sheet
Weight—5 kg (11 lb)

ETT size—4 (16 + child's age in years ÷ 4); have sizes 3.5 and 4.5 available also
Tidal volume—30 cc (6 cc/kg)
Blood volume—400 to 450 cc (8% to 9% of weight in kg)
Systolic blood pressure—80 mm Hg (80 + twice the age)
Crystalloid fluid bolus—100 cc (20 cc/kg)
Blood product infusion
        packed RBCs—50 cc (10 cc/kg)
        whole blood—100 cc (20 cc/kg)
        plasma—100 cc (20 cc/kg)
        platelets—50 cc (10 cc/kg)
        5% albumin—100 cc (20 cc/kg)
        25% albumin—20 cc (4 cc/kg)
Fluid maintenance—500 cc/24 hours (100 cc/kg/24 hours)
Defibrillation—10 watt-seconds (2 watt-seconds/kg)
Chest tube drainage concern—>22 cc/hr (>2 cc/kg/hr)
Urine output adequacy—>5 to 10 cc/hr (1 to 2 cc/kg/hour)
DPL infusion—75 cc (15 cc/kg)

Drug dosages:

Drug/concentration	Usual dose	Give
Sodium bicarbonate 1 mEq/cc	1 to 2 mEq/kg	5 to 10 mEq (5 to 10 cc)
Epinephrine 1:10,000 (0.1 mg/cc)	0.01 mg/kg (0.1 cc/kg)	0.5 cc
Atropine 0.1 mg/cc	0.02 mg/kg (0.02 cc/kg)	1 cc
Lidocaine 2% (20 mg/cc)	1 mg/kg (0.05 cc/kg)	0.25 cc

Medical diagnosis

PSYCHOSOCIAL SUPPORT OF THE CHILD

Note: *Providing appropriate quality care for the pediatric patient requires that all personnel consider the emotional as well as the physical needs of the child. Expect some degree of anxiety in any child recently traumatized. This care plan addresses anxiety in general because symptomatology varies with the specific age group and developmental maturity. Remember—the parents are an important part of the team! Provide them with emotional support and honest, complete information to decrease their anxiety.*

Nursing diagnosis

Potential for anxiety related to sudden hospitalization, separation from parents, fear of the unknown, and pain.

GOAL #1: Promote and maintain an atmosphere of trust and security.

Interventions	Rationale
1. Call the child by name whenever possible. Make sure the patient knows your name.	The first step in developing a trusting relationship is calling the child by his name or favorite nickname. He will feel more secure if he knows his nurse's name and thus who to call.
2. Approach children of any age slowly and at their eye level. Minimize the use of face masks, unless absolutely necessary.	Children can easily feel overwhelmed and threatened when approached by an adult stranger who advances rapidly and maintains a standing position. Conversations should also be held using direct eye contact. Most children respond well and feel more secure when approached by a smiling face.

GOAL #2: Minimize anxiety related to separation.

Interventions	Rationale
1. Allow the parents to remain with the child, as appropriate for injury severity.	Separation from parents is a major source of anxiety and fear. Parental presence when practical during procedures may lessen the child's anxiety. Parents should also be permitted and encouraged to participate in the child's care, as appropriate, to lessen feelings of helplessness.
2. Avoid leaving the child alone whenever possible.	Children from ages 1 to 5 can not only accomplish a significant amount of destruction when your back is turned, but generally have a great fear of physical separation.

GOAL #3: Promote the child's understanding.

Interventions	Rationale
1. Provide the child with simple explanations that he can understand, based on his age and developmental stage. Ask him questions to determine if he desires more information and to identify specific coping mechanisms in use.	Children 1 to 3 years old can understand language and simple information much better than their verbal skills would lead you to believe. The 3- to 5-year-old spends a great deal of time fantasizing and imagining. Children over the age of 5 can more fully understand information concerning procedures, injuries, and equipment. School-aged children may cope with their anxiety by avoiding or denying the situation or by becoming actively involved in their own care. The amount of information needed and desired depends on the coping strategy in use. Anxiety may decrease in younger children or in those using active coping when simple, yet honest, explanations are provided and when the child feels comfortable asking questions. Children avoiding or denying their situation may become more anxious or worried if offered too many or too-detailed explanations.
2. Avoid placing the child in an area close to more critically ill patients. Attempt to shield the child from traumatic events or sights in the patient care area.	The imagination of the young child and his limited knowledge and ability to reason may cause misinterpretation of what he sees in the emergency or intensive care areas. He may be convinced that these events will happen to him next.
3. Be alert for and limit any inappropriate conversations at the child's bedside.	Although the child is unable to comprehend the words of inappropriate conversations—such as discussions about his medical condition—he can detect and understand the tone of voice used. The active imagination of a young child may easily lead to misinterpretation and increased anxiety.
4. Eliminate or minimize unnecessary studies and examinations.	Repeated studies or examinations, especially those associated with pain, may cause the child severe anticipatory fear, making further procedures even more difficult for both the child and the caregivers.
5. Provide the child with honest answers, especially regarding pain.	The worst possible situation for any child is to have someone tell him "This will not hurt a bit" and then proceed with a painful procedure. Gentle warnings about pain promote a sense of trust in that the child begins to believe you will not lie to him. Children are sensitive to feelings of uneasiness in others and can generally sense when something is wrong. It is best to be honest with the child to maintain his trust.
6. Permit the child to participate in his own care whenever possible.	Even young children can usually perform some small task or activity; this encourages their feelings of independence and autonomy.
7. Allow the child to make choices whenever appropriate.	Patients of all ages usually experience some feelings of powerlessness, and this is true of the child as well. Helping to make plans or a decision regarding his care promotes feelings of independence.

8. Allow the child to keep a favorite toy, book, pillow, or other object in bed. Hang brightly colored objects from the side rails or as a mobile for infants.

These objects may help the child feel more secure in the strange hospital environment and offer valuable stimulation and, at times, distraction.

9. Encourage parents to bring in familiar objects, pictures, tape recordings, or cards.

These items can lessen the severity of the child's feelings of separation and loneliness.

10. Permit parents and family members to visit and call the patient frequently, as appropriate.

Visits and phone calls from family and friends strengthen the child's preexisting support systems.

Associated care plan

Psychosocial Support of the Trauma Patient

REFERENCES

PEDIATRIC TRAUMA

Carnevale, F.A. "Nursing the Critically Ill Child—A Responsive Approach," *Focus on Critical Care* 12(5):10, October 1985.

Cooney, D.R. "Splenic and Hepatic Trauma in Children," *Surgical Clinics of North America* 61(5):1165, October 1981.

Eichelberger, M.R. "Trauma," in *Life-Threatening Episodes in Infants and Children.* Kalamazoo, Mich.: Upjohn Co., 1983.

Eichelberger, M.R., and Randolph, J.G. "Complications of Pediatric Surgery and Trauma," in *Complications in Surgery and Trauma.* Edited by Greenfield, L.J. Philadelphia: J.B. Lippincott Co., 1984.

Eichelberger, M.R., and Randolph, J.G. "Pediatric Trauma: An Algorithm for Diagnosis and Therapy," *Journal of Trauma* 23(2):91-97, February 1983.

Eichelberger, M.R., and Randolph, J.G. "Thoracic Trauma in Children," *Surgical Clinics of North America* 61(5):1181, October 1981.

Elkins, R.C. "Complications of Intubation, Tracheal Surgery, and Trauma," in *Complications in Surgery and Trauma.* Edited by Greenfield, L.J. Philadelphia: J.B. Lippincott Co., 1984.

Haller, J.A., et al. "Trauma and the Child," in *The Management of Trauma,* 4th ed. Edited by Zuidema, G.D., et al. Philadelphia: W.B. Saunders Co., 1985.

Herrin, J.T., et al. "Neonatal and Pediatric Emergencies," in *MGH Textbook of Emergency Medicine,* 2nd ed. Edited by Wilkins, E.W. Baltimore: Williams & Wilkins Co., 1983.

Hoover, D.L. "Genitourinary Trauma," *Topics in Emergency Medicine* 4(3):55-60, October 1982.

Jastremski, M.S., et al. "Pediatrics," in *The Whole Emergency Medicine Catalog.* Philadelphia: W.B. Saunders Co., 1985.

Jennings, C. "Children's Understanding of Death and Dying," *Focus on Critical Care* 13(1):41-45, February 1986.

Kim, S.H. "Pediatric Surgical Emergencies," in *MGH Textbook of Emergency Medicine,* 2nd ed. Edited by Wilkins, E.W. Baltimore: Williams & Wilkins Co., 1983.

LaMontagne, L.L. "Facilitating Children's Coping—Preoperative Assessment Interviews," *AORN Journal* 42(5):718, November 1985.

Raphaely, R.C., et al. "Management of Severe Pediatric Head Trauma," *Pediatric Clinics of North America* 27(3), August 1980.

Rowe, M.I., and Marchildon, M.B. "Pediatric Trauma," in *Critical Care State of the Art* vol. 2. Society of Critical Care Medicine, 1981.

Schraeder, B.D., and Donar, M.E. "The Child with Chronic Respiratory Failure: A Special Challenge," in *Neonatal and Pediatric Critical Care Nursing.* Edited by Stahler-Miller, K. New York: Churchill Livingstone, 1983.

Slota, M.C., and Beerman, L.B. "Congenital Heart Disease: Perioperative Nursing Management," in *Neonatal and Pediatric Critical Care Nursing.* Edited by Stahler-Miller, K. New York: Churchill Livingstone, 1983.

Surgical Staff—The Hospital for Sick Children—Toronto. *Care for The Injured Child.* Baltimore: Williams & Wilkins Co., 1975.

Ward, J.D. "Central Nervous System Trauma," *Topics in Emergency Medicine* 4(3):11-18, October 1982.

Weber, T.R., and Grosfeld, J.L. "Abdominal Injuries in Children," *Topics in Emergency Medicine* 4(3):41-53, October 1982.

Weibley, R.E., and Holbrook, P.R. "Airway Management in the Traumatized Child," *Topics in Emergency Medicine* 4(3):1-7, October 1982.

STUDIES AND
PROCEDURES

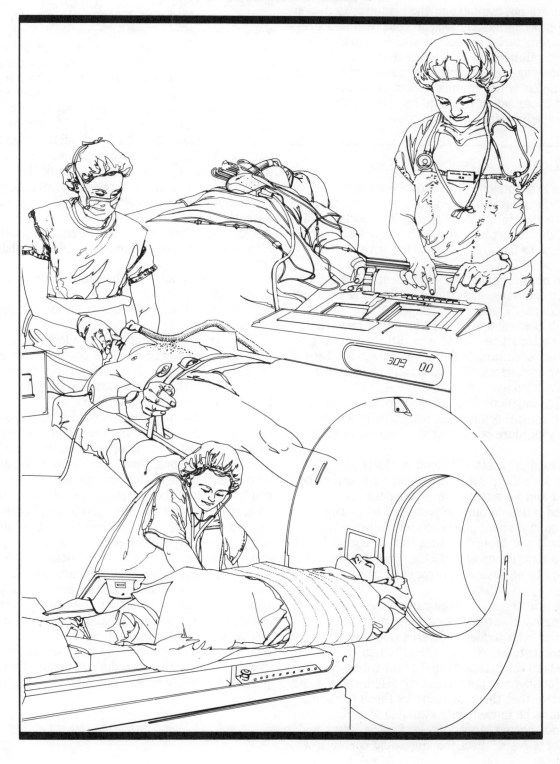

Procedure

INTRAHOSPITAL TRANSPORT OF THE SHOCK TRAUMA PATIENT

Indications

Evaluation of the traumatized patient may require procedures that are not available in the acute resuscitation area. These procedures may include computed tomography scans, angiography, nuclear medicine scans, echocardiography, multiple-gated acquisition scans, magnetic resonance imaging, and myelography among others.

Transportation of the trauma patient requires forethought and coordination if it is to be accomplished safely and expeditiously.

Preparation

1. Verify the appointment time with the technician or physician performing the procedure.
2. If the patient is intubated, find out if a ventilator is available in the department to which you are traveling. If not, arrange to have one transported with the patient.
3. Assemble or arrange for the equipment and supplies necessary to continue patient care while away from the resuscitation area. These may include:
• portable ECG monitor—During the initial resuscitation phase, each patient should have ECG monitoring regardless of his condition. If the monitor does not have an AC power cord, start off with a fully charged battery and take a spare.
• arterial line monitor—This allows continuous monitoring of the critical or unstable patient without interrupting the procedure or risking staff exposure to radiation.
• blood or blood products—If blood products are to be transported with the patient, a method for keeping the blood cooled and for monitoring its temperature is required. Blood products may be protected by placing them over ice in a small plastic cooler. Adhesive temperature labels are applied to each unit to ensure blood remains at a safe temperature. This type of transport system needs to be designed in cooperation with the blood bank.
• surgically oriented emergency cart—Most "crash" carts are geared toward the medical arrest. The trauma patient who suddenly deteriorates may require surgical interventions, such as the initiation of additional large-bore lines, insertion of chest tubes, surgical cricothyroidotomy, and open chest cardiac compression. It is imperative that the equipment for these resuscitative procedures be immediately available wherever this patient is transported. Appendix 3, "Sample Trays and Specialty Carts Lists," lists the suggested contents of this type of cart.

• patient-specific drugs—If the patient requires any nonemergency drugs, such as sedatives, neuromuscular blockers, or antibiotics, during transport, include them on the emergency cart.
• portable suction—Suction capability during transport is essential, as is backup suction equipment in the event that equipment at the patient's destination fails.
• sufficient portable oxygen supply—The trauma patient may need to be away from the resuscitation area for a prolonged period. Portable oxygen cylinders on the stretcher and emergency cart provide oxygen during transport. (Remember: An E cylinder oxygen tank running at 10 liters/minute will last approximately 50 minutes.) Arrange for a large oxygen tank (H or M cylinder) to be available if one is not routinely kept in the destination department or if wall oxygen is not available.
• immediate elevator access—Several possibilities exist for ensuring that an elevator is readily available. Among these are:
☐ calling ahead if the hospital staffs patient elevators with elevator operators
☐ sending a staff member to obtain an elevator in advance
☐ carrying emergency keys to lock the elevator.
• orthopedic equipment—This could include either splints or traction devices for fractures or equipment to aid in moving the patient, such as long wooden backboards and breakaway stretchers.
4. Assemble the personnel needed to transport the patient safely. At a minimum, the trauma patient should be accompanied by a nurse and physician familiar with the patient and proficient in trauma resuscitation and airway management. Support personnel necessary to safely transport the patient and equipment should accompany the patient. These people will be needed to assist with transfer of the patient from stretcher to table while protecting the patient's airway and cervical spine. Additional personnel may include a CRNA or anesthesiologist to manage the patient's airway and ventilator and a second nurse to assist with patient care. The patient's primary nurse should coordinate all team members to ensure that all personnel are readily available at the departure time.
5. When the patient is ready to travel, call the technician performing the procedure to ensure that the department is ready for the patient.

Contraindications

Absolute contraindication to transporting the patient out of the resuscitation area:
- unstable airway.

Relative contraindications to transporting the patient out of the resuscitation area (to anywhere except the operating room) include:
- unstable hemodynamic status
- use of high levels of positive end-expiratory pressure (PEEP) where equipment is not available to maintain PEEP during transport
- inadequate staff to safely transport the patient.

Nursing interventions
(During transport and procedures)

1. Assess the patient frequently while in transit and during procedures. This assessment should be performed as dictated by the patient's condition and should include:
- respiratory status
- cardiovascular status
- neurologic status
- allergic reactions to contrast materials
- neurovascular status of fractured extremities.

2. Verify that the patient understands the procedure to be performed. Provide additional explanations, as necessary. This will promote patient compliance and protect his right to informed consent.

3. Maintain communications with the resuscitation area or operating room concerning patient needs upon arrival.

4. Prepare for and coordinate return to the resuscitation area in the same manner as departure.

THERAPEUTIC EMBOLIZATION (T.E.)

Indications

Posttraumatic, postsurgical hemorrhage:
- bleeding associated with pelvic injury
- intraabdominal bleeding.

Preparation

The trauma patient needing transcatheter TE is critically unstable and bleeding uncontrollably. Transportation of such a patient to the radiography suite requires careful planning and coordination by all team members responsible for his care. Refer to "Intrahospital Transport of the Shock Trauma Patient" in Section VII for guidelines on safely transporting such a patient.

Description of procedure

1. The puncture site (usually femoral artery) is surgically prepared and draped.
2. The arterial puncture is performed by the physician.
3. A guide wire is inserted through a needle, then the needle is removed.
4. A catheter is threaded over the guide wire and positioned in the area of suspected bleeding.
5. An angiographic study with contrast material is done to locate the bleeding site.
6. The catheter is positioned at the bleeding site.
7. Embolic material is injected through the catheter.
8. An angiographic study with contrast material is done to confirm embolization.
9. The catheter is removed after procedure completion.
10. Pressure is applied to the arterial puncture site for at least 10 minutes, after which a dressing is applied.

Potential complications

- recurrence of bleeding owing to failure of embolization
- nausea and vomiting after contrast material injection
- bleeding and hematoma formation at catheter insertion site
- development of pseudoaneurysm at arterial puncture site
- arteriovenous fistula
- subintimal dissection
- allergic reaction to contrast material
- vascular occlusion distal to arterial puncture site caused by thrombi dislodgement during catheter insertion

Nursing interventions

1. Assist in positioning the patient supine on the radiography table.
2. Explain all procedures to the patient; warn him about the "flushed" feeling he will experience after the contrast material injection as well as about possible nausea and vomiting.
3. Ensure placement of a gastric tube connected to suction for a patient who cannot protect his own airway.
4. Monitor and document vital signs, including intake and output, before, during, and after the procedure. Contrast material will cause diuresis.
5. Monitor the patient after the procedure for recurrent bleeding from failure of embolization.
6. Monitor the catheter insertion site for bleeding and hematoma formation and assess and document the quality of pulses distal to the catheter insertion site as follows:
- every 15 minutes for the next 4 hours
- every hour for the next 8 hours
- then every 8 hours.

AORTOGRAPHY

Indications

Determination of structural integrity of the aorta when:
• a widened mediastinum is evident on a true erect chest radiograph
• findings suggest an injured aorta.

Preparation

The shock trauma patient undergoing aortography may be critically unstable. Transportation of such a patient to the radiography suite requires careful planning and coordination by all team members responsible for his care. Refer to "Intrahospital Transport of the Shock Trauma Patient" in Section VII for guidelines on safely transporting such a patient.

Description of study

1. The selected arterial puncture site (usually femoral) is surgically prepared and draped.
2. An arterial puncture is performed by the physician.
3. A guide wire is inserted through the needle.
4. A catheter is threaded over the guide wire; the distal end is positioned next to the aortic valve.
5. Contrast medium is injected through the catheter.
6. Radiographs are taken during the injection period.
7. The catheter is removed after the procedure.
8. Pressure is applied to the arterial puncture site for a minimum of 10 minutes.
9. The patient is kept on bed rest 8 to 12 hours post-study to reduce the risk of bleeding at the arterial puncture site.

Potential complications

• nausea and vomiting after contrast injection
• bleeding and hematoma formation at arterial puncture site
• pseudoaneurysm
• arteriovenous fistula
• subintimal dissection
• vascular occlusion distal to arterial puncture site, resulting from thrombi material dislodged during catheter insertion
• allergic reaction to contrast medium
• guide wire or catheter breakage
• vascular compromise of extremity if arterial compression results from hematoma formation around arterial puncture site

Nursing interventions

1. Assist with supine positioning of the patient on the aortography table. Further position the patient during the study; for example, turn him from side to side or position his arms over his head, as required.
2. Explain the procedure to the patient, especially the "flushed" feeling that occurs after contrast medium injection and the possibility of nausea and vomiting.
3. Monitor and document vital signs (including intake and output) before, during, and after the study. Expect the contrast medium to have a diuretic effect.
4. Ensure insertion and proper placement of the gastric tube; connect tube to the suction if the patient is unable to protect his airway.
5. Monitor the arterial puncture site for poststudy bleeding and hematoma formation, and assess and document the quality of pulses distal to the puncture site as follows:
• every 15 minutes for 1 hour
• every 30 minutes for the next 2 hours
• every hour for the next 8 hours
• then every 8 hours.
6. Explain to the patient why he will need to maintain bed rest after the study.

POSITIVE CONTRAST STUDY

Indications

Determination of the structural integrity of organs or vessels.

Preparation

The study determines the preparations needed. Many contrast studies can be performed in the emergency department with portable radiographic equipment. Studies include one-shot arteriography, intravenous pyelography, esophagography, cystography, and urethrography. Intrathecal contrast medium injections for myelographic studies can be given while the patient is in the emergency department before he is taken to the radiographic department.

If the patient must be transported out of the unit, see "Intrahospital Transport of the Shock Trauma Patient" in Section VII. Ask the patient about his allergies to contrast dyes. Determine the contrast material to be used, its potential adverse reactions, and the procedural precautions required (contrast studies using intrathecal injection of iohexol or metrizamide require discontinuing any neuroleptic drugs 48 hours before injection).

Description of study

Positive contrast materials are introduced into the region being studied via an intravenous, intraarterial, intrathecal, or oral route. The contrast medium increases or decreases the structural density in relation to surrounding tissue, permitting visualization and evaluation.

Potential complications

Reaction to contrast material, including:
- anaphylactic shock
- seizures
- hypotension with peripheral vascular collapse
- cardiac arrest

Nursing interventions

1. Explain the procedure to the patient.
2. Closely monitor the patient for a reaction to contrast material during and after the procedure; some reactions may be delayed.
3. Monitor the patient's vital signs and intake and output. Many contrast materials have a diuretic effect, and the patient may need fluid replacement.
4. Ensure that poststudy patient management is performed according to the physician's orders and your institution's policy. Special attention must be given to a patient receiving an intrathecal injection of iohexol or metrizamide for at least 12 hours following the myelogram. Actions include the following:
- Strictly monitor the patient's position and movement—he should be supine, the head of the bed elevated or in reverse Trendelenburg position, and his movements kept passive for the first 6 to 8 hours.
- Avoid the use of phenothiazines.
- Ensure adequate hydration.
- Promote patient and family understanding of the need to maintain head elevation.

Study

NUCLEAR MEDICINE IMAGING

Indications

Determination of organ structural abnormalities, perfusion, and function.

Preparation

No specific preparation is required for nuclear medicine imaging. See "Intrahospital Transport of the Shock Trauma Patient" in Section VII for instructions on transporting the patient out of the unit.

Description of study

A radiopharmaceutical containing a radioisotope is administered—most often by I.V. route. Through detection devices, images are produced showing the radioisotope's distribution within the organ being studied. The time between injecting the radioisotope and imaging varies according to the study. Typically, the patient is studied in the supine position, but renal and pulmonary imaging may be performed with the patient sitting up.

Nursing interventions

1. Explain the procedure to the patient.
2. Assist in positioning the patient as necessary.
3. Monitor the patient's vital signs during the procedure.
4. Follow the nuclear medicine department's guidelines for proper handling and disposal of the patient's radioactive blood and urine.

Procedure

DIAGNOSTIC PERITONEAL LAVAGE (D.P.L.)

Indications

Diagnostic peritoneal lavage is a safe, highly accurate, and rapid diagnostic procedure to confirm or rule out intraperitoneal bleeding. Results reflect the severity of injury and confirm or negate the need for an exploratory laparotomy. Previously, this procedure was reserved for patients with blunt abdominal trauma and associated injuries. However, DPL use has gained acceptance for certain types of penetrating abdominal trauma. A DPL should be performed in patients with:

- a history of blunt abdominal trauma
- a tender or painful abdomen
- thoracic or lumbar spine fractures
- pelvic fractures
- alteration in levels of consciousness or sensation
- unexplained shock state
- a penetrating abdominal injury with stable hemodynamics and an intact peritoneal cavity.

Preparation

Equipment
- sterile tray with surgical instruments
- trocar-reinforced dialysis catheter
- suture material: chromic, vicryl, gut, or nylon, as requested
- preparation razor
- 1-liter bottle or bag of Ringer's lactate (RL) solution or normal saline solution (NSS) and I.V. tubing
- red-top blood sample tube (without anticoagulant or preservative)
- gastric decompression tube/suction apparatus
- urinary catheterization equipment

Description of procedure

1. Insert an indwelling urinary catheter and gastric decompression tube before the procedure.
2. The abdomen is surgically prepared and draped.
3. A local anesthetic (lidocaine containing epinephrine) is injected into the subcutaneous tissue lateral to the umbilicus or, if a pelvic fracture is suspected, above the umbilicus.
4. The physician incises to the peritoneum, assuring hemostasis to prevent false-positive results.
5. A peritoneal puncture is made with the trocar-reinforced catheter.
6. After trocar removal, the catheter is gently advanced down toward the pelvis.
7. The catheter may be *gently* aspirated, as needed.
Note: *Aspiration may cause omentum to clog the small catheter holes and impede fluid return.*

8. If 10 cc or more of frank blood is aspirated, the catheter is removed and the patient taken to the operating room for an exploratory laparotomy.
9. If no blood is aspirated, infuse 1 liter of RL or NSS into the peritoneal cavity and allow the fluid to return by gravity.
10. Send a sample of returned fluid for RBC and WBC counts.
11. If lavage results are positive, the wound is temporarily packed; if negative, the wound is sutured and a dressing applied.

Interpretation of results

Absolute positive results:
- 10 cc or more of frank blood aspirate
- RBC count 100,000/mm^3 or more
- WBC count 500/mm^3 or more
- bile, feces, or bacteria in return fluid

Potential complications

- puncture of stomach, bladder, vasculature, or intestine
- false-positive/false-negative results
- infection

Nursing interventions

1. Promote patient understanding before the procedure.
2. Ensure that all personnel observe sterile procedure policy (wear mask, hat, and gloves).
3. Prepare the diagnostic peritoneal lavage tray.
4. Ensure urinary catheter and gastric decompression tube insertion prior to beginning the procedure.
5. Position the patient as required:
- supine during procedure
- slight Trendelenburg during infusion (unless contraindicated)
- reverse Trendelenburg during fluid return (unless contraindicated).
6. Tell the patient the sensations he may feel during the procedure (fullness or pressure during infusion) are normal.
7. Monitor respiratory status during infusion.
8. Send a return-fluid sample for laboratory analysis.
9. Apply a sterile dressing.
10. Note the volume of any retained lavage fluid in intake record.
11. Document the procedure and its effects on the patient.
12. Prepare the patient for surgery as appropriate.

ENDOSCOPY

Indications

Situations requiring visualization of, or access for aspiration and biopsy of, the esophagus, stomach, and duodenum—most commonly used for suspected:
- peptic ulcer disease
- upper GI bleeding
- hiatal hernia.

Also used prior to upper GI surgery and to augment diagnosis of:
- chest or abdominal pain of unknown etiology
- esophageal varices
- gastric outlet obstruction
- neoplasms of the esophagus, stomach, or duodenum.

Contraindications

- patient refusal or uncooperativeness
- shock state
- suspected visceral perforation
- myocardial infarction
- pneumonia
- thoracic aneurysm
- active bleeding that precludes visualization

Preparation

Equipment
- sedatives, anesthetics, as ordered
- topical anesthetic
- oral airway or bite block
- suction apparatus
- endoscope with light source

Adjunctive equipment
- ECG monitor, defibrillator
- emergency intubation equipment, drugs (see "Endotracheal Intubation" in Section VII)
- emergency crash cart

Description of study

1. Sedation or a mild anesthetic is administered prior to the study.
2. The oropharynx is anesthetized with topical anesthetic spray to reduce discomfort and block the gag reflex.
3. The endoscope is lubricated and passed through the nose or mouth.
4. The esophagus, stomach, and duodenum are visualized in turn.
5. Biopsy material or washing specimens are obtained after visualization.

Potential complications

- esophageal tear, rupture, perforation
- aspiration
- respiratory distress or arrest
- cardiac irritability, such as ventricular tachycardia, atrial fibrillation, cardiac arrest
- increased GI bleeding

Nursing interventions

1. Confirm that patient has been NPO for at least 6 hours prior to the study.
2. Promote patient understanding and verify consent.
3. Position the patient as requested by the physician:
- supine with head hyperextended
- left lateral recumbent
- semi-Fowler's.
4. Remove dentures.
5. Reassure the patient concerning sensations associated with local oropharyngeal anesthesia and cramping pain as the scope enters the pylorus.
6. Have emergency equipment and suction readily available at the bedside; turn the equipment on.
7. Monitor the patient's ECG rhythm continuously.
8. Monitor the patient's cardiopulmonary status closely throughout the study.
9. Monitor and report signs indicating complications immediately; these include:
- dyspnea
- chest or midepigastric pain
- epigastric spasms
- abdominal pain
- tachycardia
- cyanosis
- diaphoresis
- mediastinal air evident on chest radiograph.

The incidence of complications has been significantly reduced with the development of smaller, more flexible endoscopes. Poststudy patient observation is necessary, however, as signs and symptoms of complications may not manifest themselves for 24 hours.
10. Maintain NPO status until the patient's gag reflex is intact.
11. Administer analgesics after the study, as ordered, for oropharyngeal discomfort.
12. Document effects of the study, patient responses, and all nursing interventions.

BRONCHOSCOPY (FIBEROPTIC)

Indications

Upper airway structures and bronchi may be directly visualized for diagnostic evaluation or intubation in structural damage. Smoke inhalation, burns, direct trauma, or posttraumatic respiratory complications may require evaluative or diagnostic bronchoscopy. Deep suctioning of the lungs may be required for cultures and pulmonary hygiene. Also, bronchial washings or biopsies can be performed for cytologic studies. Some aspirated objects are retrievable by bronchoscopic means.

Preparation

Equipment
- flexible bronchoscope
- light source
- sterile normal saline solution (NSS), for irrigation
- lidocaine jelly or lubricant
- 2% lidocaine for local anesthesia
- two small cups for saline and lidocaine solutions
- two 10-cc syringes
- swivel adapter for endotracheal tube
- suction tubing
- topical lidocaine spray
- sterile gloves
- ten 4 × 4 sponges
- table drape

Description of study

1. Preoperative sedation is given as ordered.
2. Ventilatory patients are placed on 100% oxygen for 5 minutes.

3. Nonintubated patients' throats are anesthetized with a topical lidocaine spray.
4. As the bronchoscope is introduced and advanced, lidocaine is locally applied through it.
5. NSS is used for irrigation, pulmonary hygiene, or obtaining bronchial washings.
6. Biopsy specimens may also be obtained.

Nursing interventions

1. Explain the procedure to the patient.
2. Place the patient on an ECG monitor.
3. Record vital signs taken before the procedure.
4. Administer supplemental oxygen for nonintubated patients as ordered; patients on ventilators are placed on 100% oxygen for 5 minutes.
5. Vital signs are taken and monitored as the patient's condition warrants during and after the procedure.
6. Blood gases may be obtained.
7. Culture and specimens are labeled and sent to the appropriate laboratory.
8. Nonintubated patients are monitored for the return of the gag reflex and kept NPO until it returns.

PULMONARY ARTERY CATHETERIZATION

Indications

Measurement and management of hemodynamic parameters in the following:
- shock states
  - ☐ hemorrhagic
  - ☐ cardiogenic
  - ☐ vasogenic
- adult respiratory distress syndrome
- pulmonary thromboembolus
- pulmonary edema.

Preparation

Equipment (skin preparation and drape phase)
- multiuse tray (see Appendix 3)
- accepted scrub and solution
- masks
- sterile gloves
- sterile laparotomy sheet

Equipment (insertion phase)
- ECG monitor
- 100-mg lidocaine bolus
- transducers and related monitoring equipment
- sterile gloves and gown(s)
- 14G or 16G needle with 5-cc or 10-cc syringe for venipuncture
- introducer and guide wire set
- pulmonary artery catheter
- 3-cc syringe for balloon (usually supplied with catheter)
- 3-0 nylon suture
- sterile dressing supplies
- I.V. solution and tubing for venous infusion port and/or introducer

Description of procedure

1. The site is chosen by the physician (subclavian, brachial, external jugular, femoral).
2. The site is surgically prepared and draped.
3. A venipuncture is made.
4. The guide wire is passed through the needle and the needle removed over the guide wire.
5. A small incision is made in the skin to allow for the size of the pulmonary artery (PA) introducer.
6. The PA introducer is passed over the guide wire and into the vein; the guide wire is removed.
7. The catheter is passed through the introducer and passed to the 20-cm mark.
8. The balloon on the catheter is inflated and the catheter further inserted while the monitor is observed for PA wedge waveform.
9. The balloon is deflated to allow the catheter to float

back into the pulmonary artery.
10. The line is sutured in place and a sterile occlusive dressing applied.
11. A chest radiograph confirms correct catheter position and rules out pneumothorax.

Potential complications

- hematoma/bleeding at site of insertion
- premature ventricular contractions (PVCs), ventricular tachycardia, or fibrillation
- knotting of the catheter during insertion
- floating of the catheter into jugular or hepatic veins
- pneumothorax

Nursing interventions

1. Explain the procedure and the catheter's purpose to the patient, if appropriate.
2. Assess the patient before the procedure begins, paying particular attention to his cardiovascular system.
3. Assemble the necessary transducers and monitoring equipment. Balance the monitoring system before insertion.
4. Connect monitoring ports to transducers and flush the system.
5. Position the patient as follows:
- supine—for insertion in brachial or femoral vein.
- Trendelenburg (to promote venous distention during venipuncture), then supine (unless contraindicated)—for insertion in subclavian or jugular vein.
6. Assess the patient's vital signs every 5 minutes during the procedure. (The patient, under most circumstances, should have an arterial line in place before PA catheter insertion.)
7. Continually monitor the ECG for PVCs during catheter insertion. (Because you will need to watch the monitor and the patient during this stage of the procedure, you should have no other responsibilities.)
8. Provide emotional support to the patient during insertion. Expect him to experience pain during the initial venipuncture and, possibly, palpitations as the catheter passes through the heart.
9. Rebalance the system; obtain and document initial pressure readings.
10. Prepare to measure cardiac output according to institutional procedure.
11. Apply a sterile occlusive dressing to the insertion site.
12. Reassess the patient after the procedure, again paying particular attention to his cardiovascular system and comfort needs.
13. Arrange for a postinsertion chest radiograph to evaluate catheter placement and to rule out pneumothorax.

INTRACRANIAL PRESSURE MONITORING (BOLTS, I.V.C.)

Indications

Altered mentation or increased intracranial pressure as demonstrated by clinical presentation or computed tomography scan may necessitate monitoring intracranial pressures. Hydrocephalus may also necessitate monitoring as well as periodic fluid removal by an intraventricular catheter (IVC).

Description of procedure

Intracranial monitor insertion is usually done in the operating room.
1. Under local anesthesia, a small burr hole is made and either a bolt is inserted into the subarachnoid space or an IVC is threaded into a lateral ventricle.
2. The system is connected to a transducer system and balanced, and pressure readings are taken.
3. A sterile dressing is applied.

Potential complications

- dislodgement
- infection
- hemorrhage
- blockage

Nursing interventions

1. Monitor and document pressure readings.
2. Report prolonged elevated pressures (> 15 mm Hg for more than 5 minutes when the patient is at rest) to the neurosurgeon.
3. According to institutional policy:
- irrigate the bolt
- drain specified amounts of cerebrospinal fluid as ordered
- rebalance the system every 12 hours or when indicated.
4. Maintain aseptic technique during dressing changes.

INTRACOMPARTMENT PRESSURE MEASUREMENT

Indications

Measurement of fascial compartment pressure when risk or suspicion of compartment syndrome exists because of:
- decrease in fascial compartment size from fascial defects, external pressure
- increase in compartment volume from bleeding
- increase in compartment tissue edema from trauma, burns, surgical procedures, exercise, ischemia.

Preparation

Equipment

Continuous pressure monitoring
- skin preparation solution
- local anesthesia
- continuous indwelling monitoring catheter
- transducer-monitoring equipment
- sterile heparinized saline solution
- suture
- sterile dressing supplies

One-time pressure measurement
- skin preparation solution
- local anesthesia
- 18G, 3½" spinal needle
- water manometer
- sterile saline solution
- centimeter tape measure
- small sterile dressing

Note: *Hand-held battery-operated devices, which contain all the necessary items for actual pressure measurement, are now available.*

Description of procedure

Continuous pressure monitoring
1. The extremity is positioned.
2. The skin area is prepared and anesthetized.
3. The catheter is inserted into the fascial compartment using the introducer.
4. The catheter is connected to the monitoring device (preflushed with sterile heparinized saline solution).
5. The monitor is balanced and calibrated.
6. Initial pressure is documented.
7. The catheter is sutured in place.
8. A sterile dressing is applied.

One-time pressure measurement
1. The extremity is positioned.
2. The skin area is prepared and anesthetized.
3. The spinal needle is connected to the water manometer and the system flushed with sterile saline solution
4. The needle is inserted into the fascial compartment.
5. The distance from the insertion site to the top fluid level in the manometer is measured in centimeters.

6. Centimeters of water pressure are converted to millimeters of mercury pressure (mm Hg = cm water divided by 1.36).
7. The pressure is documented.
8. The needle is withdrawn after measurement; a small dressing is applied to the insertion site.

Potential complications

- bleeding within compartment space
- infection
- hemorrhage
- nerve injury

Nursing interventions

1. Explain the procedure to the patient.
2. Assemble and prepare the necessary equipment.
3. Position the extremity to eliminate localized external pressure on fascial compartments being measured.
4. Provide psychological support during the procedure.

Continuous pressure measurement
5. Connect the system to the catheter after insertion.
6. Balance and calibrate the transducer.
7. Document the initial pressure measurement. Closely monitor compartment pressures and evaluate trends.
8. Apply a sterile dressing.
9. Secure the monitoring lines and equipment to prevent accidental catheter displacement.
10. Continue to assess the extremity for signs of compartment syndrome.

One-time pressure measurement
5. Connect the water manometer to the spinal needle.
6. Flush the system with sterile saline solution.
7. Position the water manometer at a height where the fluid level does not exceed the top of the manometer.
8. Measure and document the distance in centimeters from the needle site to the top fluid level.
9. Apply a small dressing to the insertion site after the needle is withdrawn.
10. Continue to assess the extremity for signs of compartment syndrome.
11. Prepare the patient for surgery if elevated pressures indicate the need for fasciotomies.

AUTOTRANSFUSION

Autotransfusion collects, filters, and reinfuses a patient's blood to replace intravascular volume.
Note: *This procedure refers to autotransfusion in the acute resuscitation phase utilizing a chest tube thoracostomy collection device. There are products available for intraoperative use that wash and pack blood as well as collect, filter, and reinfuse it. Also available in the postoperative phase is an underwater seal collection device.*

Indications

• blunt or penetrating chest or abdominal trauma with acute blood loss
• massive/acute blood loss with or without available homologous blood
• rare blood type or previous transfusion reactions
Advantages in comparison to banked blood
• is safe for patients who have received previous homologous transfusions and have antigen/antibody problems
• eliminates transmission of diseases, such as hepatitis, malaria, syphilis, AIDS, cytomegalovirus
• eliminates possible technical errors in type and cross matching
• involves no hemolytic, febrile, allergic, or graft vs. host reactions; no risk of isoimmunization to erythrocyte, leukocyte, platelet, or protein antigen
• is readily available; no time delay for type and cross match or for finding a compatible donor blood type
• costs significantly less than banked blood
• uses blood normally wasted
• may circumvent religious objections to homologous transfusions
• eliminates need to adjust blood to body temperature
• provides normal pH, potassium, and ammonia levels
• provides normal levels of 2,3, DPG, which promotes tissue/cell oxygenation
• contains more viable platelets and RBCs
• contains low hemolysis levels
• provides normal clotting factors except fibrinogen (if used within 4 hours)

Contraindications

• malignancy
• infection (at site or systemic)
• enteric contamination
• preexisting coagulopathy
• injury older than 3 hours or wound reexploration
• preexisting inadequate liver or kidney function
Note: *In certain circumstances, the physician may overrule contraindications.*

Preparation

Several types of autotransfusion equipment are available. We have chosen not to mention brand names or endorse a specific product. In choosing a system, an institution should consider frequency of need and the system's cost, availability, and ease of operation. The type of equipment dictates specific preparation for this procedure. This procedure focuses on the chest-tube thoracotomy method in acute resuscitation.
Equipment
• chest tube insertion tray with preparation solutions
• anticoagulant for shed blood
• suction apparatus and collection device
• reinfusion equipment; micropore blood administration set

Description of procedure

1. Connect the autotransfusion device collection tubing to the chest tube.
2. Provide chest tube suction via underwater seal. (Some products have a built-in underwater seal, and others offer an optional underwater seal.)
3. Instill anticoagulant into shed blood (usually, the physician or institution policy will determine anticoagulant use and amount).
4. Infuse shed blood, using micropore blood administration tubing.
5. After completion of blood collection, the chest tube is clamped, connected to the sterile underwater seal drainage system, then unclamped.
6. All connections should be secured.

Potential complications

- emboli (air or particulate matter)
- hemolysis
- coagulopathy
- citrate toxicity
- sepsis
- renal and pulmonary insufficiency secondary to free circulating hemoglobin

Nursing interventions

Note: *Depending on the autotransfusion system used and institution policy, the nurse's responsibility may be as limited as gathering necessary equipment or as broad as totally managing this system.*

1. Monitor vital signs, paying particular attention to cardiovascular and respiratory parameters.

2. Guard against the presence of air or particulate matter in the blood administration tubing.

3. Maintain equipment sterility. Monitor and correct breaks in the system.

4. Monitor controlled suction.

5. Ensure the proper ratio of anticoagulant to shed blood. (Refer to the manufacturer's guidelines or physician's order.)

6. Monitor laboratory data during and after autotransfusion, particularly hemoglobin/hematocrit levels, coagulation profile, ABGs, and calcium levels.

7. Document amount of blood retrieved and reinfused in intake/output.

PREPARATION FOR SURGERY

Indications

This checklist provides guidelines to minimize surgical risk. However, emergency surgery for resuscitative, diagnostic, or definitive treatment generally limits extensive preparation.

Preparation

- Explain surgical procedure.
- Explain anesthetic risks, methods.
- Obtain a surgical permit.
- Obtain the patient's past medical history.
- Obtain his past surgical history.
- Ask about any allergies.
- Discuss postoperative expectations:
  ☐ recovery room
  ☐ ventilatory assistance or oxygen supplement
  ☐ importance of turning, coughing, deep breathing
  ☐ surgical drains
  ☐ postoperative pain medications
  ☐ additional I.V. lines, urinary catheter.
- Have necessary laboratory studies done.
- Check blood availability.
- Arrange for a chest radiograph, if needed.

- Prepare the operative site.
- Maintain NPO status.
- Remove glasses, dentures, jewelry, prosthetic devices.
- Administer preoperative medications.
- Obtain intraoperative medications; send to operating room.
- Attend to special needs:
  ☐ intraoperative maintenance of traction
  ☐ transportation
  ☐ coordination with other departments for computerized tomography scan, hyperbaric oxygen, arteriography.
- Attend to family considerations.

Procedure

INTRAAORTIC BALLOON PUMP (I.A.B.P.)

Indications

Management of conditions requiring short-term circulatory assistance:
- medically refractory unstable angina (pre- and postinfarction)
- cardiogenic shock from pump failure
- perioperative hemodynamic instability
- structural defects (ventricular septal defect, valve dysfunction, acute papillary muscle rupture, ventricular aneurysm).

Less well-established indications include:
- limitation of infarct size
- treatment of refractory ventricular tachycardia
- support of recent myocardial infarction patients needing general anesthesia for noncardiac surgical procedures.

Physiologic basis of counterpulsation

- diastolic augmentation, increasing coronary perfusion pressure and improving systemic perfusion
- afterload reduction, enabling the left ventricle to eject against a lower pressure, reducing myocardial oxygen consumption and increasing stroke volume and cardiac output

Absolute contraindications

- aortic dissection
- aortic aneurysm
- aortic valvular insufficiency
- severe peripheral vascular disease of lower limbs, including prior bypass grafting to lower limbs

Relative contraindications

- marked hemorrhagic diasthesis
- uncontrolled septicemia

Preparation

Equipment
- preparation solution
- sterile gloves, mask, gowns, drapes
- sterile dressing supplies
- percutaneous insertion set
- surgical instrument tray
- local anesthetic
- contrast imaging agents
- continuous flush system/pressurized bag
- IABP console and balloon catheters
- suture material
- ECG monitor and defibrillator, pacemaker
- emergency intubation equipment, drugs
- blood and I.V. fluids, including volume expanders
- antibiotics, anticoagulants, analgesics, sedatives
- standby fluoroscopy equipment

Description of procedure

1. Meticulous attention must be paid to aseptic technique.
2. Both femoral artery insertion sites are surgically prepared and draped (so as to allow access to the contralateral artery if necessary).
3. A local anesthetic is given and an arterial puncture made.
4. The prepared balloon catheter is threaded through the percutaneous introducer and sheath into the femoral artery, advanced, and positioned in the descending aorta distal to the left subclavian artery and proximal to the renal arteries.
5. The IABP console is turned on and connected and the alarms are set.
6. The following parameters are evaluated (usually on 1:2 to facilitate comparisons of waveforms):
- balloon function
- timing
- configuration
- synchronization with R wave and arterial dicrotic notch.
7. The flush system is connected to the central aortic lumen.
8. Pulses distal to the insertion site are assessed and compared to preinsertion assessment.
9. A sterile occlusive dressing is applied.
10. I.V. anticoagulant therapy is started.
11. A supine chest radiograph is taken to confirm that the balloon is in the correct position.

Potential complications

- vascular complications (circulatory insufficiency of the extremity distal to the insertion site, thromboemboli, aortic or femoral artery damage/dissection)
- infections (at balloon insertion site)
- hematologic complications (thrombocytopenia, hemolysis, hemorrhage)
- miscellaneous complications (balloon leak or rupture, retroperitoneal hematoma, spinal cord paralysis, renal failure)

Nursing interventions

1. Provide, with the physician, appropriate explanations to the patient and family about the procedure, its purpose, and expected results.

2. Verify, before the procedure, that the patient's consent is obtained in accordance with the gravity of the situation and the hospital's policy and procedure.

3. If feasible, obtain blood studies (CBC, prothrombin time, partial thromboplastin time, bleeding time, platelet count) before the procedure to rule out serious bleeding problems.

4. Position the patient supine.

5. Before the procedure, document the location and strength of bilateral femoral, popliteal, dorsalis pedis, and posterior tibial pulses.

6. Monitor compliance with strict aseptic technique during the procedure and while the IABP is in use.

7. Monitor the patient's cardiovascular status, including:
• heart rate and rhythm (document the most appropriate ECG signal for triggering the IABP)
• arterial, central venous, pulmonary artery, and pulmonary capillary wedge pressures
• balloon synchronization with inflation cycle
• laboratory data (hematology, serum chemistry, coagulation studies)
• urine output
• mentation.

8. Administer analgesia/systemic antibiotics/anticoagulants as ordered or required.

9. Monitor the patient's respiratory status, including:
• ABGs
• breath sounds
• cough, sputum
• chest radiograph findings.

10. Check the patient's neurovascular status distal to the insertion site:
• every 15 minutes for 1 hour
• every 30 minutes for the next 2 hours, and
• every hour thereafter or as the patient's condition warrants.

11. Provide psychological support to the patient and his family.

12. Change dressings using central line procedure in accordance with the hospital's policy.

13. Monitor the insertion site for bleeding, infection, and color or temperature change.

14. Minimize hazards of patient immobility by:
• applying antiembolism stockings or Ace bandages as ordered
• changing the patient's position every 1 to 2 hours (use a partial turn, avoiding movement at the catheter site)
• encouraging coughing and deep breathing and use of an incentive spirometer if the patient is not intubated
• performing range-of-motion exercises and chest physiotherapy
• providing skin care in accordance with the hospital's policy
• monitoring maximum body temperature.

15. Prevent bleeding at the balloon insertion site by:
• keeping the head of the bed below 45°
• avoiding flexion of the affected leg (use a loose restraint if necessary)
• avoiding full turns side to side
• sedating the patient as necessary.

16. Monitor IABP function, according to the hospital's policy and procedure, by:
• determining and using the most appropriate triggering method for the patient (ECG, arterial waveform, or intrinsic pump rate)
• evaluating balloon timing every 2 to 4 hours, when cardiac output decreases, the triggering mode is changed, the patient develops dysrhythmias, or there is a 20% change in his heart rate.

17. During insertion, operation, and removal of the IABP, observe the patient for the complications previously listed.

18. Document all pertinent data and interventions.

Procedure

PACEMAKER INSERTION, TEMPORARY TRANSVENOUS PACING

Indications

Temporary transvenous pacing prevents ventricular standstill. It is used in patients with:
- a persistent bradycardia
- resistant ectopic dysrhythmias, for transient conduction disturbances after an acute myocardial infarction
- a tachycardia unresponsive to drug therapy
- a trial phase before permanent pacemaker insertion.

Preparation

Pacing equipment
- pulse generator—battery-powered source of electricity:
    - ☐ demand pulse—fires an impulse only if a QRS complex does not occur at a preset interval
    - ☐ set rate—preset or fixed rate that disregards the heart's own electrical rate (not in general use today)
- pacing catheter—insulated wire carrying the electric current to the right ventricle's endocardium; has a unipolar or a bipolar electrode tip

Insertion equipment
- basins and skin preparation solution
- sterile drapes, gowns, gloves, and dressings
- sterile instrument tray
- large-bore catheter needle with stylus and plastic sheath
- local anesthetic
- fluoroscopy equipment

Additional equipment
- crash cart and defibrillator
- portable monitoring devices

Description of procedure

1. The insertion site is surgically prepared and draped. Preferable sites are the jugular and subclavian veins because they supply the shortest, most direct routes, and there is less risk of displacement with patient movements. The antecubital and femoral veins may also be used.
2. A local anesthetic is injected.
3. A percutaneous stick or cutdown is used to secure initial venous access.

4. The pacemaker catheter is introduced through the plastic sheath, advances through the superior vena cava to the right atrium, and crosses the tricuspid valve into the right ventricle.
5. Once capture has been achieved and the pacemaker is functioning, the catheter is sutured in place at the insertion site and a sterile dressing applied.

Potential complications

- catheter-tip displacement
- sensing errors
- loss of pacing artifact
- ventricular wall perforation by catheter tip
- thrombophlebitis and skin infection at insertion site

Nursing interventions

1. Encourage the patient to ask questions or express his feelings about the pacemaker. Reinforce the physician's explanation.
2. Check the operative permit for completeness.
3. Transport the patient to the radiology department, the cardiac catheter laboratory, or the surgical suite for pacemaker insertion.
4. Assist in patient positioning.
5. Monitor the patient's vital signs before the procedure.
6. Have a 100-mg lidocaine bolus ready before the physician inserts the pacing catheter because dysrhythmias can develop as the catheter is being threaded through the heart.
7. Closely and continuously monitor the patient for dysrhythmias during insertion and as ordered after insertion.

THE PNEUMATIC ANTISHOCK GARMENT
(PASG, also known as a MAST suit)

Indications

The PASG is an inflatable three-chamber garment that envelops the legs and abdomen. Mechanisms of action include pressure application to the abdomen and legs, reduction of vessel size, and splinting of pelvic or leg fractures. A PASG is most effective when used concomitantly with other antishock measures. Indications include:

• systolic blood pressure of 80 mm Hg or less (definite indication)
• systolic blood pressure of 80 to 100 mm Hg when accompanied by signs and symptoms of shock (possible indication).

Causes of hypotension may include:
• hemorrhagic shock
• neurogenic shock
• unstable pelvic fractures
• cardiac arrest secondary to trauma
• open or closed lower extremity fractures
• bleeding from other lower extremity injuries
• traumatic amputations with hypovolemia
• open or closed abdominal injuries
• other illnesses or injuries with signs and symptoms of shock (such as drug overdose with severe hypotension).

Advantages

• controls or tamponades abdominal and lower extremity bleeding
• may translocate some volume of peripheral blood to sites of greater need by applying uniform pressure on abdomen and legs
• provides splinting for pelvic and leg fractures
• permits simultaneous performance of diagnostic or therapeutic interventions, such as radiography, ECG, I.V. line insertion, bladder catheterization
• can be used with traction splints
• can be applied to but not inflated on high-risk patients whose condition may deteriorate and who may imminently need the PASG
• a clear PASG optimizes visualization of underlying structures

Contraindications

Absolute
• pulmonary edema or other signs of fluid overload, such as excessive pulmonary secretions, rales, distended neck veins
Relative
• isolated head injury
• impaled object in abdomen or leg
• uncontrolled bleeding above the site of PASG application

In addition, abdominal section inflation is contraindicated in the pregnant patient unless absolutely necessary to save her life, and abdominal section inflation is contraindicated in evisceration.

Note: *The attending physician may order PASG application despite the contraindications just cited. Establish that the physician is fully aware of any contraindications and follow established protocols accordingly.*

Potential complications

• impaired tissue perfusion in legs causing buildup of metabolic wastes that reenter circulation after deflation
• compartment syndrome
• irritation and possible skin breakdown over pressure areas
• respiratory impairment due to increased intrathoracic pressure
• acute hypotension related to sudden deflation
• extreme hypertension

Preparation

Currently, several different types of PASGs are on the market. Their basic principles of use are the same; they differ only in design details.
Equipment
• one PASG with three valves, tubing, and foot pump
Note: *Before each application, make sure the equipment is working properly and has no air leaks.*

Description of procedure

1. Confirm that the patient meets the blood pressure criteria for PASG application as previously outlined.
2. A PASG should be applied only by certified personnel.
3. Document the patient's blood pressure before PASG application and at least every 5 minutes thereafter.
4. Remove the patient's pants to prevent tissue damage from pressure on wrinkles. Also remove any sharp objects that can cut or tear the PASG.
5. Completely unfold the PASG. Attach the tubing and foot pump to all three compartments and open all stopcocks.
6. Logroll the patient or use an orthopedic stretcher to place him on the PASG. Never release or compromise in-line traction on the cervical spine while moving the patient.
7. Position the PASG so that the abdominal section ends just below the patient's rib cage and the leg sections end at the ankles.
8. Wrap the PASG around the patient's left leg and fasten the Velcro straps; repeat for the right leg and the abdomen.
9. First, close the abdominal section valve and inflate the leg sections. Next, close the leg section valves and open the abdominal valve. Inflate the abdominal section unless contraindicated.
10. Inflate the PASG until the systolic blood pressure is 100 to 110 mm Hg, the Velcro fasteners begin to crackle, or the pressure relief valves begin to vent.
11. Close all valves when the PASG is fully inflated.
12. Closely monitor vital signs and observe the patient for evidence of respiratory impairment. Auscultate breath sounds for possible signs of pulmonary edema.
Note: *Leave the foot pump attached to the PASG in case further inflation or reinflation becomes necessary. Remember that changes in temperature or atmospheric pressure (for example, during helicopter transport, from hot or cold environmental temperatures) can change the pressure within the PASG.*

Steps in deflation of the PASG

Note: *Do not cut the PASG.*
1. Record the patient's vital signs.
2. Do not begin deflation without permission from a physician who is knowledgeable about PASG use.
3. Deflate the abdominal section slowly by removing the hose at the valve connected to the abdominal section. Place your finger over the tube coming from the abdominal section; open the control valve and use your finger to control the slow release of air. Reconnect the pump tubing after the section is completely deflated to facilitate rapid reinflation should it be necessary.
4. Closely monitor the patient's vital signs immediately after deflation and thereafter for 5 to 10 minutes. Fluid replacement as ordered may supplement a blood pressure drop of more than 5 mm Hg.
5. Slowly deflate one of the leg sections if vital signs remain stable. Follow the procedure described for abdominal section deflation.
6. Closely monitor vital signs immediately after deflation and thereafter for 5 to 10 minutes. As in step 4, fluid replacement may supplement a blood pressure drop of more than 5 mm Hg.
7. Deflate the other leg compartment after ensuring that vital signs have stabilized. Follow the deflation steps already outlined. Continue close monitoring of vital signs at 5- to 15-minute intervals either after deflation or as the patient's condition warrants.

Maintenance

Follow the manufacturer's recommendations for PASG cleaning, maintenance, and storage.

Procedure

THE MECHANICAL CHEST COMPRESSION DEVICE (M.C.C.D.)

The MCCD is designed to deliver constant, appropriate chest compressions; most devices automatically provide ventilatory support with an esophageal obturator, endotracheal tube, or airway and mask in conjunction with the compressor, using a 50-psi oxygen source.

Indications

• cardiopulmonary arrest—The patient is clinically dead (no pulse, heartbeat, or spontaneous respirations).
• potential cardiopulmonary arrest—The MCCD can be set up and positioned, but not turned on, on a patient in unstable condition before transport. The device can then be rapidly engaged should the patient develop cardiac arrest en route.

Advantages over manual cardiopulmonary resuscitation (CPR)

• delivers constant compressions with intermittent ventilations
• minimizes emergency personnel fatigue
• enables emergency personnel simultaneously to perform other lifesaving measures, such as I.V. line insertion and hemorrhage control
• permits continuous chest compressions and ventilations during defibrillation
• provides correct CPR during transport and the initial in-hospital resuscitation phase

Possible disadvantages

• It can increase the risk of blunt sternal trauma.
• It may slip out of proper chest position during transport and deliver inadequate CPR.
• Some facilities may find the cost of the device prohibitive.
• Personnel must undergo extensive training before they use the device.
• Not all geographic areas or hospital facilities have the device or the personnel familiar with its proper use.

Contraindications

• presence of pulse and spontaneous respirations
• obvious death (for example, decapitation, advanced rigor mortis)

Preparation

• Personnel must have a thorough understanding of the device and have had ample hands-on practice (approximately 15 sessions with trained, experienced personnel) to use the MCCD appropriately.
• Routine inservice training and review are required to maintain personnel skills.
• Refer to the manufacturer's instruction manual for adult and pediatric MCCD application.

Equipment

• complete mechanical chest compressor and oxygen source

Special considerations

• oxygen source—The resuscitation area should have a special quick-release pressure valve that delivers 50 psi of oxygen in each resuscitation cubicle or room; E-cylinder oxygen tanks may be used if a quick-release pressure valve is unavailable; remember that the MCCD uses about eight E cylinders/hour.
• manual ventilation—After the patient arrives in the resuscitation area with the MCCD in place and functioning, the ventilation switch may be turned off while the external chest compressions continue; this permits synchronized intermittent manual ventilations.

• MCCD placement—The transportation mode in your catchment area dictates MCCD placement on either the patient's right or left side during transport; for example, we have found, in working with the Bell Jet Ranger helicopter, that the MCCD must be placed on the patient's right side, whereas conventional ambulance design necessitates MCCD placement on the patient's left side. Proper MCCD placement before transport must conform to the demands of your particular transportation vehicles; recognizing these demands before applying an MCCD obviates the need to reposition it, preserves time during patient loading and transport, and facilitates its effective use.

• equipment monitoring—The MCCD requires close evaluation for proper compression pad positioning, adequate volume of available oxygen in the tank, and effectiveness of CPR, whether used during transport or during initial in-hospital resuscitation.

• rapid MCCD removal:
☐ turn off the master on/off valve switch
☐ loosen the arm-locking knob and swing the arm toward the patient's feet
☐ pull the release knob inside the handle on the base plate and slide the base plate out of the MCCD board pocket

☐ maintain the patient in proper head and cervical spine alignment to prevent neck hyperextension (a folded sheet or small, flat pillow can provide enough height to maintain alignment)
☐ let the patient stay on the MCCD board for the remainder of the initial resuscitation process.

Care and maintenance

When using the MCCD device, remember:
• The cost of the MCCD mandates careful use; avoid rough handling or accidental dropping.
• Make every effort to keep the equipment dry, especially the base-plate controls.
• Follow the manufacturer's recommendations for cleaning and routine maintenance.

CLOSED-TUBE THORACOSTOMY

A chest tube is inserted into the chest cavity to drain air and fluid, reinflate the lung, and reestablish normal negative pulmonary pressures.

Indications

- pneumothorax
- tension pneumothorax
- hemothorax
- hemopneumothorax
- pleural effusion
- empyema
- chylothorax

Preparation

Equipment
- surgical cap, mask, gown, scrub attire
- sterile gloves
- preparation solution and sponges
- local anesthetic, needles, syringes
- thoracostomy tray, including:
  - ☐ sterile drapes
  - ☐ scalpel with #10 blade
  - ☐ needle holder
  - ☐ Kelly clamp
  - ☐ assorted hemostats
- assorted chest tubes
  - ☐ 28 to 32 French, to evacuate air
  - ☐ 36 to 40 French, to evacuate blood, clots, and fluid
- petrolatum gauze
- dressing materials and 3″ adhesive tape
- suction apparatus
  - ☐ disposable underwater-seal chest drainage device
  - ☐ three-bottle system
  - ☐ one- or two-bottle water-seal system

Description of procedure

1. Once the insertion site is determined (second or third intercostal space midclavicular line for air evacuation and fourth to sixth middle or posterior intercostal space midaxillary line for air, blood, or fluid evacuation), the area is surgically prepared and draped and the skin and intercostal space are locally anesthetized. The skin is incised and the appropriate tube is inserted into the chest cavity.
2. The chest tube is connected to either an underwater-seal suction drainage device or possibly an autotransfusion device for hemothorax evacuation. (See "Autotransfusion" in Section VII.)
3. The chest tube is sutured in place with 0 silk or 2 nylon suture material; petrolatum gauze and a sterile dressing are then applied.
4. Secure all tube connections with tape, wire, or plastic fasteners.

5. Obtain an upright chest radiograph to evaluate tube placement, lung reexpansion, and fluid evacuation.

Potential complications

- intercostal vessel laceration
- pulmonary laceration
- tube placed in the lung or soft tissue rather than in the pleural space

Nursing interventions

1. Explain the procedure to the patient.
2. Sedate the patient as ordered.
3. Place him in a supine, semi-Fowler's, or lateral decubitus position. The patient's position is determined by associated injuries (for example, cervical spine injury) and tube placement.
4. Monitor the patient's vital signs before, during, and after the insertion.
5. Record initial chest tube drainage. Monitor and record drainage from every 5 minutes to once an hour, depending on the amount of drainage. This step is especially important in a patient with a large hemothorax because massive and continued bleeding may require a thoracotomy to locate and control it.
6. Observe for signs of tube occlusion from kinks, clots, or mucous plugs. Maintain chest tube patency by milking or stripping the tube, in short sections, from the patient to the closed drainage system. This step helps maintain tube patency, preventing blood and clot occlusion, and does not create a severe increase in intrapleural pressure, which can damage lung tissue.
7. Monitor the closed drainage system for fluctuation in respiration in the water-seal chamber; turn off the suction and observe. The fluctuation will stop if the tubing is obstructed or the lung reexpanded. If air bubbles develop, check the chest tube from the patient to the closed drainage system to ensure the system's integrity. If the system is intact, a persistent air leak may reflect a tracheobronchial tree rupture.
8. Monitor the suction chamber for continuous bubbling; lack of bubbling may indicate suction failure.
9. If the chest tube becomes disconnected from the suction device, reconnect it. If reconnecting is not possible, let the chest tube act as an open pneumothorax until it can be connected to another underwater suction device. *Clamping the chest tube can cause a tension pneumothorax.* Notify the physician immediately.
10. If the chest tube is accidentally pulled out, cover the site with petrolatum gauze and a dry dressing. Notify the physician. Order a chest radiograph immediately to assess chest cavity air or fluid levels. Closely monitor the patient for signs of a tension pneumothorax.

Procedure

ORGAN DONATION

Criteria

Note: *The recommendations described in this text are general; specific conditions vary both from state to state and according to the particular procurement team.*

General considerations

• The donor should be older than age 5 and younger than age 65.
• The donor should be negative for hepatitis, AIDS, syphilis, malignancy, renal disease, sepsis, prolonged hypotension, diabetes (relative), and hypertension (defined as chronic diastolic pressure >100 mm Hg).

Specific considerations

Cornea
• negative history of previous eye surgery, corneal disease, rabies
Heart/lungs
• donor age 0 to 35 years
• negative history of cardiovascular disease
• no previous tracheostomy
(A cardiac consultation may be requested.)
Kidney
• donor age 0 to 65 years
• negative history of renal disease
Liver
• donor age 0 to 55 years
• negative history of hepatobiliary disease, alcoholism
Pancreas
• negative history of alcoholism
• negative history of diabetes in either the donor or any first-generation relative

Evaluation

Brain-death criteria vary from state to state; documentation of persistent cessation and irreversibility of brain function, however, is mandatory. If your state has no brain-death legislation, we recommend adherence to standards established by the President's Commission for the Study of Ethical Problems in Medicine and Biomedical and Behavioral Research (see Table 7.1). Contact the procurement team, and obtain samples for the following laboratory studies:
• urinalysis and urine for culture/sensitivity tests
• blood for tissue typing and culture/sensitivity tests
• blood type classification
• blood urea nitrogen, creatinine, hepatitis-associated antigen, serology (VDRL, RPR).

Donor maintenance

General considerations
1. Ensure adequate oxygenation and ventilation; continue optimal pulmonary hygiene (suction, chest physiotherapy); monitor ABG levels.
2. Continue fluid resuscitation and infusion to maintain a normotensive state and maximize perfusion:
• Control bleeding sources.
• Monitor trends in hemoglobin/hematocrit values.
• Transfuse blood, if necessary.
• Adjust volume therapy to maintain a systolic pressure of 100 to 110 mm Hg.
• If hypotension persists after adequate volume administration, inotropic agents may be ordered; dopamine and dobutamine are the drugs of choice; *metaraminol, norepinephrine, and epinephrine are contraindicated.*
• In a heart or lung donor, closely monitor volume status and control fluid balance by using a central venous pressure line.
3. Monitor the donor's core body temperature; institute measures to maintain normothermia:
• for hypothermia—warm blankets, hyperthermia blanket, warming lights, warming cascade on respirator, and fluids warmed through coils and warmers
• for hyperthermia—cooling blanket, cool packs.
4. Monitor the donor's electrolyte balance; add potassium to I.V. fluids as ordered.
5. Monitor the donor's urinary output:
• Regulate I.V. fluid rates to maintain urinary output within a 50- to 200-cc/hour range.
• Give diuretics, if ordered, if you are unable to maintain adequate urinary output with volume infusion.
• If the donor develops diabetes insipidus, give vasopressin (20 units in I.V. fluid titrated to 0.2 to 0.5 units/hour to achieve adequate urine output) as ordered. (Although vasopressin may be given subcutaneously, the preferred route is I.V. because it provides more controlled regulation; therapeutic effect may be achieved with lower doses.)
6. Use strict aseptic technique when changing dressings, suctioning, and caring for wounds. Administering prophylactic antibiotics to a donor is not recommended.
7. Prepare the donor for surgery.
Specific considerations
• corneas—Keep the donor's eyes moist with normal saline solution and tape eyelids closed.
• heart—Weigh the donor with a bedside scale; a patient needing more than 8 mcg/kg/minute of dopamine may be excluded as a potential donor.

• liver—Weigh the donor and measure his abdominal girth; check his coagulation profile and serum bilirubin concentration.

• skin—You may need to perform a special wrapping process according to your hospital's protocol, after washing the donor's trunk and legs.

• lung—An adult donor should be placed on positive end-expiratory pressure preoperatively.

• pancreas—Check the donor's serum glucose and amylase levels.

Family interaction

1. Family members may be approached by a team of health care providers, including a physician, an RN, and an organ procurement team member.

2. Ensure that the family members clearly understand the brain-death concept, if applicable.

3. Explain organ donation; give family members ample time for private discussion.

4. Obtain the family's consent in cooperation with other organ donation team members, using as the order of priority: spouse, adult son or daughter, parent, adult brother or sister, guardian of deceased, and medical examiner (after a reasonable but unsuccessful search for the next of kin).

5. Accept and support the family in their decision.

6. Facilitate family visit(s) to the donor before harvesting.

Additional considerations

If the donor undergoes cardiopulmonary arrest, resuscitation should be exactly like that for any other patient (cardiopulmonary resuscitation, fluid and drug therapy). If his circulation stops, the heart, pancreas, lungs, and bones should be harvested immediately. Kidneys and corneas must be harvested within 30 minutes and 12 hours, respectively; skin within 12 to 24 hours. Patients who are dead on arrival may be utilized as tissue donors.

Table 7.1 Brain-Death Criteria

Brain function cessation
• Unreceptivity and unresponsivity: The patient must be unresponsive to sensory input (pain and voice).
• Absent brain stem reflexes: Pupillary, corneal, and oropharyngeal responses are absent; testing doll's eyes and calorics fails to elicit eye movement; apnea test is positive (no spontaneous respirations even after the patient's $PaCO_2$ reaches 60 mm Hg).

Brain function irreversibility
• Coma: The cause must be known and adequate to explain the clinical picture.
• Absence of other causes of coma: Sedative drug intoxication, hypothermia (less than 32.2° C. [90° F.]), neuromuscular blockade, and shock must be ruled out as causes.

Criteria persistence
• The brain-death criteria just described must persist for an appropriate time, for example:
  ☐ 6 hours with a confirmatory isoelectric EEG
  ☐ 12 hours without a confirmatory isoelectric EEG
  ☐ 24 hours for anoxic brain injury without a confirmatory isoelectric EEG.
• Exercise caution when making the diagnosis of brain death in a child younger than age 5.

Reproduced, with permission, from J. Mills et al., eds. *Current Emergency Diagnosis and Treatment,* 2nd ed. © 1985 by Lange Medical Publications, Los Altos, CA.

Procedure

THE CRITICALLY ILL OR INJURED PATIENT REQUIRING SPECIAL CARE
(Patients with AIDS, hepatitis, or gross infection)

Note: *All prehospital and acute resuscitation area personnel should be alert and cautious because emergency care is often rendered long before diagnostic testing confirms that a patient has a communicable disease or an infectious process.*

As of this writing, panic remains high among members of the lay public about AIDS transmission. Well-informed health care providers can help eliminate misunderstandings while rendering quality care to AIDS patients. When caring for infected patients:
* *Their presence should not disrupt hospital protocol or routine.*
* *Protection of these patients, other patients, and health care providers from acquiring a patient-related infection or communicable disease is a high priority.*
* *Patient confidentiality must be maintained.*

Indications

AIDS
Members of high-risk groups:
* homosexual men
* hemophiliacs
* I.V. drug users
* blood recipients
* infants born into high-risk AIDS families

Infection, non-AIDS-related
Any patient with:
* gram-negative or gram-positive microorganisms
* necrotizing fasciitis
* gas gangrene
* any overwhelming or synergistic infectious process

Hepatitis
Members of high-risk groups:
* blood recipients
* dialysis patients
* I.V. drug users
* infants of mothers with preexisting hepatitis

Infection, AIDS-related
History or presence of:
* Kaposi's sarcoma (patient younger than age 60)
* opportunistic infections
* fever of unexplained origin, weight loss, lymphadenopathy, general malaise

Preparation

1. Determine the precautions needed for individual patient care; that is, confirm the need for and type of isolation:
* protective
* blood/body fluid
* respiratory
* skin/wound.

2. Assemble all necessary equipment.

3. Prepare a cubicle or room as necessary.

General considerations

1. Isolate the patient according to your hospital's policy:
* Gloves should be worn when suctioning or handling the patient's blood, body fluids, dressings, and excreta or if the caregiver has a break in the skin on hands.
* Gowns are recommended to protect the caregiver from being soiled with the patient's body fluids.
* A mask or goggles are recommended if a potential exists for contamination with the patient's sputum or mucus.

Note: *AIDS patients are particularly susceptible to infection and may well require protective isolation.*

2. Minimize traffic into the patient-care area to reduce the risk of further infection to the patient and of cross contamination. You may designate one person as caregiver to remain inside the room and one person outside to procure equipment and supplies, run laboratory samples, and so on.

3. Wash your hands before and after rendering patient care.

4. Remove all unnecessary equipment from the patient's cubicle or room. Cover or place in a cabinet those items that cannot be removed.

Note: *A kit or specialized isolation tray with disposable articles and emergency equipment should be available in the acute resuscitation area and should accompany the patient during his transport to any hospital department or room. (See "Isolation Trays" in Appendix 3.)*

5. Label the following with the precaution "Blood/Body Fluid Precautions":
- the patient's room, chart, and cardex
- any disposable or reusable equipment used in caring for the patient (linen, dishes, utensils)
- laboratory samples
- trash.

6. Double-wrap or bag all material leaving the patient's room for reprocessing or disposal. Many hospitals designate specially colored linen and trash bags for contaminated patients.

7. Exercise extreme caution when handling contaminated needles, syringes, scalpel blades, or any other sharp objects.

Note: *Do not replace caps on needles since this increases the risk of an inadvertent needle stick. Needles should be placed in an impervious container and disposed of according to the hospital's policy.*

8. Immediately clean up all spills of AIDS victims' blood or body fluids with a 1:10 solution of chlorine bleach.

9. Follow the hospital's policy or protocol if accidental exposure or wounding occurs.

10. Ensure and monitor total compliance with isolation precautions by family and visitors. Give clear, concise explanations about why and how to follow these precautions.

11. When caring for an infected patient, anticipate the need for blood, sputum, urine, and wound cultures. Have equipment, as well as accompanying laboratory slips, ready.

12. The patients described in this procedure should not be considered as potential candidates for organ donation.

13. Many institutions prohibit a pregnant staff member from caring for an AIDS patient with cytomegalovirus.

Note: *Every hospital should establish department-specific standards and protocols on care of AIDS, hepatitis, and grossly infected patients. Housekeeping protocols usually require more time than usual after contaminated cases, which can result in a slower turnaround time in emergency rooms or acute resuscitation areas.*

ENDOTRACHEAL INTUBATION (ORAL AND NASAL)

Note: *Many shock trauma patients require emergency endotracheal intubation early in the resuscitation phase for effective airway management. This procedure is not performed without risk, however, as several problems commonly associated with trauma render this patient a less than ideal candidate for intubation and anesthesia. These problems include:*

- *incomplete history of accident*
- *inadequate patient history of current medication, preexisting disease processes, drug allergies*
- *delayed gastric emptying, starting from the time of the accident*
- *potential chemical intoxication (from drugs and alcohol)*
- *existing, or potential, hypovolemic shock*
- *multisystem injuries with extensive physiologic derangements.*

Indications

General
- Maintain a patent airway in an unresponsive patient or a patient with a depressed or absent gag reflex.
- Assist or maintain adequate ventilation.
- Provide high fraction of inspired oxygen and positive end-expiratory pressure.
- Treat a decreased PaO_2 not amenable to supplemental oxygen therapy by mask or nasal prongs.
- Anticipate the need for intense pulmonary hygiene (oral intubation).
- Anticipate the need for surgical intervention requiring general anesthesia.
- Provide hyperventilation as emergent therapy for increased intracranial pressure caused by an expanding-mass lesion.
- Treat pulmonary contusion, aspiration pneumonitis, flail chest.

Orotracheal route
- suspected or confirmed mid- or upper-third facial injury
- suspected or confirmed basilar skull fractures

Nasotracheal route
- suspected or confirmed cervical spine injury
- intraoral access needed for surgical procedures (arch bar application, dental impressions, suturing of intraoral lacerations)
- plastic or maxillofacial surgical evaluation of oral occlusion in patients with midface fractures (patient initially intubated by orotracheal route, then nasotracheally intubated for actual examination)

Possible contraindications

General
- extensive maxillofacial injuries
- complete airway obstruction or airway trauma

Orotracheal
- suspected or confirmed cervical spine injury (head cannot be manipulated for adequate cord visualization)

Nasotracheal
- apnea
- suspected or confirmed basilar skull fractures (tube may enter the cranium through a fracture of the cribriform plate or posterior wall of the sinus)
- suspected or confirmed cerebrospinal fluid leaks (increased risk for meningitis)
- need for long-term intubation (increased risk for sinusitis)
- need for extensive pulmonary hygiene (small tube size and the multiple curves the nasal tube must follow impair optimal pulmonary hygiene, for example, in the patient requiring long-term ventilation or with excessive secretions from a pulmonary contusion or aspiration pneumonitis)

Preparation

Equipment
- laryngoscope with curved and straight blades
- extra batteries for handle, extra bulbs for blades
- endotracheal tubes in various sizes—usually 7, 8, and 9 mm for adults (see also "Pediatric Airway Obstruction" in Section VI)
- stylet
- Magill forceps
- water-soluble lubricant
- topical anesthetic (for the conscious patient)
- vasoconstrictive spray (for nasal intubation)
- 12-cc syringe
- naso- and oropharyngeal airways or bite blocks
- adhesive spray
- adhesive or twill tape

Adjunctive equipment
- suction apparatus with tonsillar tip and tracheal catheter
- bag and mask with oxygen source preattached
- drugs for rapid-sequence induction (see Table 7.2)
- gastric decompression tube with gastric suction apparatus

- mechanical ventilator
- emergency airway tray (see Appendix 3)
- needle cricothyroidotomy set (see "Needle Cricothyroidotomy" in Section VII)
- fiberoptic bronchoscope (for fiberoptic intubation)

Patient position

- supine

Note: *One team member must assume responsibility for maintaining manual in-line traction when cervical spine integrity is unconfirmed or altered.*

Description of procedure

Note: *Never remove an esophageal obturator airway (EOA) before performing endotracheal intubation; the risk of vomiting is extremely high. Intubate with the EOA in place and remove the EOA only after the endotracheal tube is secured.*

Orotracheal intubation

1. The endotracheal (ET) tube's cuff is inflated. The syringe is removed and the cuff and pilot balloon are checked for leaks. The cuff is then completely deflated.
2. The ET tube is lubricated with a water-soluble lubricant. The stylet is lubricated and placed inside the ET tube. Lubrication facilitates rapid stylet removal after intubation.
Note: *The distal end of the stylet should stop approximately 1" from the end of the ET tube. It must never extend beyond the ET tube or through Murphy's eye (an opening at the distal end between the cuff and the tube's distal end, which prevents lodging of the tube opening against the tracheal wall) as it can cause extensive lacerating injuries during intubation.*
3. Manual in-line traction is applied on the patient's head and cervical spine, and the anterior portion of the cervical collar is removed. Traction must be maintained during the entire procedure, until the cervical collar can be reapplied.
4. The patient is preoxygenated for 1 to 2 minutes with bag and mask and 100% oxygen.
5. Anesthetics, sedatives, neuromuscular blockers, and other specified medications are administered. (See Table 7.2 for rapid-sequence induction.)
Note: *Cricoid pressure (posterior compression of the cricoid cartilage that compresses the cervical esophagus between the cricoid cartilage and the 6th cervical vertebra) is applied the moment the patient loses consciousness. This must be maintained throughout the entire procedure, until the patient has been successfully intubated and the cuff is inflated. This prevents possible aspiration of gastric contents, which may reflux during anesthesia induction.*
6. After adequate muscular relaxation, direct laryngoscopy is performed for visualization of the glottis and vocal cords.
7. The stylet-enforced tube is gently inserted and advanced through the cords into the trachea until the balloon has passed below the cords.

8. The stylet is quickly removed and the cuff is inflated to 14 to 24 cm water pressure, or until the air leak during ventilation stops. The patient is manually ventilated with 100% oxygen.
9. Breath sounds are auscultated in five spots: the right and left upper chest, the right and left midaxillary line, and the abdomen, with simultaneous visualization of chest and abdominal expansion to confirm proper placement of the ET tube.
10. Adhesive spray is applied to the tube, cheeks, and upper lip; tape is applied to secure the tube's position.
11. A bite block or oral airway is inserted to prevent the patient's teeth from accidentally tearing the tube.
12. A gastric decompression tube is inserted to minimize the risk of aspiration should the patient vomit.
Note: *Aspiration, commonly associated with increased morbidity/mortality rates, can still occur despite the presence of the cuffed ET tube and the gastric decompression tube.*
13. A chest radiograph and ABG sampling after intubation confirm proper tube placement and evaluate ventilation effectiveness.

Nasotracheal intubation

1. The ET tube cuff is inflated, and the cuff and the pilot tube are checked for leaks. The cuff is then deflated and the tube is lubricated with a water-soluble anesthetic lubricant.
2. Manual in-line traction is applied to the patient's head and cervical spine, and the anterior portion of the cervical collar is removed. Traction must be maintained during the entire procedure, until the collar can be reapplied.
3. The patient is preoxygenated with a bag and mask and 100% oxygen for 1 to 2 minutes.
4. The nasal passage is sprayed with a vasoconstrictor to constrict the mucosa. Conscious patients usually require anesthetic spray as well. (Cocaine or Neo-Synephrine 10 mg in 5 cc of 2% xylocaine jelly may be used.)
5. Anesthetic agents, muscle relaxants, or sedatives are administered as necessary. (Neuromuscular blocking agents should not be used if the patient is ventilating spontaneously as the patient's ventilations are used as a guide for proper tube placement. These agents should not be used if it is felt that orotracheal intubation, the alternative route, would be difficult.)
6. The tube is gently inserted into the anesthetized nostril and slowly and carefully advanced through the posterior choana. With the patient hyperventilating, the tube is passed through the oropharynx and into the trachea. The intubator places his left hand on one side of the trachea and can feel if the ET tube is entering the piriform fossa or the glottis. Manipulation of the trachea facilitates passage of the ET tube through the cords during inspiration. Use of Magill forceps and the laryngoscope permits tube visualization and aids direction and insertion of the tube into the trachea if blind placement fails.

7. After tube placement in the trachea, the cuff is inflated and the patient is manually ventilated with 100% oxygen.

8. Breath sounds are auscultated (in the right and left upper chest, the right and left midaxillary line, and over the stomach) with simultaneous inspection of chest and abdominal expansion. These measures confirm proper tube placement.

9. Adhesive spray is applied to the tube, upper lip, and cheek. The tube is then taped in place. (Twill tape can be used to tie the tube in position if preferred.)

10. A gastric decompression tube is inserted to prevent possible aspiration should the patient vomit.

11. A postintubation chest radiograph and ABG sampling confirm proper tube position and oxygenation.

Potential complications

General
- esophageal intubation (causes hypoxia and possible vomiting and aspiration)
- right main stem bronchus intubation (ventilates right lung only, leading to left lung atelectasis and ventilation/perfusion mismatch)
- inability to intubate (hypoxia and possible death)
- airway trauma or hemorrhage (usually from improperly placed stylet; can also lead to pneumothorax)
- vocal cord trauma (evulsion of cords or trauma to recurrent laryngeal nerve; may not be evidenced until extubation, when the patient develops stridor and ventilation difficulty)
- endotracheal tube cuff tear or rupture (causes leak and requires reintubation)
- laryngeal, vocal cord, or tracheal damage (from prolonged tube placement, which may cause stenosis, pressure-related necrosis, or fistula formation)

Orotracheal
- loosened or chipped teeth (from laryngoscope blade) with possible aspiration of tooth
- lip, tongue, mouth, oral mucosa, or pharyngeal injury (such as a laceration from the laryngoscope blade)
- cervical strain or dislocation (from hyperextension)
- neurologic deficit (in a patient with a cervical spine injury)

Nasotracheal
- introduction of the tube into the brain (with basilar skull fracture)
- trauma to the epiglottis or piriform fossa (from ET tube)
- fracture of nasal turbinates with severe hemorrhage (impairs further attempts at intubation)
- introduction of nasal bacteria into the trachea (resulting in infection)
- nasal mucosa necrosis (from prolonged pressure)
- sinusitis

Nursing interventions

1. Ensure availability and proper functioning of necessary equipment, as listed above. (This equipment and its function should be checked routinely at the beginning of every shift.)

2. Provide the patient with a brief, simple explanation of the procedure, as appropriate. Thoroughly prepare the patient for the use of neuromuscular blocking agents; explain that he will be paralyzed but continue to hear and feel. The effects of this frightening experience can be avoided through adequate sedation with an amnestic agent, for example, any of the benzodiazepines. Narcotics and tranquilizers should always be used with neuromuscular blocking agents. (See "Use of Neuromuscular Blocking Agents" in Section IV.)

3. Closely monitor and document the patient's vital signs throughout the procedure. Inform the intubator of sudden, untoward changes.

4. Administer or assist with administration of drug therapy prior to or during the procedure.

5. Apply cricoid pressure as directed.

6. Assist with cuff inflation, tube stabilization, and ventilation with 100% oxygen after insertion, as necessary.

7. After insertion, auscultate breath sounds bilaterally and over the stomach, and observe chest and abdominal expansion or movement to confirm tube position.

8. Suction the endotracheal tube after it is secured; observe and document secretion characteristics.

9. Assist with the chest radiograph and protect the security of the tube throughout the study to prevent accidental dislodgement or premature extubation.

10. Document the procedure and all nursing interventions, including auscultation of chest and abdomen and the presence and equality of breath sounds. Document the postintubation chest radiograph and ABG sampling.

11. Monitor the intubated patient every hour, or as the patient's condition warrants, for proper tube placement, patency, and ventilation. Report any air leaks from the cuff immediately. Monitor and document the patient's compliance with mechanical ventilation; administer medication as ordered and indicated to maximize ventilatory effects. (See "Use of Neuromuscular Blocking Agents" in Section IV.)

12. Suction the intubated patient every 1 to 2 hours, or as the patient's condition warrants. Perform oral or nasal care every 4 hours, or more frequently as needed. Monitor skin and mucosa in contact with the tube for signs of pressure or irritation.

Table 7.2

Rapid-Sequence Induction

Note: *Rapid-sequence induction minimizes the time between loss of consciousness and completion of endotracheal intubation.*

1. preoxygenation with 100% oxygen for 1 to 2 minutes (enables the patient to withstand the period of apnea during intubation)

2. d-tubocurarine 3 mg I.V. (reduces fasciculations, which increase intraabdominal and intragastric pressures, thus predisposing the patient to regurgitation)

3. thiopental[1] 3 to 4 mg/kg I.V. *or* ketamine[2] 2 mg/kg I.V. *or* diazepam[1] 0.2 to 0.3 mg/kg I.V.

4. succinylcholine 1 to 2 mg/kg I.V.

[1] Dose must be lowered in the hypotensive patient; preferred drug for head-injured patient as it lowers intracranial pressure and lowers cerebral perfusion pressure.
[2] Should not be used in the patient with an actual or potential closed head injury as it will increase intracranial pressure and cerebral oxygen consumption.

NEEDLE CRICOTHYROIDOTOMY

Note: *Needle cricothyroidotomy is a lifesaving procedure and must be performed with speed and precision. Nevertheless, it is only a temporary airway establishment measure and must be followed by a more formal procedure, such as a surgical cricothyroidotomy or a tracheostomy. Use this ventilation method for no more than 30 to 45 minutes because inadequate exhalation leads to a carbon dioxide buildup.*

Indications

- inability to perform endotracheal intubation or to insert an esophageal obturator airway because of:
  ☐ maxillofacial injury
  ☐ laryngeal fractures
  ☐ facial or upper airway edema
  ☐ facial or upper airway burns
  ☐ severe oropharyngeal hemorrhage
  ☐ age (preferred to surgical cricothyroidotomy in patients younger than age 12)

Contraindications

- lack of training or skill in properly performing the procedure
- availability of other airway establishment methods

Preparation

Note: *A needle cricothyroidotomy kit, with all the necessary supplies, should be readily available to avoid wasting time in gathering equipment.*
Equipment
- skin preparation solution
- 4 × 4 gauze sponges
- 12G to 14G, 8.5-cm I.V. needle and catheter
- 12-cc syringe
- 3.0-mm endotracheal tube adapter
- silk or twill tape
Adjunctive equipment
- jet insufflation setup (Y connector, oxygen tubing)
- oxygen source

Patient position

- supine

Description of procedure

1. The anterior cricothyroid membrane is identified and palpated.
2. The patient's neck is rapidly scrubbed and prepared.
3. A skin puncture is made midline directly over the cricothyroid membrane.
4. The needle is advanced inferiorly at a 45° angle through the cricothyroid membrane. (Syringe aspiration is constant during insertion: aspirating air signals entry into the trachea.)
5. Upon entry into the tracheal lumen, the needle is removed and the catheter carefully advanced downward into position.
6. The catheter hub is attached to the endotracheal adapter, which is attached to the Y connector. The oxygen tubing then fits onto one side of the Y connector.
7. Auscultate breath sounds and secure the apparatus to the patient's neck.
8. Use a 1:4-second ratio to obtain ventilation. That is, with a finger occluding the open port of the Y connector, deliver oxygen for 1 second. Then, open the occluded port and let the patient exhale for 4 seconds.

Potential complications

- esophageal, posterior tracheal, thyroid perforation
- bleeding, hematoma
- inadequate ventilation-related hypoxia

Nursing interventions

1. Assemble equipment, including cricothyroidotomy kit, oxygen source, and suction apparatus, at the patient's bedside.
2. Assist with proper patient positioning.
3. If the patient is conscious, give him a brief, simple explanation about the procedure and offer constant emotional support. (A conscious, airway-obstructed patient will be very frightened.)
4. Maintain the patient on an ECG monitor and continuously assess him throughout the procedure for cardiopulmonary instability or deterioration.
5. Auscultate breath sounds and evaluate chest expansion after the procedure.
6. Help secure the cricothyroidotomy apparatus and ventilate the patient as needed.
7. Document the procedure and all nursing interventions.
8. Monitor the patient for postprocedural complications; evaluate ABG results.
9. Anticipate the need, and prepare the patient, for surgery.

SURGICAL CRICOTHYROIDOTOMY

Note: *This is a lifesaving procedure and must be performed with speed and precision.*

Indications

- inability to perform endotracheal intubation or to insert an esophageal obturator airway because of:
  - ☐ maxillofacial injury
  - ☐ laryngeal fractures
  - ☐ facial or upper airway edema
  - ☐ facial or upper airway burns
  - ☐ severe oropharyngeal hemorrhage

Contraindications

- patients younger than age 12
- lack of training or skill in properly performing the procedure
- availability of other airway establishment methods

Preparation

Note: *An emergency airway tray with the necessary surgical instruments and equipment should be preassembled and readily available in the resuscitation area. (See Appendix 3, "Sample Trays and Specialty Carts Lists.")*
Equipment (emergency airway tray contents)
- sterile drapes
- towel clip
- Allis tissue forceps or clamp
- two rat-tooth forceps
- self-retaining retractor
- tracheal spreader
- two Army-Navy retractors
- tracheostomy hook
- #3 knife handle with #10 blade attached
- #3 knife handle with #11 blade attached
- two small solution cups with gauze sponges inside
- two 12-cc syringes
- 25G needle
- 4 × 4 gauze sponges
- lidocaine, 1%
Adjunctive equipment/supplies
- skin preparation and scrub solutions
- tracheostomy tubes, various sizes
- sterile, water-soluble lubricant
- sterile suction tubing
- suture material
- twill tape
- tracheostomy adapter
- suction apparatus
- oxygen source

- materials for sterile technique (mask, hat, gloves, scrub suits or sterile gowns)

Description of procedure

1. The patient's neck is surgically prepared.
2. If the patient is conscious, local anesthetic is infiltrated.
3. The surgeon stabilizes the thyroid cartilage with the nondominant hand while incising through the cricothyroid membrane.
4. The tracheal spreader or the knife handle is placed in the incision and either opened or turned at a 90° angle to dilate the incision and open the airway.
5. The appropriate-sized tracheostomy tube is inserted through the incision and directed downward and posteriorly into the trachea.
6. Inflate the tracheostomy tube cuff, manually ventilate the patient, and evaluate his chest expansion and bilateral breath sounds.
7. Secure the tube with twill tape when it is properly positioned (sutures may be employed as needed).
8. A postprocedural chest radiograph confirms proper tube placement.

Potential complications

- aspiration
- hemorrhage or hematoma
- esophageal or posterior tracheal laceration
- laryngeal stenosis
- vocal cord paralysis
- cellulitis

Nursing interventions

1. Assemble equipment, including an emergency airway tray, oxygen source, and suction apparatus, at the patient's bedside.
2. Assist with supine patient positioning.
3. If the patient is conscious, give him a brief, simple explanation about the procedure and offer emotional support. (A conscious, airway-obstructed patient will be very frightened.)
4. Maintain the patient on an ECG monitor and continuously assess him for cardiopulmonary instability or deterioration.
5. Inflate the tracheostomy tube cuff after insertion.
6. Auscultate bilateral breath sounds and chest expansion.
7. Help secure the tube and ventilate the patient as needed.
8. Send a blood sample for ABG analysis.
9. Document the procedure and all nursing interventions.
10. Monitor the patient for postprocedural complications.

REFERENCES

STUDIES & PROCEDURES

Therapeutic Embolization/Aortography

Snopek, A.M. *Fundamentals of Special Radiographic Procedures,* 2nd ed. Philadelphia: W.B. Saunders Co., 1984.

Positive Contrast Study

Patient Management—Intrathecal Use of Iohexol. New York: Winthrop-Breon Laboratories, 1984.
Patient Management—Intrathecal Use of Metrizamide. New York:

Winthrop-Breon Laboratories, 1984.
Snopek, A.M. *Fundamentals of Special Radiographic Procedures,* 2nd ed. Philadelphia: W.B. Saunders Co., 1984.

Nuclear Medicine Imaging

Mettler, F.A., and Guiberteau, M.J. *Essentials of Nuclear Medicine Imaging,* 2nd ed. New York: Grune & Stratton, 1986.

Diagnostic Peritoneal Lavage

American College of Surgeons Committee on Trauma. *Advanced Trauma Life Support.* Student Manual, 1984.
McLellan, B.A., et al. "Analysis of Peritoneal Lavage Parameters in Blunt Abdominal Trauma," *Journal of Trauma* 25(5):393-99, May 1985.

Myers, R.A.M., et al. "A Safe, Semi-Open Procedure for Diagnostic Peritoneal Lavage," *Surgery, Gynecology and Obstetrics* 153:738-40, November 1981.

Intracranial Pressure Monitoring

Cooper, P.R., ed. *Head Injury.* Baltimore: Williams & Wilkins Co., 1982.

Davis, J.E., and Mason, C.B. *Neurologic Critical Care.* New York: Van Nostrand Reinhold Co., 1979.

Autotransfusion

Davidson, S.J. "Emergency Unit Autotransfusion," *Surgery* 703-07, November 1978.
Emminizer, S., et al. "Autotransfusion: Current Status," *Heart & Lung* 10(1):83, January/February 1981.
Lockhart, C., and Mattox, K. "Autotransfusion—A Technique for the Trauma Patient," *Nursing Clinics of North America* 13:235-45, June 1978.

Lockhart, C., et al. "A Review of Autotransfusion," *Journal of Emergency Nursing* 38-41, March/April 1979.
Mattox, K. "Comparison of Techniques of Autotransfusion," *Surgery* 700-02, November 1978.

Intraaortic Balloon Pump

Arvesty, J. "Percutaneous Intraaortic Balloon Insertion," in *Cardiac Catheterization and Angiography.* Edited by Grossman, W. Philadelphia: Lea & Febiger, 1986.
Ford, P.J., et al. "Intraaortic Balloon Pump Management," in *AACN Procedure Manual for Critical Care.* Edited by Millar, S.,

et al. Philadelphia: W.B. Saunders Co., 1985.
Yee, B.H. "Mechanical Interventions," in *Cardiac Critical-Care Nursing.* Edited by Zorb, S., and Yee, B. Boston: Little, Brown & Co., 1986.

Pacemaker Insertion

Lyon, L.J. *Basic Electrocardiography Handbook.* New York: Van Nostrand Reinhold Co., 1977.

Meltzer, L.E., et al. *Intensive Coronary Care: A Manual for Nurses,* 4th ed. Bowie, Md.: Robert J. Brady Co., 1983.

The Pneumatic Antishock Garment

American College of Surgeons Committee on Trauma. *Advanced Trauma Life Support.* Student Manual, 1984.
Caroline, N.L. *Emergency Medical Treatment.* Boston: Little, Brown & Co., 1982.

Hafen, B.Q., and Karren, K.J. *Prehospital Emergency Care and Crisis Intervention.* Englewood, Colo.: Morton Publishing, 1983.

The Mechanical Chest Compression Device

Hafen, B.Q., and Karren, K.J. *Prehospital Emergency Care and Crisis Intervention.* Englewood, Colo.: Morton Publishing, 1983.

Thumper. *CPR Minimal Operating Standards.* Distributed by Dixie, USA, Inc., Houston.

Closed-Tube Thoracostomy

Mills, J., et al., eds. *Current Emergency Diagnosis and Treatment,* 2nd ed. Los Altos, Calif.: Lange Medical Pubns., 1985.

Organ Donation

Gaul-Minkowski, P. Personal Communication, 1986.

Reiley, P.J. "Organ Donation," in *AACN Procedure Manual for Critical Care.* Edited by Millar, S., et al. Philadelphia: W.B. Saunders Co., 1985.

Simon, R.P. "Coma," in *Current Emergency Diagnosis and Treatment.* Edited by Mills, J., et al. Los Altos, Calif.: Lange Medical Pubns., 1985.

The Critically Ill or Injured Patient Requiring Special Care

Brick, P.D. "Multisystem Emergencies—AIDS," in *Emergency Care—The First 24 Hours.* Edited by O'Boyle, C.M., et al. East Norwalk, Conn.: Appleton-Century-Crofts, 1985.

Canada Diseases Weekly Report 10s:1-4, March 1984.

Garner, J.S., and Simmons, B.P. "CDC Guidelines for Isolation Precautions in Hospitals," *Infection Control* 4:245-325, 1983.

Haber, S.L. "What Every Laboratorian Should Know about AIDS, Part 1," *Medical Laboratory Observer* 17(11):32-38, November 1985.

Hnatko, S.I. "Royal Alexandra Develops AIDS Infection Control Protocol," *Dimensions in Health Service* 62(8):25-28, September 1985.

Maryland Institute for Emergency Medical Services Systems, Department of Infectious Disease. *MIEMSS Infection Control Policy Manual,* January 1986.

Williams, W.W., et al. "Guideline for Infection Control in Hospital Personnel," *American Journal of Infection* 12(1):34-63, February 1984.

Endotracheal Intubation

American College of Surgeons Committee on Trauma. *Advanced Life Support.* Student Manual, 1984.

Giesecke, A.H. "Anesthesia for Trauma Surgery," in *Anesthesia,* vol. 1. Edited by Miller, R.D. New York: Churchill Livingstone, 1981.

Stoetling, R.K. "Endotracheal Intubation," in *Anesthesia,* vol. 1. Edited by Miller, R.D. New York: Churchill Livingstone, 1981.

Needle Cricothyroidotomy

American College of Surgeons Committee on Trauma. *Advanced Life Support.* Student Manual, 1984.

Surgical Cricothyroidotomy

American College of Surgeons Committee on Trauma. *Advanced Life Support.* Student Manual, 1984.

Appendix 1

APPROVED NURSING DIAGNOSES APRIL 1986

NORTH AMERICAN NURSING DIAGNOSIS ASSOCIATION
3525 Caroline Street, St. Louis, MO 63104;
(314) 577-8954

Activity Intolerance
Activity Intolerance, Potential
Adjustment, Impaired†
Airway Clearance, Ineffective
Anxiety
Body Temperature, Potential Alteration in†
Bowel Elimination, Alteration in: Constipation
Bowel Elimination, Alteration in: Diarrhea
Bowel Elimination, Alteration in: Incontinence
Breathing Pattern, Ineffective
Cardiac Output, Alteration in: Decreased
Comfort, Alteration in: Chronic Pain†
Comfort, Alteration in: Pain
Communication, Impaired: Verbal
Coping, Family: Potential for Growth
Coping, Ineffective Family: Compromised
Coping, Ineffective Family: Disabling
Coping, Ineffective Individual
Diversional Activity, Deficit
Family Process, Alteration in
Fear
Fluid Volume, Alteration in: Excess
Fluid Volume Deficit, Actual
Fluid Volume Deficit, Potential
Gas Exchange, Impaired
Grieving, Anticipatory
Grieving, Dysfunctional
Growth and Development, Altered†
Health Maintenance, Alteration in
Home Maintenance Management, Impaired
Hopelessness†
Hyperthermia†
Hypothermia†
Incontinence, Functional†
Incontinence, Reflex†
Incontinence, Stress†
Incontinence, Total†
Incontinence, Urge†
Infection, Potential for†

Injury, Potential for: (poisoning, potential for; suffocation, potential for; trauma, potential for)
Knowledge Deficit (specify)
Mobility, Impaired Physical
Neglect, Unilateral†
Noncompliance (specify)
Nutrition, Alteration in: Less than Body Requirements
Nutrition, Alteration in: More than Body Requirements
Nutrition, Alteration in: Potential for More than Body Requirements
Oral Mucous Membrane, Alteration in
Parenting, Alteration in: Actual
Parenting, Alteration in: Potential
Post-Trauma Response†
Powerlessness
Rape Trauma Syndrome
Self-Care Deficit: feeding, bathing/hygiene, dressing/grooming, toileting
Self-Concept, Disturbance in body image, self-esteem, role performance, personal identity
Sensory-Perceptual Alteration: visual, auditory, kinesthetic, gustatory, tactile, olfactory
Sexual Dysfunction
Sexuality Patterns, Altered†
Skin Integrity, Impairment of: Actual
Skin Integrity, Impairment of: Potential
Sleep Pattern Disturbance
Social Interaction, Impaired†
Social Isolation
Spiritual Distress (distress of the human spirit)
Swallowing, Impaired†
Thermoregulation, Ineffective†
Thought Processes, Alteration in
Tissue Integrity, Impaired†
Tissue Perfusion, Alteration in: cerebral, cardiopulmonary, renal, gastrointestinal, peripheral
Urinary Elimination, Alteration in Patterns
Urinary Retention†
Violence, Potential for: self-directed or directed at others

† Diagnoses accepted in 1986

Source: Classification of Nursing Diagnoses: Proceedings of the Seventh Conference. Edited by McLane, Audrey M. (to be published by C.V. Mosby Co., St Louis.)

Appendix 2

SUPPLEMENTAL NURSING DIAGNOSES

Decreased tissue perfusion, carbon dioxide retention, life-threatening dysrhythmias, and metabolic acidosis, potential for

Extension of myocardial infarct, potential for

Fetal distress, potential for

Fluid and electrolytes imbalance, potential for

Hyperkalemia, potential for

Hypoxia, potential for

Ineffective breathing patterns and impaired motor, sensory, and cognitive function, potential for

Level of consciousness, sensation, and motor function, potential for altered

Loss of vision, potential for

Motor and sensory deficit, potential for

Muscle ischemia, potential for

Muscle tissue death, potential for

Neurologic function, alteration in

Paralytic ileus, potential for

Premature labor and delivery, potential for

Renal dysfunction, potential for

Respiratory function, potential for alteration in

Sensory perception and motor function, potential for decreased

Soft tissue necrosis, potential for

Spontaneous abortion, potential for

Appendix 3

SAMPLE TRAYS AND SPECIALTY CARTS LISTS

Multiuse Tray

Use:
Percutaneous or cutdown I.V. or arterial line insertion; chest tube insertion; minor laceration repair

Contents:
Instruments
- 1 rat-tooth pickup with teeth
- 1 Crile clamp
- 1 mosquito clamp
- 1 long Kelly clamp
- 1 needle holder
- 1 suture scissors
- 1 #3 knife handle
- 2 small cups

Miscellaneous
- 4 towels
- 2 35-cc syringes
- 1 12-cc syringe

- 1 #10 knife blade
- 1 23G needle
- 1 18G needle
- 1 20-cc vial 1% Xylocaine (plain)
- 20 4×4 gauze sponges
- 5 gauze sponges in each cup

Have available at bedside:
- preparation and scrub solution
- sterile drape to cover tray
- sutures appropriate for procedure
- chest tube, I.V. catheters appropriate for procedure
- topical antibiotic ointment
- sterile dressing, tape

Instrument Set

Use:
Added to multiuse tray as a supplement for chest tube insertion, cutdown procedures

Contents:
Instruments
- 1 Kelly clamp
- 1 Crile clamp
- 3 mosquito clamps
- 1 Metzenbaum scissors
- 1 #3 knife handle
- 1 #11 knife blade

Miscellaneous
- 4 towels

Peritoneal Lavage Tray

Use:
Diagnostic peritoneal lavage

Contents:
Instruments
- 1 suture scissors
- 1 Metzenbaum scissors
- 1 needle holder
- 4 mosquito clamps
- 2 Crile clamps
- 1 pickup with teeth
- 1 #4 knife handle
- 2 large cups
- 2 Army-Navy retractors
- 1 self-retaining retractor

Miscellaneous
- 1 #20 blade

- 1 12-cc syringe
- 1 18G needle, 1½″
- 1 25G needle, ⅝″
- 4 towels
- 20 4×4 gauze sponges
- 5 4×4 gauze sponges in each cup

Have available at bedside:
- 1-liter bottle normal saline solution/Ringer's lactate
- I.V. infusion set
- Xylocaine with epinephrine
- sutures per request

Gardner-Wells Tong Tray

Use:
Application of cervical traction

Contents:
Instruments
- 1 Gardner-Wells tongs
with s-hooks
- 2 small cups

Miscellaneous
- 4 towels
- 1 vial 1% Xylocaine (plain)
- 1 12-cc syringe
- 1 23G needle
- 1 18G needle
- 1 #15 blade
- 20 4×4 gauze sponges
- 5 4×4 gauze sponges in each cup

Have available at bedside:
- traction apparatus
- traction cord, weights
- shaving razor, blades
- topical antibiotic ointment

Plastics Tray

Use:
Minor plastic surgery repairs

Contents:
Instruments

- 4 small Crile or mosquito clamps
- 1 Blister needle holder
- 2 Adson pickups
- 1 small Metzenbaum or Stevens scissors
- 1 #3 knife handle
- 2 small cups

Miscellaneous

- 1 #11 blade
- 1 #15 blade
- 1 25G needle
- 1 23G needle
- 1 18G needle

- 1 10-cc syringe
- 4 towels
- 20 4×4 gauze sponges
- 5 4×4 gauze sponges in each cup

Have available at bedside:

- 1 vial 1% Xylocaine with epinephrine
- 1 vial 1% Xylocaine (plain)

- sutures per surgeon's request
- topical antibiotic ointment
- large (16G) butterfly for drain
- red-top blood tube for drain
- cautery machine and equipment

Isolation Trays

Use:
Initial care of a grossly infected or contaminated patient†

Contents:
Tray I

- sterile gloves sizes 6½, 7, 7½, and 8—two pairs each
- sterile 4×4 gauze sponges
- sterile abdominal pads
- 1 box of unsterile examining gloves
- 2 sterile tracheal suction kits
- 2 sterile oropharyngeal suction catheters
- 1 gastric decompression tube

- 2 blood culture sets
- 2 anaerobic culture sets
- 2 aerobic culture sets
- 2 microbiology slides
- 1 sterile specimen cup for slides
- 2 plastic isolation linen bags
- medication labels

Tray II

- sterile 2×2 gauze sponges
- 3 5-cc containers of normal saline solution (NSS) for endotracheal tube instillation
- 1 5% vial of injectable NSS
- 1 5% vial of injectable sterile water

- 2 ABG syringes
- 2 intracatheters of each size (14G, 16G, 18G, 20G)
- 2 silk tape rolls of each size (½", 1", 2")
- 1 cloth tape (3" size)
- 1 elastoplast tape (3" size)
- disposable tourniquets
- 12-cc syringes
- oropharyngeal airways
- shaving razors
- straight razor blades
- alcohol swabs
- antibiotic ointment
- lubricant
- thermometers
- 18G needles
- 5-in-1 plastic connectors
- blood tubes (at least two of each—red, purple, blue, gray)
- cotton-tipped applicators
- tongue depressors
- Kerlix rolls
- stopcocks
- Band-Aids
- disposable blood pressure cuffs

†Predesigned isolation trays are most important when a dedicated "isolation" cubicle is unavailable in the emergency care area. Large plastic trays with several dividers are preferable to a specific cart as they are much easier to clean properly. These trays prove invaluable during the initial resuscitation phase; their use eliminates contaminating an entire cubicle and its disposable supplies. The large plastic bags that line the trays are used to wrap any remaining supplies for transfer with the patient to the appropriate patient care area. Keep an ample supply of disposable blood pressure cuffs, in sizes small, medium, and large, so you can send the disposable cuff with the patient when he transfers.

Emergency Transportation Cart

Note: *This cart is used for the transportation of the unstable, or potentially unstable, critically injured trauma patient to other locations in the hospital. The trauma patient may require several diagnostic and therapeutic interventions outside of the resuscitation area or operating room, and he may be absent from these areas for several hours. As an example, a patient may require head, cervical, and facial computed tomography scans followed by aortography, pelvic angiography, and therapeutic embolization of pelvic arterial bleeders. This cart is stocked to provide equipment and supplies for on-site medical and surgical management. The following list suggests appropriate equipment and supplies for a mobile cart, but the cart must be chosen and stocked according to institution needs. Remember, all equipment should be readily accessible and clearly labeled. A preestablished system for regular checking and restocking of this cart ensures immediate availability of needed equipment.*

Cardiovascular:
Drugs

- 5 each of:
  - ☐ sodium bicarbonate, 50 mEq
  - ☐ atropine, 1 mg
  - ☐ calcium, 1 g
  - ☐ epinephrine, 1 mg
  - ☐ lidocaine, 100 mg
- 2 each of:
  - ☐ lidocaine, 2 g
  - ☐ verapamil HCl
  - ☐ nitroprusside sodium, 50 mg
  - ☐ propranolol, 1 mg
  - ☐ furosemide, 100 mg
  - ☐ dobutamine, 250 mg
  - ☐ Solu-Medrol, 125 mg
  - ☐ potassium chloride, 40 mEq
  - ☐ sodium chloride and sterile water, 10 cc
  - ☐ heparin sodium, 1,000 units/cc
- 4 mannitol 25% (12.5 g)
- 4 dopamine, 200 mg
- 4 phenytoin, 250 mg
- 2 phenytoin, 100 mg
- 2 dexamethasone, 4 mg/cc, 30-cc vial
- 2 each of:
  - ☐ sodium thiopental, 500 mg
  - ☐ naloxone, 0.4 mg
  - ☐ succinylcholine chloride, 20-mg vial
  - ☐ pancuronium bromide, 4 mg/cc, 5-cc ampul
  - ☐ diphenhydramine (Benadryl), 50 mg

Additional sedative, hypnotic, or analgesic medications are added to the cart as indicated for individual patients.

- 12 ECG electrodes
- Cooler for blood and blood products
- Portable defibrillator with extra battery
- 2 pressure bags for rapid I.V. infusion or arterial line flush
- Thoracoabdominal tray (see Appendix 3 for tray contents)
- I.V. solutions:
  - ☐ 2 normal saline, 500 cc
  - ☐ 4 Ringer's lactate, 500 cc
  - ☐ 2 dextrose 5% in 0.45% normal saline solution (D$_5$½NSS)
  - ☐ 2 D$_5$W, 250 cc
  - ☐ 2 D$_5$W, 50 cc
  - ☐ 1 normal saline with heparin sodium, 1,000 units
  - ☐ 2 Plasmanate, 500 cc
- 1 arterial line setup
- 3 each of 14G, 16G, 18G, and 20G peripheral intravenous catheters
- 2 each of:
  - ☐ I.V. administration sets
  - ☐ blood administration sets
  - ☐ volume-limiting sets (Buretrol, Vol-u-trol)
  - ☐ guide wires
  - ☐ introducer/guide wire sets
  - ☐ #10 French (F) feeding tubes
  - ☐ extension sets
  - ☐ subclavian catheters
  - ☐ tourniquets
  - ☐ Xylocaine 1% plain, 20 cc

Respiratory:
- 2 each of 7.0, 8.0, and 9.0 endotracheal tubes
- 1 each of 30-mm, 33-mm, and 36-mm tracheostomy tubes
- 1 laryngoscope handle with extra batteries
- 1 each straight and curved laryngoscope blades
- 1 light bulb for laryngoscope blades
- 1 each of nasopharyngeal airways, sizes 8, 9, 10, and 11 mm
- 1 each of small, medium, and large adult oropharyngeal airways
- 1 stylet
- 1 resuscitation bag with mask and tubing
- 2 each of #28, #32, #36, and #40 F chest tubes
- 1 underwater-seal chest drainage system
- 1 bottle sterile water to fill chest drainage system
- 1 portable suction machine
- 4 tracheal suction catheter sets
- 2 rigid oropharyngeal suction tubes

- 1 extra E cylinder oxygen tank

Gastrointestinal:
- 2 #16 F Salem gastric tubes

Miscellaneous:
- syringes/needles
- chest tube connectors
- scalpel blades, 2 each of sizes 10, 11, 15, and 20
- preparation razors
- three-way stopcocks
- alcohol swabs
- Band-Aids
- water-soluble lubricant
- blood specimen tubes (two each of red, blue, gray, purple)
- medication labels
- tracheal irrigation solution
- antibiotic ointment
- antiseptic solution and scrub
- multiuse tray (see Appendix 3 for tray contents)
- sterile drapes
- sterile gloves, two each of sizes 6½, 7, 7½, 8
- 4 × 4 gauze pads (packages of 2 and 10)
- 2 × 2 gauze pads
- suture removal kit
- tongue blades
- cotton swabs
- sutures, 3-0 nylon, 2-0 nylon, 3-0 silk ties, 3-0 double-armed prolene
- tape for dressings and endotracheal/gastric tubes

Pediatric Admission Cart

Note: *Copies of the pediatric manual used in your facility, premade drug and fluid charts according to weight, names and telephone numbers of appropriate pediatric or neonatal consultants, and notice of where additional supplies are stored or can be obtained should also be on this specialty cart. A preestablished system for periodic cart checks should be instituted to ensure availability and proper functioning of all equipment.*

Respiratory supplies:
- endotracheal tubes—uncuffed (two of each size)
  - ☐ 2.5 mm
  - ☐ 3.0 mm
  - ☐ 3.5 mm
  - ☐ 4.0 mm
  - ☐ 4.5 mm
  - ☐ 5.0 mm
  - ☐ 5.5 mm
  - ☐ 6.0 mm
  - ☐ 6.5 mm
- endotracheal tubes—cuffed (two of each size)
  - ☐ 5.5 mm
  - ☐ 6.0 mm
  - ☐ 6.5 mm
- tracheostomy tubes (at least one of each size)
  - ☐ 0
  - ☐ 1
  - ☐ 2
  - ☐ 3
  - ☐ 4
  - ☐ 6
  - ☐ 4.5 silastic
- laryngoscope and blades (one of each size)
  - ☐ 0 Miller
  - ☐ 1 Miller
  - ☐ 2 Miller
  - ☐ 1 Mackintosh
  - ☐ 2 Mackintosh
- batteries—two AA replacement bulbs for laryngoscope
- twill tape
- lubricant
- tape
  - ☐ ½″ silk
  - ☐ 1″ adhesive
- manual resuscitator bags (two)
- stylets (various thicknesses)
- suction catheters (six of each size)
  - ☐ #5 French (F)
  - ☐ #8 F
  - ☐ #10 F
- oral airways (all sizes)
- black oxygen masks
- disposable oxygen supplies
- bulb syringe

Cardiovascular supplies:
- syringes (four to six of each size)
  - ☐ tuberculin
  - ☐ 3 cc
  - ☐ 3 cc with 21G needle
  - ☐ 3 cc with 23G needle
  - ☐ 6 cc
  - ☐ 12 cc
  - ☐ 35 cc
- needles (all sizes) spinal needles (two to four of each size)
  - ☐ 25G
  - ☐ 22G
  - ☐ 20 G
  - ☐ 18G
- intravenous catheters (six of each size)
  - ☐ *Long lines*
    - 8″, 22G
    - 8″, 19G
    - 8″, 16G
  - ☐ *Short lines*
    - 20G
    - 22G
  - ☐ *Butterflies*
    - 25G, ¾″ with 12″ tubing
    - 25G, ⅜″ with 3½″ tubing
    - 23G, ¾″ with 12″ tubing
- intravenous infusion sets (at least two of each type)
  - ☐ extension tubing
  - ☐ volume-limited chambers
  - ☐ solution sets

- intravenous solutions (at least two of each type)
  - ☐ D₅W—250 cc
  - ☐ D₅¼NSS—250 cc
  - ☐ D₅W—500 cc
  - ☐ NSS—500 cc
  - ☐ D₅¼NSS—500 cc
  - ☐ LR—500 cc
- chest tubes (two to three of each size)
  - ☐ #12 F
  - ☐ #16 F
  - ☐ #20 F
  - ☐ #24 F
  - ☐ #28 F
- blood pressure cuffs (various sizes)
- external defibrillator paddles
- pediatric pneumatic antishock garment
- wooden cardiopulmonary board
- emergency cardiac drugs (at least two of each)
  - ☐ sodium bicarbonate
  - ☐ epinephrine
  - ☐ atropine
  - ☐ lidocaine
  - ☐ calcium
  - ☐ 5% dextrose bolus
  - ☐ dopamine/dobutamine

Miscellaneous:
- adhesive spray
- tape (all widths/types)
- antibiotic ointment
- heparin
- medication labels
- straight blades
- sterile 5-cc vials of injectable water/saline (two of each)
- alcohol swabs
- suture removal kits

- suture—4-0 silk ties, 3-0 silk on curved needle (four of each type)
- stopcocks (four)
- armboards—long and short
- blood sampling tubes—purple, red, blue, gray

Gastrointestinal:
- feeding tubes (four of each size)
  - ☐ #5 F
  - ☐ #8 F
  - ☐ #10 F
  - ☐ #12 F

Musculoskeletal:
- pediatric cervical collars—hard and soft (various sizes)
- pediatric arm and leg splints
- pediatric Hare traction device

Genitourinary:
- urinary catheters (three of each size)
  - ☐ #8 F
  - ☐ #10 F
  - ☐ #12 F
  - ☐ #14 F
  - ☐ #5 F feeding tube (may be used in newborns)
- urine collector bags (10)
- diapers (various sizes)
- lubricant

Sterile surgical trays:
- thoracotomy tray
- vascular tray
- emergency airway tray
- internal defibrillator paddles

Burn Cart

Use:
- Initial care of the burned patient

Contents:
Drawer 1
- intracatheters
- needles
- arterial catheters
- syringes
- knife blades—six of each size #20, #15, #11
- blood tubes

Drawer 2
- extension tubing
- stopcocks
- culture tubes
- gastric tubes, #10
- eye drops/ lubricant
- sterile barriers
- antibiotic ointment
- tape
- razors

Drawer 3
- masks and sterile gloves; burn charts

Drawer 4
- gauze rolls (10); 4 × 4 gauze sponges (eight boxes)

Drawer 5
- sterile burn sheets; sterile gowns

Drawer 6
- preparation solution and scrub (two bottles each)
- Ringer's lactate (10 bags)
- Silvadine cream
- NSS pour bottles (five)
- buretrols (four)
- infusion administration sets (four)

Emergency Airway Tray

Use:
Emergency cricothyroidotomy

Contents:
Instruments
- 1 towel clip
- 1 Allis tissue forceps (clamp)
- 2 rat-tooth forceps
- 1 self-retaining retractor
- 1 tracheal spreader
- 2 Army-Navy retractors
- 1 tracheostomy hook
- 1 #3 knife handle with #10 blade attached
- 1 #3 knife handle with #11 blade attached
- 2 small cups

Miscellaneous
- 1 12-cc syringe

- 20 4 × 4 gauze sponges
- 5 gauze sponges in each cup

Have available at bedside:
- preparation and scrub solution
- tracheostomy tubes in various sizes

- sterile water-soluble lubricant for tracheostomy tube
- sterile suction tubing
- suture per surgeon's request
- twill tape
- tracheostomy adapter for ventilator

Thoracoabdominal Tray

Use:
Emergency thoracotomy, emergency laparotomy

Contents:
Instruments

Note: *Arrange instruments in orderly fashion and cover with layers of laparotomy sponges.*
- 4 long Kelly clamps
- 2 short Kelly clamps
- 4 Crile clamps
- 2 #4 knife handles
- 2 Mayo needle holders
- 1 rib cutter
- 1 long, curved Mayo scissors
- 1 short, curved Mayo scissors
- 1 straight Mayo scissors
- 1 long Metzenbaum scissors
- 1 short Metzenbaum scissors
- 2 pickups with teeth
- 1 long pickup with teeth
- 2 Deaver or large Richardson retractors
- 1 Finochietto self-retaining rib spreaders
- 2 vascular clamps (DeBakey aortic clamp, Satinsky clamp)

Miscellaneous
- 2 #20 blades
- 8 laparotomy sponges

Place the following instruments on top of laparotomy sponges:
- 1 #4 knife handle with #20 blade on, keeping knife blade pack on for protection
- 1 long, straight vascular clamp
- 1 Metzenbaum scissors

Add to tray after it is opened:
- 10 laparotomy sponges
- 1 fenestrated straight suction catheter
- 1 pack of sterile suction tubing
- 1 bulb syringe
- 1 metal pitcher (100 cc)

- internal defibrillation paddles as needed
- cardiac double-armed suture as needed
- various sizes of precut Telfa pledgets

Have available at bedside:
- Lebsche sternum knife and mallet
- separate suction source for chest suction
- warmed sterile NSS for irrigation
- pour bottles of iodine-based preparation solution
- equipment necessary for pleural drainage

Halo Tray

Use:
Application of Halo apparatus for cervical spine traction

Contents:
Miscellaneous

- Halo rings—sizes #2, #3, #4, #5
- 1 bucket handle with two hooks
- 5 positioning plates (round bottom)
- 5 positioning plates (rounded-end screws)
- 5 skull pins (pointed-end screws)
- 5 locking devices
- 1 Allen wrench
- 4 towels
- 1 vial 1% Xylocaine (plain)
- 20 plain 4 × 4 gauze sponges
- 1 12-cc syringe without needle
- 1 18G needle
- 1 25G needle
- 1 crescent wrench (⁷⁄₁₆″, ⁹⁄₁₆″)
- 4 bolts
- 4 washers
- 1 #11 blade
- preparation cups

Have available at bedside:

- traction apparatus, cord
- weights (rule of thumb is 5 lb/vertebra; for example, C5 fracture requires 25 lb)
- shaving razor, blades
- topical antibiotic ointment

Neuroarteriogram Tray

Use:
One-shot carotid arteriogram when computerized tomography scanner is unavailable or contraindicated; provides visualization of extravasation due to active bleeding and variance in intracerebral or extracerebral vessels due to edema or hematoma formation

Contents:
Instruments

- 1 medium cup
- 2 small cups
- 1 #3 knife handle

Miscellaneous

- 20 4 × 4 gauze sponges
- 5 4 × 4 gauze sponges in small cup only
- 2 35-cc syringes
- 1 #15 blade
- 1 10-cc syringe
- 1 23G needle
- 1 22G needle
- 1 18G needle
- 1 vial 1% Xylocaine (plain)
- 4 towels

Have available at bedside:

- injectable contrast medium
- sterile NSS, 150-cc bag/infusion set
- 35-cc syringe
- preparation solution
- Potts-Cournand needle
- roentgenography extension set
- radiographer with portable radiography equipment

Appendix 4

HOSPITAL RESOURCES DOCUMENT CARING FOR THE INJURED PATIENT

The following table shows levels of categorization and their essential (E) or desirable (D) characteristics.

	LEVELS		
	I	**II**	**III**
A. HOSPITAL ORGANIZATION			
1. Trauma Service	E	E	E
a) Specified delineation of privileges for the trauma service must be made by the medical staff credentialing committee.			
b) Trauma team—organized and directed by a general surgeon who is an expert in and committed to care of the injured. All patients with multiple-system or major injury must be initially evaluated by the trauma team, and the surgeon who will be responsible for overall care of a patient (the team leader) must be identified. A team approach is required for optimal care of patients with multiple-system injuries.			
2. Surgery Departments/Divisions/Services/Sections			
(each staffed by qualified specialists)			
Cardiothoracic Surgery	E	D	
General Surgery	E	E	E
Neurologic Surgery	E	E	
Obstetrics-Gynecologic Surgery	D	D	
Ophthalmic Surgery	E	D	
Oral Surgery—Dental	D	D	
Orthopaedic Surgery	E	E	
Otorhinolaryngologic Surgery	E	D	
Pediatric Surgery	E	D	
Plastic and Maxillofacial Surgery	E	D	
Urologic Surgery	E	D	
3. Emergency Department/Division/Service/Section *(staffed by qualified specialists[1])*	E	E	E
4. Surgical Specialties Availability[2]			
In-house 24 hours a day:			
General Surgery	E	E[3]	
Neurologic Surgery	E[4]	E[4]	
On call and promptly available from inside or outside hospital:			
Cardiac Surgery	E	D	
General Surgery			E
Neurologic Surgery			D
Microsurgery Capabilities	E	D	
Gynecologic Surgery	E	D	
Hand Surgery	E	D	

	LEVELS		
	I	II	III
Ophthalmic Surgery	E	E	D
Oral Surgery—Dental	E	D	
Orthopaedic Surgery	E	E	D
Otorhinolaryngologic Surgery	E	E	D
Pediatric Surgery	E	D	
Plastic and Maxillofacial Surgery	E	E	D
Thoracic Surgery	E	E	D
Urologic Surgery	E	E	D

5. Nonsurgical Specialty Availability

In-hospital 24 hours a day:

	I	II	III
Emergency Medicine	E[5]	E[5]	E
Anesthesiology	E[6]	E[6,7]	E[7]

On call and promptly available from inside or outside hospital:

	I	II	III
Cardiology	E	E	D
Chest Medicine	E	D	
Gastroenterology	E	D	
Hematology	E	E	D
Infectious Diseases	E	D	
Internal Medicine	E	E	E
Nephrology	E	E	D
Neuroradiology	D		
Pathology	E	E	D
Pediatrics	E	E	D
Psychiatry	E	D	
Radiology	E	E	D

B. SPECIAL FACILITIES/RESOURCES/CAPABILITIES

1. Emergency Department

a) Personnel

	I	II	III
1. Designated physician director	E	E	E
2. Physician with special competence in care of the critically injured who is a designated member of the trauma team and physically present in the emergency department 24 hours a day	E	E	E
3. RNs, LPNs, and nurse's aides in adequate numbers	E	E	E

b) Equipment for resuscitation and to provide life support for the critically or seriously injured shall include but not be limited to:

	I	II	III
1. Airway control and ventilation equipment including laryngoscopes and endotracheal tubes of all sizes, bag-mask resuscitator, pocket masks, oxygen, and mechanical ventilator	E	E	E
2. Suction devices	E	E	E
3. Electrocardiograph-oscilloscope-defibrillator	E	E	E

		LEVELS	
	I	**II**	**III**
4. Apparatus to monitor central venous pressure	E	E	E
5. All standard intravenous fluids and administration devices, including intravenous catheters	E	E	E
6. Sterile surgical sets for procedures standard for the emergency department, such as thoracostomy, cutdown, etc.	E	E	E
7. Gastric lavage equipment	E	E	E
8. Drugs and supplies necessary for emergency care	E	E	E
9. Radiography capability, 24-hour coverage by in-house technician	E	E	E
10. Two-way radio linked with vehicles of emergency transport system	E	E	E
11. Skeletal traction device for cervical injuries	E	E	E

2. Intensive Care Units (ICUs) for Trauma Patients
ICUs may be separate specialty units.

a) Designated medical director	E	E	E
b) Physician on duty in ICU 24 hours a day or immediately available from in-hospital	E	E	D
c) Nurse-patient minimum ratio of 1:2 on each shift	E	E	E
d) Immediate access to clinical laboratory services	E	E	E

e) Equipment:

1. Airway control and ventilation devices	E	E	E
2. Oxygen source with concentration controls	E	E	E
3. Cardiac emergency cart	E	E	E
4. Temporary transvenous pacemaker	E	E	E
5. Electrocardiograph-oscilloscope-defibrillator	E	E	E
6. Cardiac output monitoring	E	E	D
7. Electronic pressure monitoring	E	E	D
8. Mechanical ventilator-respirators	E	E	E
9. Patient-weighing devices	E	E	E
10. Pulmonary function measuring devices	E	E	E
11. Temperature control devices	E	E	E
12. Drugs, intravenous fluids, and supplies	E	E	E
13. Intracranial pressure monitoring devices	E	E	D

3. Postanesthetic Recovery Room *(surgical ICU is acceptable)*

a) Registered nurses and other essential personnel 24 hours a day	E	E	E
b) Appropriate monitoring and resuscitation equipment	E	E	E

4. Acute Hemodialysis Capability *(or transfer agreement)*	E	D	D

5. Organized Burn Care	E	E	E

    a) Physician-directed Burn Center staffed by nursing personnel trained in burn care and equipped properly for care of the extensively burned patient,
    or
    b) Transfer agreement with nearby burn center or hospital with a burn unit

	LEVELS		
	I	II	III
6. Acute Spinal Cord/Head Injury Management Capability a) In circumstances where a designated spinal cord injury rehabilitation center exists in the region, early transfer should be considered; transfer agreements should be in effect. b) In circumstances where a head injury center exists in the region, transfer should be considered in selected patients; transfer agreements should be in effect.	E	E	E
7. Radiological Special Capabilities a) Angiography of all types	E	E	D
b) Sonography	E	D	
c) Nuclear scanning	E	D	
d) In-house computerized tomography with technician	E	E	
8. Rehabilitation Medicine a) Physician-directed rehabilitation service staffed by nursing personnel trained in rehabilitation care and equipped properly for care of the critically injured patient, **or** b) Transfer agreement when medically feasible to a nearby rehabilitation service.	E	E	E

C. OPERATING SUITE SPECIAL REQUIREMENTS
Equipment-instrumentation

	I	II	III
1. Operating room adequately staffed in-house and immediately available 24 hours a day	E	E	D
2. Cardiopulmonary bypass capability	E	D	
3. Operating microscope	E	D	
4. Thermal control equipment: a) for patient	E	E	E
b) for blood	E	E	E
5. X-ray capability	E	E	E
6. Endoscopes, all varieties	E	E	E
7. Craniotome	E	E	D
8. Monitoring equipment	E	E	E

D. CLINICAL LABORATORY SERVICE *(available 24 hours a day)*

	I	II	III
1. Standard analyses of blood, urine, and other body fluids	E	E	E
2. Blood typing and cross matching	E	E	E
3. Coagulation studies	E	E	E
4. Comprehensive blood bank or access to a community central blood bank and adequate hospital storage facilities	E	E	E
5. Blood gases and pH determinations	E	E	E
6. Serum and urine osmolality	E	E	D†
7. Microbiology	E	E	E
8. Drug and alcohol screening	E	E	D†

	LEVELS		
	I	II	III
E. QUALITY ASSURANCE			
1. Organized quality assurance program	E	E	E
2. Special audit for all trauma deaths and other specified cases	E	E	E
3. Morbidity and mortality review	E	E	E
4. Trauma conference, multidisciplinary[8]	E	E	
5. Medical nursing audit, utilization review, tissue review	E	E	E
6. Trauma registry review[9]	E	E	E
7. Review of prehospital and regional systems of trauma care	E	D	D
F. OUTREACH PROGRAM	E	D	
Telephone and on-site consultations with physicians of the community and outlying areas			
G. PUBLIC EDUCATION	E	E	D
Injury prevention in the home, in industry, and on the highways and athletic fields; standard first aid; problems confronting the public, the medical profession, and hospitals regarding optimal care for the injured			
H. TRAUMA RESEARCH PROGRAM	E	D	D
I. TRAINING PROGRAM			
1. Formal programs in continuing education provided by hospital for:			
a) Staff physicians	E	E	D
b) Nurses	E	E	D
c) Allied health personnel	E	E	D
d) Community physicians	E	E	D

[1]The emergency department staff should ensure immediate and appropriate care for the trauma patient. The emergency department physician should function as a designated member of the trauma team and the relationship between emergency department physicians and other participants of the trauma team must be established on a local level, consistent with resources but adhering to established standards and ensuring optimal care.

[2]Requirements may be fulfilled by senior residents capable of assessing emergent situations in their respective specialities. They must be capable of providing surgical treatment immediately and providing control and surgical leadership for the care of the trauma patient. When residents are used to fulfill availability requirements, staff specialists must be on call and promptly available.

[3]The established trauma system should ideally ensure that the trauma surgeon will be present in the emergency department at the time of the patient's arrival. When sufficient prior notification has not been possible, a designated member of the trauma team will immediately initiate the evaluation and resuscitation. Definitive surgical care must be instituted by the trauma surgeon in a timely manner that is consistent with established standards.

[4]An attending neurosurgeon must be promptly available and dedicated to that hospital's trauma service. The in-house requirement may be fulfilled by an in-house neurosurgeon or surgeon (or physician in Level II facilities) who has special competence, as judged by the chief of neurosurgery, in the care of patients with neural trauma, and who is capable of initiating measures directed toward stabilizing the patient and initiating diagnostic procedures.

[5]In Level I and Level II institutions, requirements may be fulfilled by senior level emergency medicine residents capable of assessing emergency situations in trauma patients and providing any indicated treatment. When residents are used to fulfill availability requirements, the staff specialist on call will be advised and be promptly available.

[6]Requirements may be fulfilled by anesthesiology residents capable of assessing emergent situations in trauma patients and providing any indicated treatment. When anesthesiology residents are used to fulfill availability requirements, the staff anesthesiologist on call will be advised and be promptly available.

[7]Requirements may be fulfilled when local conditions assure that the staff anesthesiologist will be in the hospital at the time of or shortly after the patient's arrival in the hospital. During the interim period, prior to the arrival of the staff anesthesiologist, a certified nurse anesthetist (CRNA) capable of assessing emergent situations in trauma patients and of initiating and providing any indicated treatment will be available.

[8]Regular and periodic multidisciplinary trauma conferences that include all members of the trauma team should be held. These conferences will be for the purpose of quality assurance through critiques of individual cases.

[9]Documentation of severity of injury (by trauma score, age, and injury severity score) and outcome (survival, length of stay, and ICU length of stay), with monthly review of statistics, is essential.

†Toxicology screens need not be immediately available but are desirable. If not available, results should be included in all quality assurance reviews.

Reprinted from Committee on Trauma—American College of Surgeons, *ACS Bulletin*, October 1986, with permission of the publisher.

Appendix 5

TRAUMA SCORE

The score is composed of the Glasgow Coma Scale (reduced to approximately one-third value) and measurements of cardiopulmonary function. Severity of injury is estimated by totaling the numbers. The lowest score is 1; the highest score is 16.

Glasgow Coma Scale (GCS)

		Points
Eye Opening	Spontaneous	4
	To voice	3
	To pain	2
	None	1
Best Verbal Response	Oriented	5
	Confused	4
	Inappropriate words	3
	Incomprehensible words	2
	None	1
Best Motor Response	Obeys commands	6
	Localizes (pain)	5
	Withdraws (pain)	4
	Flexion (pain)	3
	Extension (pain)	2
	None	1
Total	Apply this score to the GCS portion of the Trauma Score below.	**3 to 15**

Trauma Score

	Points	Score
Glasgow Coma Scale (GCS) (Total points from above)	**14 to 15**	5
	11 to 13	4
	8 to 10	3
	5 to 7	2
	3 to 4	1

		Points/score
Respiratory Rate	10 to 24/min	4
	25 to 35/min	3
	36/min or more	2
	0 to 9/min	1
	None	0
Respiratory Expansion	Normal	1
	Reactive/None	0
Systolic Blood Pressure	90 mm Hg or more	4
	70 to 89 mm Hg	3
	50 to 69 mm Hg	2
	0 to 49 mm Hg	1
	No pulse	0
Capillary Refill	Normal	2
	Delayed	1
	None	0
Total Trauma Score†		**1 to 16**

† Since outcome can be correlated with initial trauma score, a patient with a trauma score of 12 or less should optimally be managed at a Level I or II trauma center.
Reprinted from American College of Surgeons Committee on Trauma, *Advanced Trauma Life Support*. Student Manual, 1984, with permission of the publisher.

Appendix 6

TETANUS PROPHYLAXIS

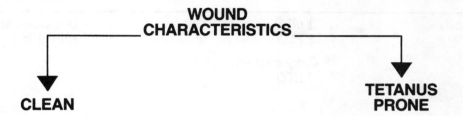

WOUND CHARACTERISTICS

CLEAN

- Less than 6 hours old
- Abrasion, simple laceration (with neat, straight edges)
- Caused by glass, knife blade, or other sharp surface
- No contaminants present or suspected
- Tissue appears clean and well vascularized, perfused
- No obvious signs of infection

TETANUS PRONE

- 6 or more hours old
- Avulsion, puncture, stellate laceration
- Caused by burn, crush, cold, gunshot, farm or industrial equipment, bite (human or animal)
- Contaminants present (soil or dirt, feces, saliva)
- Tissue appears devitalized
- Signs of infection present

PROPHYLACTIC THERAPY

No toxoid booster needed if patient has been fully immunized and had toxoid booster within the past *10 years.*

Give toxoid booster (0.5 cc absorbed toxoid) if last booster was more than 10 years ago or if immunization history is uncertain or unknown.

No toxoid booster needed if patient has been fully immunized and has had toxoid booster within the past 5 years.

Give toxoid booster (0.5 cc absorbed toxoid) if last booster was more than 5 years ago.

Give toxoid booster (0.5 cc absorbed toxoid) and 250 units tetanus immune globulin, human, if the patient has not been fully immunized or if the immunization history is uncertain or unknown.

Note: *When injections of both absorbed toxoid and tetanus immune globulin are required, the injections should be given via different syringes and in different, distant sites. Tetanus immune globulin should be administered intramuscularly.*

References: 1) Odling-Smee, G.W. *"Infections Following Trauma,"* in *Trauma Care.* Edited by Odling-Smee, G.W., and Crockard, A. New York: Grune & Stratton, 1981. 2) Burke, J.F., and Bondoc, C.C. "Wound Sepsis: Prevention and Control," in *The Management of Trauma,* 4th ed. Edited by Zuidema, G.D., et al. Philadelphia: W.B. Saunders Co., 1985. 3) Committee on Trauma, American College of Surgeons. *Advanced Trauma Life Support Course Manual.* American College of Surgeons, 1984.

Appendix 7

ACID-BASE IMBALANCES

Disorder	ABG Results	Physiologic Basis
Respiratory acidosis	↓ pH ↑ $PaCO_2$ Compensatory: ↑ HCO_3^-	Decreased alveolar ventilation, resulting in carbon dioxide retention
Respiratory alkalosis	↑ pH ↓ $PaCO_2$ Compensatory: ↓ HCO_3^-	Increased alveolar ventilation, resulting in carbon dioxide loss
Metabolic acidosis	↓ pH ↓ HCO_3^- Compensatory: ↓ $PaCO_2$	HCO_3^- loss, ↑ acid formation
Metabolic alkalosis	↑ pH ↑ HCO_3^- Compensatory: ↑ $PaCO_2$	↑ HCO_3^-, and acids or potassium loss

Potential Causes	Signs and Symptoms	Compensatory Mechanisms
Depression of medullary respiratory center due to drugs, injury, or disease Pulmonary diseases Inadequate tidal volume (TV) or respiratory rate on ventilator	Decreased mentation, restlessness, combativeness, headache, diaphoresis, anxiety, tachycardia	Renal compensation by HCO_3^- retention, acid elimination, and increased ammonia production
Hyperventilation from anxiety, pain, excessive TV or respiratory rate on ventilator Respiratory-center stimulation by drugs, injury, or disease Fever or high ambient temperature Sepsis	Increased rate and depth of respirations, "tingling" or numb feeling, light-headedness or syncope, anxiety	Renal compensation by HCO_3^- elimination, acid retention, and decreased ammonia production
Diarrhea, diabetes, shock, renal failure, azotemia, small-bowel fistulas	Increased rate and depth of respirations, fatigue/lethargy, acetone odor to breath, unconsciousness	Rapid pulmonary compensation by hyperventilation, renal metabolic compensation by HCO_3^- retention, acid elimination, increased ammonia production
Vomiting, gastric suctioning, prolonged use of diuretics, excessive HCO_3^- ingestion	Decreased rate and depth of respirations, hypertonicity, twitching to tetanus, convulsions, irritability, restlessness/combativeness, unconsciousness	Rapid pulmonary compensation by hypoventilation, renal metabolic compensation by HCO_3^- elimination, acid retention, decreased ammonia production

References

Palmer, L. "Arterial Blood Gas Analysis," in *Diagnostics*. Springhouse, Pa.: Springhouse Corp., 1983.

Shires, G.T., et al. "Fluid, Electrolyte, and Nutritional Management of the Surgical Patient," in *Principles of Surgery*, 4th ed. Edited by Schwartz, S.I. New York: McGraw-Hill Book Co., 1984.

Appendix 8

FLUID-ELECTROLYTE IMBALANCES

Causes	Signs and Symptoms/ Laboratory Results	Treatment
1. Hypovolemia: Hemorrhage, diabetes insipidus (DI), renal disease, vagal stimulation, drug reactions, hyperglycemic hyperosmolar nonketotic coma	Tachycardia, weak pulse, hypotension, oliguria, ↓ central venous pressure (CVP), ↓ level of consciousness (LOC), pallor, ↓ hematocrit/hemoglobin	Correct the cause; administer appropriate I.V. fluids.
2. Hypervolemia: Excessive I.V. fluid administration	Hypertension, edema, bounding pulse, ↑ CVP, pulmonary edema, venous distention, ↓ hemoglobin/hematocrit, ↓ blood urea nitrogen (BUN)	Treat with diuretics, dialysis phlebotomy; no treatment may be needed; prevention is the best treatment.
3. Intravascular/Interstitial Shift: Hemorrhage, ↓ water intake, concentrated tube feedings, vomiting/diarrhea, burns, prolonged gastric suctioning, soft tissue injury, intestinal obstruction, fever	Shock state, tachycardia, weak pulse, oliguria, ↓ LOC, dry mucous membranes, ↑ hemoglobin/hematocrit, ↑ BUN, hypotension	Correct the cause; administer appropriate I.V. fluids.
4. Interstitial/Intravascular Shift: Burns, soft tissue injury, excessive colloid or hypertonic I.V. administration	Hypertension, bounding pulse, venous distention, ↑ CVP, weakness, ↓ hemoglobin/hematocrit, ↓ BUN, hyponatremia	No treatment is usually needed except in patients with abnormal heart, liver, or kidney function; they are usually treated with diuretics.
5. Hyponatremia: Excessive sweating or water intake, ↓ salt intake, congestive heart failure (CHF), renal failure, diuretic therapy, freshwater near drowning, vomiting, diarrhea, burns	Confusion, headache, abdominal cramps, apathy, hypotension, weakness, hyperactive reflexes, convulsions, oliguria, ↓ serum sodium, ↓ chloride, ↓ specific gravity	Decrease water intake or increase sodium intake.
6. Hypernatremia: ↓ water intake, ↓ sodium intake, prolonged watery diarrhea, prolonged hyperventilation, saltwater near drowning, DI	Dehydration; thirst; dry mucous membranes; weakness; fever; warm, flushed skin; muscle pain; ↑ serum sodium level; ↑ serum chloride level; ↑ specific gravity	Correct the cause, if possible; restrict sodium intake; increase fluid intake.

Causes	Signs and Symptoms/Laboratory Results	Treatment
7. Hypokalemia: ↓ potassium intake, diuretics, vomiting or diarrhea, burns, CHF, fistulas, colitis, steroids	Diminished reflexes, irregular pulse, thirst, hypotension, ECG changes, muscular weakness or irritability, ↓ serum potassium level, ↓ serum chloride level	Increase dietary potassium intake; administer P.O. or I.V. potassium supplements.
8. Hyperkalemia: ↑ potassium intake, burns, soft tissue injury, advanced kidney disease, adrenal insufficiency, hemorrhagic shock, excessive I.V. administration	Irritability, nausea, diarrhea, confusion, flaccid muscles, ECG changes, hypotension, abdominal cramping, ↑ serum potassium level	Decrease intake; treat with dialysis; give a sodium polystyrene sulfonate enema; give sodium bicarbonate, glucose, and insulin together I.V.
9. Hypocalcemia: Diarrhea, burns, renal failure, draining wounds, citrated blood administration, acidosis overcorrection, vitamin D deficiency	Carpopedal spasms; tetany; convulsions; tingling in fingers, toes, lips; muscle cramps; ECG changes; ↓ serum calcium level	Administer calcium P.O. or I.V.
10. Hypercalcemia: Vitamin D overdose, renal disease, excessive antacid use, excessive calcium intake	Pathologic fractures, deep-bone or flank pain, lethargy, nausea, vomiting, ECG changes, osteoporosis, kidney stones, kidney infections, ↑ serum calcium level	Correct the cause; administer disodium phosphate, sodium sulfate, diuretics.
11. Hypomagnesemia: Alcohol abuse, vomiting, ↓ intake, malnutrition, diuretics, prolonged GI suctioning, diarrhea, pancreatitis, kidney disease	Tetany, lethargy, nausea, vomiting, tachydysrhythmias, hypotension, confusion, hyperactive reflexes, ↓ serum magnesium level	Increase dietary intake, administer I.V. magnesium.
12. Hypermagnesemia: Excessive intake, kidney disease, severe dehydration, repeated magnesium-containing enemas, magnesium antacids in renal failure	Lethargy, flushing, depressed respirations, hypotension, flaccid muscles or paralysis, dysrhythmias, ↑ serum magnesium level	Decrease intake; administer I.V. 10% calcium gluconate; treat renal-failure patients with dialysis.

Adapted from: Neel, C.J., and Wallerstein, M.B. "Fluid and Electrolyte Imbalances," in *A Pocket Guide for Medical-Surgical Nursing*. Bowie, Md.: Brady Communications Co., 1985.

Appendix 9

TRIAGE DECISION SCHEME

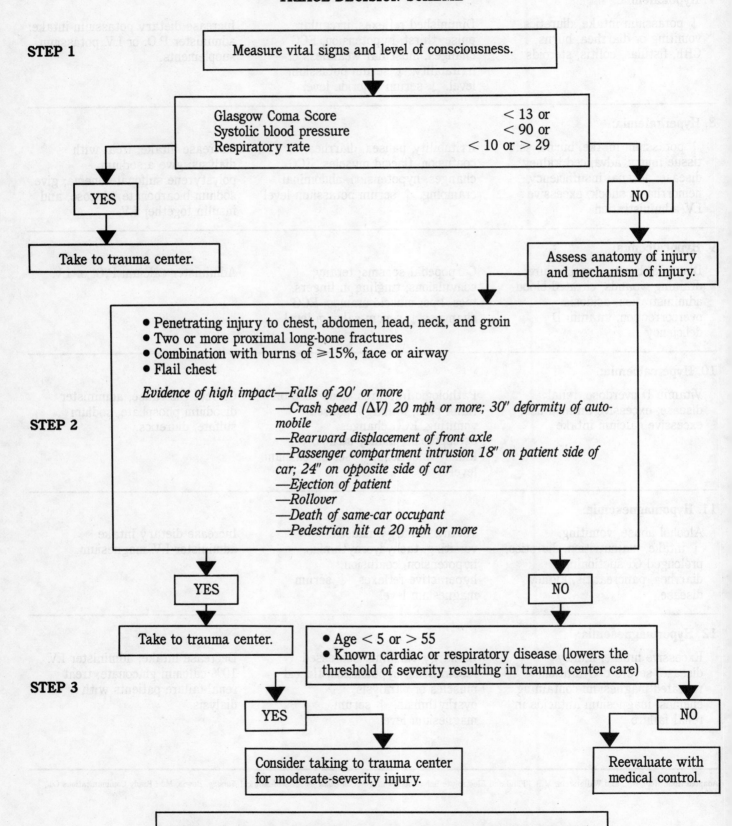

STEP 1 — Measure vital signs and level of consciousness.

Glasgow Coma Score   < 13 or
Systolic blood pressure   < 90 or
Respiratory rate   < 10 or > 29

YES → Take to trauma center.

NO → Assess anatomy of injury and mechanism of injury.

STEP 2

- Penetrating injury to chest, abdomen, head, neck, and groin
- Two or more proximal long-bone fractures
- Combination with burns of ≥15%, face or airway
- Flail chest

Evidence of high impact—*Falls of 20′ or more*
    —*Crash speed (ΔV) 20 mph or more; 30″ deformity of automobile*
    —*Rearward displacement of front axle*
    —*Passenger compartment intrusion 18″ on patient side of car; 24″ on opposite side of car*
    —*Ejection of patient*
    —*Rollover*
    —*Death of same-car occupant*
    —*Pedestrian hit at 20 mph or more*

YES → Take to trauma center.

NO →
- Age < 5 or > 55
- Known cardiac or respiratory disease (lowers the threshold of severity resulting in trauma center care)

STEP 3

YES → Consider taking to trauma center for moderate-severity injury.

NO → Reevaluate with medical control.

WHEN IN DOUBT, TAKE THE PATIENT TO A TRAUMA CENTER.

Reprinted from Committee on Trauma—American College of Surgeons, *ACS Bulletin*, October 1986, with permission of the publisher.

INDEX

A

Abdominal trauma during pregnancy, blunt and penetrating, 99-105
  abruptio placentae, 101-102
  airway clearance, ineffective, potential for, 99
  anxiety, potential for, 104-105
  assessment, 99
  diagnostic studies, 99
  fetal distress, potential for, 104
  fetal/maternal tissue perfusion, decreased, potential for, 100-102
  fluid volume deficit, 100-101
  functional residual capacity, decreased, 100
  gas exchange, decreased, potential for, 99-100
  infection, potential for, 103
  nasal and upper airway engorgement, 99
  peritoneal contamination, 103
  premature labor, potential for, 102-103
  ruptured membranes, 103
  uterine damage, 101-102
  vomiting and aspiration, 100
Acid–base imbalances, 372-373t
Acid ingestion, effects of, 176t
Acute myocardial infarction, 90-92
  assessment, 90
  bradykinin activation, 90-91
  cardiac output, decreased, potential for, 91-92
  cardiac pain receptors, stimulation of, 90-91
  comfort, alteration in, 90-91
  diagnostic studies, 90
  dysrhythmias, 91-92
  extension of, potential for, 92
  myocardial contractility, changes in, 90-92
  myocardial oxygen supply, inadequate, 92
  myocardial tissue edema, 90-91
Acute pancreatitis, 248-251
  antidigestion of pancreatic enzymes, 250-251
  assessment, 248
  bowel permeability, increased, 251
  breathing patterns, ineffective, potential for, 249
  diagnostic studies, 248
  fluid volume deficit, 250
  gas exchange, decreased, potential for, 249
  infection, potential for, 250-251
  pain, 249
  paralytic ileus, 249
  pulmonary effusions, 249
  tissue perfusion, decreased, potential for, 250
Acute pericardial tamponade, 87-89
  assessment, 87
  cardiac compression, 87, 88
  cardiac output, decreased, 88
  diagnostic studies, 87
  tissue perfusion, decreased, potential for, 87-89

Acute renal failure, 259-263
  assessment, 259
  catabolism, increased, 262-263
  diagnostic studies, 260
  fluid volume deficit, potential for, 261-262
  fluid volume excess, potential for, 260-261
  GI bleeding, 261-262
  hyperkalemia, potential for, 161
  inability of kidneys to eliminate body fluid, 260-261
  infection, potential for, 262-263
  level of consciousness, altered, potential for injury related to, 262
  potassium excretion, decreased, 261
  uremia, 261-262
Acute upper gastrointestinal bleeding, 107-112
  assessment, 107
  blood loss, 108-109
  control of, 109-110
  diagnostic studies, 107
  fluid volume deficit, 108-109
  identification of site, 109
  infection, potential for, 110-111
  peritonitis, 110-111
  symptoms, 112t
  tissue perfusion, impaired, potential for, 107-110
Acute whole-body radiation exposure, 166-169
  anxiety, potential for, 168-169
  assessment, 166
  coagulopathy, 167
  diagnostic studies, 166
  dosage effects, 166t
  electrolyte imbalance, potential for, 168
  excessive diarrhea, 168
  fluid volume deficit, potential for, 167-168
  hematopoietic syndrome, 167
  infection, potential for, 167
  knowledge deficit of patient about health effects, 168-169
  leukocyte/granulocyte formation, diminished, 167
  neurologic deterioration, 168
  sensory perception, altered, potential for, 168
Adult respiratory distress syndrome, 229-231
  assessment, 229
  cardiac output, decreased, potential for, 231
  diagnostic studies, 229
  fluid accumulation, 229-230
  gas exchange, impaired, potential for, 229-230
  pneumothorax, 230
Airway obstruction. See Lower airway obstruction and Upper airway obstruction.
Alcohol abuse, 205t
Alkali ingestion, effects of, 176t
Amphetamine abuse, 204t
Amputation. See Traumatic amputation.
Anaphylactic shock. See Vasogenic shock.
Anticipation, as component in trauma care, 3-4
Antidiuretic hormone secretion, inappropriate, in trauma, 46
Aorta, traumatic rupture of. See Traumatic rupture of aorta or great vessels.
Aortography, 325
Approved nursing diagnoses, April 1986, 357
Autotransfusion, 334-335

Brain/brain stem injury, findings in, 42t
Brain-death criteria, 346
Bronchoscopy (fiberoptic), 330
Burn care considerations, general, 170-172
  additional required care, 171
  analgesic administration, 171
  assessment factors, 170
  associated injuries, 170
  infection, 171
  pediatric/geriatric patients, special needs of, 171
  psychosocial aspect, 172
  surgical intervention, 171
  tetanus immunization, 171
  transfer to regional burn center, 170
  volume replacement, 170
Burn cart, 363
Burn depth, classification of, 180t

C

Cannabis abuse, 205t
Carbon monoxide inhalation. See Inhalation injuries.
Cardiogenic shock, 24-27
  assessment, 24
  diagnostic studies, 24
  inadequate cardiac output, 25t, 25-27
  left ventricular failure, 25-27
  tissue perfusion, decreased, potential for, 25-27
  vicious cycle of, 25i
Caustic chemical ingestion, 176-178
  airway clearance, ineffective, potential for, 177
  assessment, 176
  bowel elimination, altered, potential for, 177-178
  corrosive chemical damage, 177
  diagnostic studies, 176
  fluid and electrolyte imbalance, potential for, 178
  GI tract perforation, potential for, 177-178
  nutrition, altered, potential for, 177-178
Cervical spine injury, 28-35
  aspiration of vomitus, 32
  assessment, 28
  autonomic nervous system, loss of, 32-33
  breathing patterns, ineffective, potential for, 32
  deep vein thrombosis, 33-34
  diagnostic studies, 28
  diaphragmatic elevation, 32
  fluid volume deficit, potential for 30-31
  gas exchange, impaired, potential for, 29-30
  gastric distention from paralytic ileus, 32
  mechanical ventilatory control, decreased, 29-30
  neurogenic bladder, 31-32
  pulmonary thromboembolism, 34
  sensorimotor deficit, potential for, 28-29
  skin integrity, impaired, potential for, 33
  sympathetic vasomotor tone, loss of, 30-31
  thermoregulation, ineffective, potential for, 32-33
  tissue perfusion, altered, potential for, 33-34
  urinary elimination, alteration in, 31-32
  urinary tract infections, 32

B

Barbiturate abuse, 205t
Battle's sign, 42
Bladder injury. See Renal system injury.
Blood requirements, 14t

Chemical burns, 173-175
  assessment, 173
  burning process, discontinuation of, 173-174
  diagnostic studies, 173
  gas exchange, impaired, potential for, 174-175
  infection, potential for, 174-175
  lower airway obstruction, 174-175
  skin integrity, potential for additional loss of, 173-174
Closed-tube thoracostomy, 344
Cocaine abuse, 204t
Communication systems, as component in trauma care, 4
Compartment syndrome, 267-269
  assessment, 267
  diagnostic studies, 268
  indicators of involvement, 267-268t
  minimizing risk of, 269
  muscle tissue perfusion, decreased, potential for, 269
  renal dysfunction, potential for, 269
  tubular necrosis, 269
Core body temperature, measurement of, 18
Critically ill/injured patient requiring special care, 347-348
Cyanide/hydrogen cyanide inhalation. See Inhalation injuries.

D

Deep vein thrombosis, 232-235
  assessment, 232
  blood loss from anticoagulant therapy, 234-235
  diagnostic studies, 232
  fluid volume deficit, potential for, 234-235
  onset of, 233-234
  peripheral tissue perfusion, altered, potential for, 232-234
  risk factors in formation of, 232-233
  risk of pulmonary thromboembolus from fragmentation of, 234
Diabetes insipidus, 222-223
  assessment, 222
  diagnostic studies, 222
  fluid volume deficit, potential for, 222-223
  urinary elimination patterns, alteration in, 223
  urine output, increased, 222-223
Diagnostic peritoneal lavage, 328
Diaphragmatic rupture. See Ruptured diaphragm.
Dislocations, 140-141
  assessment, 140
  diagnostic studies, 140
  neurovascular compromise, 141
  physical mobility, impaired, potential for, 140-141
  reduction, 140-141
  sensorimotor function, impaired, potential for, 141
  tissue integrity, potential for further impairment of, 140
  tissue perfusion, decreased, potential for, 141
Disseminated intravascular coagulation, 278-281
  assessment, 278
  blood loss, control of, 279-280
  coagulopathy, 279
  comfort, alteration in, 281
  diagnostic studies, 278
  laboratory values in, 278t
  oxygen availability and utilization, 280
  tissue necrosis, 281
  tissue perfusion, decreased, potential for, 279-280

E

Ectopic pregnancy, ruptured. See Ruptured ectopic pregnancy.
Electrical burns, 189-192
  assessment, 189
  breathing patterns, ineffective, potential for, 189
  circulatory blood volume, decreased, 189-190
  diagnostic studies, 189
  level of consciousness, altered, potential for, 190
  myocardial dysfunction, 189-190
  physical mobility, impaired, potential for, 191
  respiratory paralysis, 189
  sensorimotor function, altered, potential for, 190
  tissue perfusion, decreased, potential for, 189-190, 191
  venous thrombosis, 191
Emergency airway tray, 363
Emergency Medical Services (EMS) systems, development of, 8
Emergency transportation cart, 361
Endoscopy, 329
Endotracheal intubation (oral and nasal), 349-351
Endotracheal tube, selection of, for children, 304t
Esophageal varices. See Acute upper gastrointestinal bleeding.
External genitalia injury, 123-124
  assessment, 123
  body image, altered, 123-124
  comfort, alteration in, 124
  self-concept, disturbance in, 123-124
  skin and tissue integrity, impaired, 123
  urinary elimination, altered patterns of, potential for, 124
  urinary obstruction or retention, 124
Extraocular movement testing, 217t
Eye examination, 217-218t
Eye injuries, 211-218
  assessment, 211
  burn injury, presence of, 215
  comfort, altered, potential for, 211-213
  corneal epithelial defects, 212-213
  diagnostic studies, 211
  extension of, potential for, 214
  foreign body, presence of, 211-212
  ocular pressure, increased, 216
  vision loss, potential for, 216
  visual perception, altered, potential for, 212-213, 215-216

F

Facial fractures, types of, 199t
Fat embolism syndrome, 264-266
  assessment, 264
  diagnostic studies, 264
  fat globule release, increased, 265
  fat metabolism, altered, 265
  minimizing risk of, 264-265
  neurologic deterioration, 266
  pulmonary blood flow, increased resistance to, 266
  tissue perfusion, decreased, potential for, 264-266
Fetal maturity, classification of, 104

Flail chest, 76-78
  assessment, 76
  breathing patterns, ineffective, potential for, 76-77
  chest pain, 77
  diagnostic studies, 76
  gas exchange, impaired, potential for, 77-78
  infection, potential for, 77-78
  mechanical dysfunction of chest wall, 76-77
  multiple rib or sternal fractures, 76-77
  retained secretions, 77-78
Fluid–electrolyte imbalances, 374-375t
Fluid requirements, 14t
Fractures, open/closed, 134-139
  arterial occlusion, 136-137
  assessment, 134
  blood loss, 135t
  comfort, alteration in, 139
  compartment syndrome, 137-138
  diagnostic studies, 134
  edema, 135
  fat embolism syndrome, 138
  fluid volume deficit, potential for, 135
  immobilization of fractured bone ends, 135
  infection, potential for, 136
  nerve damage, 137
  physical mobility, impaired, 139
  sensorimotor deficit, potential for, 137-138
  soft tissue disruption, 134-135
  tetanus, 136
  tissue integrity, potential for further impairment of, 134-135
  tissue perfusion, decreased, potential for, 136-138
  wound contamination, 136

G

Gardner-Wells tong tray, 359
Gas gangrene, 270-271
  assessment, 270
  clostridial infection, potential for, 270-271
  diagnostic studies, 270
  fluid volume deficit, potential for, 270
Genitalia injury, external. See External genitalia injury.
Glasgow Coma Scale, 370
Great vessels, rupture of. See Traumatic rupture of aorta or great vessels.

H

Hallucinogen abuse, 205t
Halo tray, 364
Hand injuries, 145-151
  assessment, 145
  compartment syndrome, 150
  diagnostic studies, 145
  infection, potential for, 148-149
  mobility, impaired, potential for, 150
  muscle ischemia, potential for, 150
  nerve/tendon damage, 145-147
  rabies, 148-149
  sensorimotor deficit, potential for, 145-147
  tetanus, 148
  tissue perfusion, decreased, potential for, 147-148
  vascular impairment, 147-148
  wound contamination, 149
  wound healing, 149

Head injury, 42-50
  antidiuretic hormone secretion, disruption in, 46
  aspiration, 44
  assessment, 42
  atelectasis, 44
  blood loss, 45
  breathing patterns, ineffective, 44
  cardiac output, decreased, potential for, 45
  cerebral oxygenation, 44
  coagulopathy, 46
  diagnostic studies, 43
  dysrhythmias, 45
  fluid and electrolyte imbalance, potential for, 46
  fluid volume deficit, potential for, 45, 46
  gas exchange, impaired, potential for, 44
  hypothalamic malfunction, 48-49
  infection, potential for, 49
  intracranial pressure, increased, 46-48
  lower airway obstruction, 44
  neurologic deterioration, potential for, 46-47
  neurologic function, altered, potential for, 48
  nutrition, altered, potential for, 49-50
  retained secretions, 44
  seizure activity, 48
  septic shock, 49
  sympathetic vasomotor activity, heightened, 45
  thermoregulation, altered, potential for, 48-49
  thromboplastin, release of, from damaged tissue, 46
  upper airway obstruction, 44
  urine output, increased, 46
Hematomas from head injury, findings in, 43t
Hemolytic transfusion reaction. See Transfusion reactions.
Hemorrhagic shock, 14-18
  assessment, 14
  coagulopathy, 17-18
  diagnostic studies, 14-15
  fluid volume deficit, 15-18
  hypothermia, potential for, 18
  rapid infusion of I.V. fluids, 18
  tissue perfusion, decreased, potential for, 15-17, 18
Hemothorax, 69-72
  assessment, 69
  atelectasis, 71
  cardiac output, decreased, potential for, 69, 71
  diagnostic studies, 69, 70, 71
  fluid volume deficit, 70
  gas exchange, impaired, potential for, 69-72
  hypoxia, 69, 70
  infection, potential for, 71-72
  pleural cavity compression and pressure, 71
  retained secretions, 71-72
  tissue perfusion, decreased, potential for, 69, 70
Heparin, 34
Homans' sign, 34
Hospital resources to care for injured patient, 365-369
Hypercalcemia, 375t
Hyperkalemia, 375t
Hypermagnesemia, 375t
Hypernatremia, 374t
Hypervolemia, 374t
Hypocalcemia, 375t
Hypokalemia, 375t
Hypomagnesemia, 375t
Hyponatremia, 364t

Hypothermia, 156-159
  assessment, 156
  carbon dioxide retention, 158-159
  core temperature restoration, 158-159
  dysrhythmias, 159
  findings, 157t
  metabolic acidosis, 158-159
  neurologic problems, 159
  potential for, related to environmental exposure, 156, 158
  tissue perfusion, decreased, potential for, 158-159
Hypovolemia, 374t

I
Inevitable abortion, 117
Inhalation injuries, 193-198
  airway clearance, ineffective, 194
  assessment, 193
  breathing patterns, ineffective, potential for, 196-197
  cardiac output, decreased, potential for, 196
  cognitive function, impaired, potential for, 196-197
  diagnostic studies, 193
  gas exchange, impaired, potential for, 194-196
  myocardial compromise, 196
  oxygen availability, 194-195
  physical findings in, 198t
  respiratory irritation, 194
  sensorimotor function, impaired, potential for, 196-197
Instrument set, 359
Interstitial/intravascular shift, 374t
Intraabdominal trauma, blunt and penetrating, 95-98
  abdominal distention, 98
  assessment, 95
  bowel elimination, alteration in, 98
  diagnostic studies, 95
  disruption in intraabdominal organ, 96
  evisceration, 96-97
  fluid volume deficit, potential for, 96-97
  infection, potential for, 97
  paralytic ileus, 98
  peritoneal inflammation, 97, 98
  vascular integrity, 96, 97
  wound contamination, 97
Intraaortic balloon pump, 337-338
Intracompartment pressure measurement, 333
Intracranial pressure monitoring, 332
Intrahospital transport of shock trauma patient, 322-323
Intravascular/interstitial shift, 374t
Isolation trays, 360

K
Kidney injury. See Renal system injury.

L
Laboratory values, changes in, during shock, 15t
Laryngeal fracture, 57-59
  airway clearance, ineffective, potential for, 57-58
  assessment, 57
  diagnostic studies, 57
  difficulty in breathing, fear related to, potential for, 58
  displacement of fractured cartilage, 58
  risk factors, 57
  soft tissue edema, 58
  verbal communication, impaired, potential for, 59

Lower airway obstruction, 55-56
  assessment, 55
  atelectasis, 56
  diagnostic studies, 55
  gas exchange, impaired, potential for, 55
  infection, potential for, 56
  retained secretions, 56
Lund and Browder burn chart, 184i

M
Malnutrition in trauma patient, 240-243
  assessment, 240
  diagnostic studies, 240
  hypermetabolic, hypercatabolic responses, 240-241
  nutrition, altered, potential for, 240-243
  nutritional support, 241-242
  therapy complications, 242-243
Massive pelvic injury, 129-133
  assessment, 129
  coagulopathy, 130
  compartment syndrome, 131-132
  diagnostic studies, 129
  fluid volume deficit, 129-131
  fracture site disruption, 130-131
  sciatic nerve involvement, 133
  sensorimotor deficit, potential for, 131-132
  sensory perception, decreased, potential for, 133
  tissue perfusion, decreased, potential for, 129-130
  urinary elimination, altered, potential for, 132
  urinary tract injury and disruption, 132
MAST suit, 340-341
Maxillofacial injuries, 199-203
  airway clearance, ineffective, 199-200
  assessment, 199
  body image, altered, 202-203
  concomitant neurologic injury, 201
  diagnostic studies, 199
  fear, potential for, 202-203
  fluid volume deficit, potential for, 201
  hemorrhage, 201
  infection, potential for, 202
  sensorimotor function, altered, potential for, 201
  upper airway obstruction, 51-52, 199-200
Mechanical bowel obstruction, 256-258
  accumulation of intestinal secretions, 257
  assessment, 256
  barium inpaction, 256
  bowel elimination, alteration in, 256-257
  diagnostic studies, 256
  electrolyte imbalance, 257
  extracellular fluid depletion, 257
  fluid volume deficit, potential for, 257
  gastric/intestinal distention, 256-257
  infection, potential for, 258
  intestinal strangulation, 258
Metabolic acidosis, 372-373t
Metabolic alkalosis, 372-373t
Multiuse tray, 359
Myocardial contusion, 93-94
  assessment, 93
  cardiac output, decreased, potential for, 93-94
  comfort, altered, potential for, 94
  diagnostic studies, 93
  dysrhythmias, 94
  pain, 94
  pump failure, 93-94

N

Near drowning, freshwater/saltwater, 160-165
  airway clearance, ineffective, potential for,
    160-161
  aspiration of foreign material, 161
  assessment, 160
  cardiac output, decreased, potential for, 163
  cerebral edema, 163
  cerebral perfusion, decreased, potential for,
    163
  diagnostic studies, 160
  dysrhythmias, potential for, 163
  electrolyte imbalance, potential for, 161
  fluid volume deficit, potential for, 164
  fluid volume excess, potential for, 161
  gas exchange, impaired, potential for, 160-
    162
  hemolysis, 164
  hypothermia, potential for, 162
  infection, potential for, 165
  intrapulmonary shunting, 161-162
  metabolic acidosis, 162
  myocardial ischemia, 163
  redistribution of intravascular fluids, 164
  tissue perfusion, decreased, potential for,
    164
Needle cricothyroidotomy, 353
Neuroarteriogram tray, 364
Neurogenic shock. *See* Vasogenic shock.
Neuromuscular blocking agents, use of, 236-
    239
  comfort, altered, potential for, 239
  elimination patterns, alteration in, 238-239
  fear of total paralysis, potential for, 236-237
  mobility, impaired, 237-238
  respiratory function, alteration in, 237
  skin integrity, impaired, potential for, 238
Nonhemolytic transfusion reactions. *See* Trans-
    fusion reactions.
Nuclear medicine imaging, 327
Nursing diagnoses
  approved, 357
  supplemental, 358
Nursing process during acute resuscitation, 6-7

O

Open pneumothorax, 65-66
  assessment, 65
  breathing patterns, ineffective, potential for,
    65-66
  diagnostic studies, 65
  gas exchange, impaired, potential for, 65-66
  infection, potential for, 66
  lung collapse, 65
  thoracic bellows, loss of, 65
  wound contamination, 66
Opioid abuse, 204t
Organ donation, 345-346

P

Pacemaker insertion, temporary transvenous
    pacing, 339
Pancreatitis. *See* Acute pancreatitis.
Paralytic ileus, 252-255
  aspiration of vomitus, 255
  assessment, 252
  bowel elimination, alteration in, 252-253
  diagnostic study, 252
  diaphragmatic elevation, 254
  fluid absorption in bowel, decreased, 253-254
  fluid volume deficit, potential for, 253-254
  pain, 253
  peristalsis, decreased/absent, 252-253, 254
  respiratory function, impaired, potential for,
    254-255

Parkland formula for calculating volume re-
    placement, 184
Patient, effect of trauma on, 2
Pediatric admission cart, 362
Pediatric airway obstruction, 300-304
  airway clearance, ineffective, 300-302
  assessment, 300
  bacterial growth
    in cricothyroidotomy site, 303
    in lungs, 303
  diagnostic studies, 300
  gas exchange, impaired, potential for, 302-
    303
  infection, potential for, 303
Pediatric care considerations, 313-315
  age and weight, 313
  cardiovascular considerations, 314-315
  drug dosages, 313, 314t
  equipment, 313
  gastrointestinal considerations, 315
  mechanism of injury, 313
  neurologic considerations, 315
  resources and referrals, 315
  respiratory considerations, 314
Pediatric gastric distention, 312-313
  aspiration, 312
  assessment, 312
  breathing patterns, ineffective, 312
  diagnostic studies, 312
Pediatric hypothermia, 310-311
  assessment, 310
  body heat loss, 310-311
  core temperature restoration, 311
  diagnostic studies, 310
  patients at risk for, 310
Pediatric hypovolemic shock, 305-309
  assessment, 305
  blood loss, minimization of, 307-308
  diagnostic studies, 305
  fluid balance, maintenance of, 308
  fluid volume deficit, 305-309
  oxygenation, maximization of, 306-307
  tissue perfusion, decreased, potential for,
    305-309
Pediatric trauma, 299-320
Pelvic injury. *See* Massive pelvic injury.
Penetrating chest trauma, 81-83
  assessment, 81
  diagnostic studies, 81
  fluid volume deficit, 82-83
  gas exchange, impaired, 82
  hemorrhage, 82-83
  hypoxia, 82
  infection, potential for, 83
  tissue perfusion, decreased, potential for, 81-
    83
  wound contamination, 83
Peptic ulcer. *See* Acute upper gastrointestinal
    bleeding.
Peritoneal lavage tray, 359
Peritonitis, 244-247
  assessment, 244
  bowel elimination, alteration in, 246-247
  diagnostic studies, 244
  fluid volume deficit, 244-245
  gas exchange, impaired, potential for, 245
  hemorrhage, 244-245
  infection, potential for, 245-246
  paralytic ileus, 246-247
  respiratory reserve, decreased, 245
Phencyclidine abuse, 205t
Plastics tray, 360
Pneumatic antishock garment, 340-341

Pneumothorax, 67-68
  air accumulation in pleural space, 67
  assessment, 67
  diagnostic study, 67
  gas exchange, impaired, potential for, 67-68
  infection, potential for, 68
  lung collapse, 67
  retained secretions, 68
Polyvinyl chloride inhalation. *See* Inhalation in-
    juries.
Positive contrast study, 326
Pregnancy, findings in, 106t
Prehospital care, as component in trauma care,
    4, 8-11
Protocols, as component in trauma care, 4-5
Psychosocial support of a child, 317-319
  alleviating fear of unknown, 318-319
  anxiety related to sudden hospitalization, po-
    tential for, 317-319
  separation from parents, 317
  trust and security, 317
Psychosocial support of the trauma patient,
    286-297
  anxiety/fear, potential for, 286-287
  defense mechanisms, use of, 287
  family processes, altered, potential for, 296-
    297
  individual coping, ineffective, 289-290
  powerlessness, potential for, 291-292
  self-concept, disturbance in
    related to change in body image, 293-294
    related to change in role performance,
      294-295
  spiritual distress, potential for, 295
  verbal communication, impaired, 188
Pulmonary artery catheterization, 331
Pulmonary contusion, 73-75
  acidosis, 74
  airway clearance, ineffective, potential for,
    75
  assessment, 73
  atelectasis, 73
  breathing patterns, ineffective, potential for,
    75
  diagnostic studies, 73
  gas exchange, impaired, potential for, 73-74
  hypoxia, 73-74
  infection, potential for, 73
  lower airway obstruction, 73
  painful ventilatory effort, 75
  retained secretions, 74-75
Pulmonary edema, 227-228
  assessment, 227
  cardiac output, decreased, potential for, 228
  diagnostic studies, 227
  fluid accumulation in alveoli and pulmonary
    interstitium, 227-228
  fluid volume excess related to overhydration,
    228
  gas exchange, impaired, 227-228
  myocardial action, diminished, 228
Pulmonary thromboembolus, 224-226
  activity intolerance, potential for, 226
  assessment, 224
  atelectasis, 224-225
  blood loss, minor, potential for, 225-226
  cardiac output, decreased, potential for, 225
  diagnostic studies, 224
  fluid volume deficit, potential for, 226
  gas exchange, impaired, 224-225
  hypoxemia, 226
  occult blood loss, 226
  pulmonary circulation, blockage in, 225
  pulmonary perfusion, decreased, 224-225
Pupillary light reflex, testing of, 218t

Q

Quality assurance, as component in trauma care, 4

R

Radiation dosage, effects of, 166t
Radiation exposure. *See* Acute whole-body radiation exposure.
Rapid-sequence induction for endotracheal intubation, 352
Receiving facilities, as component in trauma care, 4
Renal system injury, 120-122
  assessment, 120
  diagnostic studies, 120
  disruption in organ integrity, 121-122
  fluid volume deficit, potential for, 120-121
  hemorrhage, 120-121
  infection, potential for, 122
  urinary elimination, altered, potential for, 121-122
Respiratory acidosis, 372-373t
Respiratory alkalosis, 372-373t
Resuscitation reminders sheet, sample, for children, 316t
Rule of Nines, 183i
Ruptured diaphragm, 79-80
  abdominal viscera herniation, 79-80
  assessment, 79
  cardiac output, decreased, potential for, 79-80
  diagnostic studies, 79, 80
  gas exchange, impaired, potential for, 79-80
  lung compression, 79, 80
  mediastinal shift, 79, 80
  tissue perfusion, decreased, potential for, 79-80
  vena cava compression, 79
Ruptured ectopic pregnancy, 113-115
  anxiety, potential for, 114
  assessment, 113
  diagnostic studies, 113
  extrauterine bleeding, 114
  fluid volume deficit, potential for, 113-114
  hemorrhage, 113-114
  infection, potential for, 114

S

Sensorimotor testing of eye, 218t
Septic shock. *See* Vasogenic shock.
Skull fractures, findings in, 42t
Smoke inhalation. *See* Inhalation injuries.
Soft tissue injuries, 142-144
  assessment, 142
  delayed wound healing, 144
  diagnostic studies, 142
  fluid volume deficit, potential for, 142-143
  hemorrhage, 142-143
  infection, potential for, 143-144
  soft tissue necrosis, potential for, 143
  tetanus, 144
  tubular necrosis, 143
  urinary elimination, impaired, potential for, 143
  wound contamination, 143-144
Spinal cord injury. *See* Cervical spine injury.

Spontaneous abortion, 116-119
  anxiety, potential for, 119
  assessment, 116
  diagnostic studies, 116
  fluid volume deficit, potential for, 117-118
  hemorrhage, 117, 118
  infection, potential for, 118-119
  potential for, 116-117
Subarachnoid hemorrhage, findings in, 43t
Substance abuse in trauma patient, 204-205t
"Sucking" chest wound. *See* Open pneumothorax.
Suction catheter, selection of, for children, 304t
Supplemental nursing diagnosis, 358
Surgery, preparation for, 336
Surgical cricothyroidotomy, 354

T

Team approach to trauma, 2-5
Tension pneumothorax, 62-64
  assessment, 62
  cardiac output, decreased, potential for, 62-63
  diagnostic studies, 62
  diastolic filling, decreased, 62-63
  gas exchange, decreased, potential for, 62, 63-64
  hypoxia, potential for, 62-63
  infection, potential for, 63-64
  intrapleural pressure, increased, 62, 63
  mediastinal shift, 62, 63
  retained secretions, 64
  tissue perfusion, decreased, potential for, 62-63
  vena cava compression, 62
Tetanus prophylaxis, 371
Therapeutic embolization, 324
Thermal burns, 179-188
  assessment, 179
  burning process, discontinuation of, 181
  carbon monoxide inhalation, 181
  comfort, altered, potential for, 186
  compartment syndrome, 185
  contractures, 187-188
  diagnostic studies, 179
  fluid volume deficit, potential for, 182-183
  gas exchange, impaired, potential for, 181-182
  hypothermia, potential for, 185
  infection, potential for, 186-187
  laryngeal edema, 181-182
  Lund and Browder burn chart, 184i
  paralytic ileus, potential for, 186
  Parkland formula for calculating volume replacement, 184
  peripheral perfusion, decreased, potential for, 185
  physical mobility, impaired, potential for, 187-188
  redistribution of fluid, 182
  Rule of Nines, 183i
  skin barrier, loss of, 182, 185, 186
  skin integrity, potential for additional loss of, 181
  smoke inhalation, 181, 182
  tissue perfusion, decreased, potential for, 182-183

Thoracic, lumbar, and sacral spine injury, 36-41
  aspiration of vomitus, 39
  assessment, 36
  autonomic nervous system control, loss of, 38
  breathing patterns, ineffective, potential for, 39
  deep vein thrombosis, 40
  diagnostic studies, 36
  diaphragmatic elevation, 39
  fluid volume deficit, potential for, 38
  gas exchange, impaired, potential for, 37
  gastric distention from paralytic ileus, 39
  mechanical ventilatory control, decreased, 37
  pulmonary thromboembolism, 41
  sensorimotor deficit, potential for, 37
  skin integrity, impaired, potential for, 39-40
  sympathetic vasomotor tone, 38
  thermoregulation, altered, potential for, 38
  tissue perfusion, altered, potential for, 40-41
Thoracoabdominal tray, 363
Threatened abortion, 116-117
Toxic inhalation. *See* Inhalation injuries.
Tracheobronchial tree rupture, 60-61
  assessment, 60
  diagnostic studies, 60, 61
  gas exchange, impaired, potential for, 60-61
  infection, potential for, 61
  lower airway obstruction, 61
  pneumothorax, 60
Transfusion reactions, 272-277
  allergic
    airway clearance, ineffective, 275
    signs, 277t
    tissue perfusion, decreased, potential for, 274-275
  assessment, 272
  diagnostic studies, 272
  febrile
    hyperthermia, 274
    signs, 277t
  hemolytic
    gas exchange, impaired, 273
    signs, 277t
    tissue perfusion, decreased, potential for, 272-273
  septic
    infection, potential for, 275-276
    signs, 277t
Transportation, as component in trauma care, 4
Trauma score, 370
Traumatic amputation, 125-128
  anxiety, potential for, 128
  assessment, 125
  fluid volume deficit, potential for, 125-126
  infection, potential for, 126
  muscle tissue death, potential for, 127
  tetanus, 126
  tissue perfusion, decreased, 127
  vascular injury, 127
  wound contamination, 126
Traumatic rupture of aorta or great vessels, 84-86
  assessment, 84
  diagnostic studies, 84
  fluid volume deficit, 85-86
  tissue perfusion, decreased, potential for, 84-86
Triage decision scheme, 376
Turning frame for spinal cord injury, 29

U

Upper airway obstruction, 51-54
  airway clearance, ineffective, 51-52
  aspiration of foreign objects into lungs, 53
  assessment, 51
  bacterial growth
    in cricothyroidotomy site, 53-54
    in lungs, 53
  diagnostic studies, 51
  gag reflex, stimulation of, 51-52
  gas exchange, impaired, potential for, 53
  infection, potential for, 53-54
Ureter injury. *See* Renal system injury.
Urethra injury. *See* Renal system injury.

V

Vasogenic shock, 19-23
  accumulation of fluid in alveoli and pulmo-
    nary interstitium, 21
  assessment, 19
  bacterial/fungal invasion, 22-23
  diagnostic studies, 19
  fatigue of respiratory muscles, 22
  fluid volume deficit, potential for, 20-21
  gas exchange, impaired, potential for, 21
  ineffective breathing patterns, potential for,
    22
  peripheral vasodilation, 20-21
  signs, 19t
  systemic infection, potential for, 22-23
Venomous snakebites, 206-210
  assessment, 206
  coagulopathy, 208-209
  coral snake envenomation, 206-207
  diagnostic studies, 206
  fluid volume deficit, potential for, 208-209
  neurologic function, altered, potential for,
    206-207
  pit viper envenomation, 208-209
  skin integrity, alteration in, 208, 210
  systemic reactions to venom, 207
  tissue perfusion, decreased, potential for,
    209
  vascular compromise, 209
Visual acuity testing, 217t
Visual field testing, 218t

NOTES

NOTES

NOTES

NOTES

NOTES

NOTES